Head and Neck Pathology

Editor

RAJA R. SEETHALA

SURGICAL PATHOLOGY CLINICS

www.surgpath.theclinics.com

Consulting Editor
JASON L. HORNICK

March 2017 • Volume 10 • Number 1

ELSEVIER

1600 John F. Kennedy Boulevard • Suite 1800 • Philadelphia, Pennsylvania, 19103-2899

http://www.theclinics.com

SURGICAL PATHOLOGY CLINICS Volume 10, Number 1
March 2017 ISSN 1875-9181, ISBN-13: 978-0-323-50988-6

Editor: Stacy Eastman
Developmental Editor: Donald Mumford

Surgical Pathology Clinics (ISSN 1875-9181) is published quarterly by Elsevier Inc., 360 Park Avenue South, New York, NY 10010. Months of issue are March, June, September, and December. Business and Editorial Office: Elsevier Inc., 1600 John F. Kennedy Blvd., Ste. 1800, Philadelphia, PA 19103-2899. Accounting and Circulation Offices: Elsevier Inc., 3251 Riverport Lane, Maryland Heights, MO 63043. Periodicals postage paid at New York, NY and at additional mailing offices. Subscription prices are $206.00 per year (US individuals), $274.00 per year (US institutions), $100.00 per year (US students/residents), $258.00 per year (Canadian individuals), $312.00 per year (Canadian Institutions), $258.00 per year (foreign individuals), $312.00 per year (foreign institutions), and $120.00 per year (international & Canadian students/residents). Foreign air speed delivery is included in all *Clinics'* subscription prices. All prices are subject to change without notice. **POSTMASTER:** Send address changes to *Surgical Pathology Clinics*, Elsevier, 3251 Riverport Lane, Maryland Heights, MO 63043. **Customer Service: 1-800-654-2452 (US). From outside the United States, call 1-314-447-8871. Fax: 1-314-447-8029. E-mail: JournalsCustomerServiceusa@elsevier.com (for print support)** and JournalsOnlineSupport-usa@elsevier.com **(for online support)**.

Reprints. For copies of 100 or more, of articles in this publication, please contact the Commercial Reprints Department, Elsevier Inc., 360 Park Avenue South, New York, NY 10010-1710. Tel. 212-633-3874; Fax: 212-633-3820; E-mail: reprints@elsevier.com.

Surgical Pathology Clinics of North America is covered in *MEDLINE/PubMed (Index Medicus)*.

Contributors

CONSULTING EDITOR

JASON L. HORNICK, MD, PhD
Director of Surgical Pathology, Director,
Immunohistochemistry Laboratory, Brigham
and Women's Hospital, Associate Professor of
Pathology, Harvard Medical School, Boston,
Massachusetts

EDITOR

RAJA R. SEETHALA, MD
Professor of Pathology and Otolaryngology,
Department of Pathology and Laboratory
Medicine, University of Pittsburgh,
Presbyterian University Hospital, Pittsburgh,
Pennsylvania

AUTHORS

**ELIZABETH ANN BILODEAU, DMD, MD,
MSEd**
Associate Professor, Department of Diagnostic
Sciences, University of Pittsburgh School of
Dental Medicine, Pittsburgh, Pennsylvania

JUSTIN A. BISHOP, MD
Associate Professor, Departments of
Pathology, Otolaryngology-Head and Neck
Surgery and Oncology, The Johns Hopkins
Medical Institutions, Baltimore, Maryland

SIMION I. CHIOSEA, MD
Department of Pathology, Presbyterian
University Hospital, University of Pittsburgh
Medical Center, Pittsburgh, Pennsylvania

BOBBY M. COLLINS, DDS, MS
Division Director, Oral and Maxillofacial
Pathology, Department of Surgical Science,
East Carolina University School of Dental
Medicine, Greenville, North Carolina

SARAH G. FITZPATRICK, DDS
Adjunct Research Assistant Professor,
Department of Oral and Maxillofacial
Diagnostic Sciences, University of Florida,
Gainesville, Florida

CHI K. LAI, MD, FRCPC
Division of Anatomical Pathology,
Department of Pathology and Laboratory
Medicine, The Ottawa Hospital, University
of Ottawa, Ottawa, Ontario, Canada

VIRGINIA A. LiVOLSI, MD
Department of Pathology and Laboratory
Medicine, Hospital of the University of
Pennsylvania, Philadelphia, Pennsylvania

KELLY R. MAGLIOCCA, DDS, MPH
Assistant Professor, Department of Pathology
and Laboratory Medicine, Emory University,
Atlanta, Georgia

JONATHAN B. McHUGH, MD
Associate Professor, Department of Pathology,
University of Michigan Health System,
Ann Arbor, Michigan

KATHLEEN T. MONTONE, MD
Department of Pathology and Laboratory
Medicine, Hospital of the University
of Pennsylvania, Philadelphia, Pennsylvania

BIBIANNA PURGINA, MD, FRCPC
Division of Anatomical Pathology,
Department of Pathology and Laboratory
Medicine, The Ottawa Hospital, University of
Ottawa, Ottawa, Ontario, Canada

LISA M. ROOPER, MD
Assistant Faculty, Department of Pathology,
The Johns Hopkins Medical Institutions,
Baltimore, Maryland

RAJA R. SEETHALA, MD
Professor of Pathology and Otolaryngology,
Department of Pathology and Laboratory
Medicine, University of Pittsburgh,
Presbyterian University Hospital, Pittsburgh,
Pennsylvania

EDWARD B. STELOW, MD
Department of Pathology, University of
Virginia, Charlottesville, Virginia

LESTER D.R. THOMPSON, MD
Department of Pathology, Southern California
Kaiser Permanente Group, Woodland Hills
Medical Center, Woodland Hills, California

AARON M. UDAGER, MD, PhD
Assistant Professor, Department of Pathology,
University of Michigan Health System, Ann
Arbor, Michigan

Contents

Video content accompanies this article at http://www.surgpath.theclinics.com.

The surgical method of margin sampling affects local control, pathologists' approach to margin sampling, and clarity of pathology reports. Studies have shown that exclusive reliance on tumor bed margins is associated with worse local control and should be avoided. En bloc resections and margins obtained from the resection specimen remain the "gold standard." Successful surgical treatment of early carcinomas of the oral cavity relies on close cooperation between surgeons and pathologists on issues of specimen orientation and margin sampling.

Squamous cell carcinoma (SCC) is a malignant epithelial tumor showing evidence of squamous differentiation. It is the most common malignancy of the larynx, with several variants (verrucous, exophytic or papillary, spindle-cell (sarcomatoid) carcinoma, basaloid, acantholytic, adenosquamous) recognized, with well-established precursor lesions. Dysplasia is now separated into only low-grade and high-grade categories. Each SCC variant has unique cytomorphologic features and histologic differential diagnoses that are important to consider, as management and outcomes are different.

Human papillomavirus (HPV) is an essential causal factor in a subset of head and neck neoplasms, most notably oropharyngeal squamous cell carcinoma, for which HPV infection has important diagnostic, prognostic, and therapeutic implications. This article summarizes the current understanding of HPV-associated neoplasms of the head and neck, including the recently described carcinoma with adenoid cystic-like features. Salient clinical, gross, and microscopic features are discussed, and the utility of specific ancillary studies is highlighted.

Immune-related disorders of the oral cavity may occur as primary disease process, secondary to systemic disease or neoplasm, or as a reaction to medications and other agents. The entities represented within this group may vary significantly by severity, clinical presentation, microscopic presentation, and special testing results. The selected immune-related conditions of the oral cavity in this article are categorized and presented by their prototypical tissue reaction patterns: vesiculobullous, including acantholytic and subepithelial separation; psoriasiform; spongiotic; and lichenoid reaction patterns.

odontogenic cyst), benign tumors (keratocystic odontogenic tumor, ameloblastoma, adenomatoid odontogenic tumor, calcifying epithelial odontogenic tumor, ameloblastic fibroma and fibroodontoma, odontoma, squamous odontogenic tumor, calcifying cystic odontogenic tumor, primordial odontogenic tumor, central odontogenic fibroma, and odontogenic myxomas), and malignant tumors (clear cell odontogenic carcinoma, ameloblastic carcinoma, ameloblastic fibrosarcoma).

Benign and malignant primary bone and soft tissue lesions of the head and neck are rare. The uncommon nature of these tumors, combined with the complex anatomy of the head and neck, pose diagnostic challenges to pathologists. This article describes the pertinent clinical, radiographic, and pathologic features of selected bone and soft tissue tumors involving the head and neck region, including angiofibroma, glomangiopericytoma, rhabdomyosarcoma, biphenotypic sinonasal sarcoma, chordoma, chondrosarcoma, and osteosarcoma. Emphasis is placed on key diagnostic pitfalls, differential diagnosis, and the importance of correlating clinical and radiographic information, particularly for tumors involving bone.

SURGICAL PATHOLOGY CLINICS

THE CLINICS ARE AVAILABLE ONLINE!
Access your subscription at:
www.theclinics.com

Preface
Head and Neck Pathology

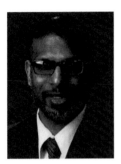

Raja R. Seethala, MD
Editor

As with many subspecialties in pathology, head and neck pathology had evolved from a hobby or interest in a generalist setting to a full-fledged nuanced discipline in a multidisciplinary subspecialized setting. The appeal and challenge of this subspecialty stem from the extreme, arguably unparalleled diversity of lesions encountered relative to the small proportion of total body volume occupied by the head and neck region. The objectives of this issue are not to cover all aspects of head and neck pathology in their entirety. The goal instead is to provide a synopsis of the core features of intraoperative margin assessment in squamous cell carcinoma, autoimmune disease manifestations in the oral cavity, odontogenic cysts and tumors, HPV-associated neoplasms, laryngeal dysplasias and carcinoma variants, salivary gland tumors, sinonasal glandular and round blue cell neoplasms, nonneoplastic and infectious disease of the sinonasal tract, and select bone and soft tissue neoplasms distinctive to the head and neck.

Head and neck pathology has been rapidly evolving over the past decade with the advancement of ancillary, particularly molecular techniques, allowing for further diagnostic refinement, though the foundation of diagnosis remains an integration of morphologic, clinical, and radiologic features. Of note, this is the second issue in *Surgical Pathology Clinics* to focus on head and neck pathology. This issue builds on the prior iteration,[1] again recruiting experts in the field who will guide the reader through the challenges, pitfalls, and recent developments in the aforementioned topics. The intent of this issue is to provide current and relevant information to a broad audience, including pathologists in training, general surgical pathologists, and head and neck pathology subspecialists.

I would like to thank all the authors for their excellent and thoughtful contributions, and Donald Mumford for facilitating the editorial process. I would like to thank all my mentors throughout my career evolution, especially Dr E. Leon Barnes, the humble giant of his era in this field,[2] who gave me the template, tools, and substrate to actually become a head and neck pathologist.

Raja R. Seethala, MD
Department of Pathology and Laboratory Medicine
University of Pittsburgh
Presbyterian University Hospital
200 Lothrop Street
Pittsburgh, PA 15213, USA

E-mail address:
seethalarr@upmc.edu

REFERENCES

1. Richardson MS, editor. Current concepts in head and neck pathology. Surg Pathol Clin 2011;No. 4.
2. Seethala RR, Chiosia SI. Tribute: E. Leon Barnes. Head Neck Pathol 2012;6(1):54–7.

http://dx.doi.org/10.1016/j.path.2016.12.001
1875-9181/17/© 2016 Published by Elsevier Inc.

Intraoperative Margin Assessment in Early Oral Squamous Cell Carcinoma

Simion I. Chiosea, MD

KEYWORDS

- Margin • Squamous cell carcinoma • Oral cavity • Frozen • Gross examination

Key points

- The approach to margin sampling affects local control. Sampling of tumor bed correlates with worse local control.

- The status (positive vs negative) of the margin obtained from the resection specimen correlates with local recurrence, and thus, resection specimen–based margin assessment is always recommended (even if tumor bed margins are submitted separately).

- Adequate margin revision should ideally be represented by one tissue fragment, characterized by size and shape that fits the revised aspect of the resection specimen.

- Resolution of frozen versus final sampling issues is possible only if the examined fragment of tissue is oriented as to the true new margin surface.

- Adequate design of studies on margins should include local recurrence as a primary endpoint, actual measurement of margin clearance, distinguish second primary carcinomas from recurrences, and comment on the source of margins (resection specimen and/or tumor bed).

- Anatomic landmarks, orientation, and approach to margin assessment in partial glossectomy, hemiglossectomy, and mandibulectomy are illustrated.

 Video content accompanies this article at http://www.surgpath.theclinics.com.

ABSTRACT

The surgical method of margin sampling affects local control, pathologists' approach to margin sampling, and clarity of pathology reports. Studies have shown that exclusive reliance on tumor bed margins is associated with worse local control and should be avoided. En bloc resections and margins obtained from the resection specimen remain the "gold standard." Successful surgical treatment of early carcinomas of the oral cavity relies on close cooperation between surgeons and pathologists on issues of specimen orientation and margin sampling.

OVERVIEW

The aim of intraoperative margin assessment is to evaluate the adequacy of tumor removal, also referred to as "margin assessment."[1] Although the need for routine intraoperative margin assessment is engrained in the minds of surgeons and pathologists, the method of margin assessment is not universally agreed on. In fact, the approach to intraoperative margin assessment (gross only vs routine microscopic examination) and its overall clinical value are questioned,[2–4] especially for advanced (pT3-4) carcinomas.[5]

Although complete tumor removal with adequate margins is a fundamental oncologic

Conflict of Interest and Disclosure: None.

Department of Pathology, Presbyterian University Hospital, University of Pittsburgh Medical Center, A610.3, 200 Lothrop Street, Pittsburgh, PA 15213, USA

E-mail address: chioseasi@upmc.edu

Surgical Pathology 10 (2017) 1–14

http://dx.doi.org/10.1016/j.path.2016.10.002

principle, there are actually no *direct* evidence-based data showing whether *intraoperative* margin assessment improves local control. Such research is difficult due to the variability in margin sampling, assessment, and reporting. Specifically, there are currently 2 ways of sampling margins.[6–8] In the specimen-driven approach, the entire resection specimen is sent for margin assessment to the pathologist. In a defect-driven scenario, the surgeon performs a resection and then samples tumor bed (ie, margins from wound, cavity, or patient). In the latter scenario, the size, location, and number of tumor bed margins is not guided by the formal margin assessment from the actual resection specimen. Most of the literature on margin assessment essentially ignores the source of margins and the relationship between the 2 margin types. Several recent studies have shown that the only prognostically relevant margins are those derived from the actual resection specimen and the mere fact of tumor bed sampling correlates with worse local control (**Fig. 1**).[9–16]

Indirectly, the need for and value of routine intraoperative margin assessment as practiced currently is highly questionable. In most cases, the margins are adequate and the only value of intraoperative margin assessment is reassurance (see **Fig. 1**, group 1). When the margins are suboptimal, they are revised (see **Fig. 1**, group 2); however, margin revision appears to be of little to no therapeutic value (**Fig. 2**).[9,12,17–20] Finally, the tumor bed margins obtained in the defect-driven approach are of no prognostic significance and the mere sampling of tumor bed margins seems to correlate with worse local control (see **Fig. 1**, group 3).[12–14] In groups 2 and 3 the intraoperative information on margins does not appear to lead to clinical benefit.

Margin status is clinically most relevant in a group of patients who are ideally cured by surgery alone, namely patients with pT1-2.[5] The intent of this review was to illustrate how to best perform intraoperative margin evaluation in early carcinomas of the oral cavity. The principles of gross examination are emphasized. The limitations of and interdisciplinary friction caused by tumor bed margins were highlighted by questionnaire-type studies by the American Head and Neck Society and North American Society of Head and Neck Pathologists[6,7] and are summarized in **Box 1**. Therefore, this review focuses on intraoperative examination of resection specimens and margin revision.

MARGIN ASSESSMENT

What is an adequate margin clearance (distance from the invasive tumor front to the margin)?

Very few studies adequately addressed the issue of the safe distance to the margins (**Box 2**).[22]

When the principles proposed in **Box 2** are followed, there appears to be a linear relationship between local recurrence and margin clearance. There is a 33% decrease in risk of local recurrence for an increase of 1 mm of margin clearance (up to 5 mm of margin clearance for oral tongue).[12,13] The confounding effect of tumor bed margins on prognostic significance of margin clearance (as measured from the resection specimen) is unclear.

ORAL CAVITY RESECTION SPECIMENS: ORIENTATION AND MARGIN ASSESSMENT

Most oral cavity resection specimens, such as segmental mandibulectomies, hemiglossectomies, partial glossectomies, and partial maxillectomies can be oriented based on anatomic landmarks. Anatomic landmarks may include uvula, maxillary tuberosity in partial maxillectomy (**Fig. 3**), tip of the tongue and curvature of the mandible (**Figs. 4** and **5**, Videos 1 and 2), and distinguishing qualities of the mucosa in dorsal and ventral aspects of oral tongue (**Figs. 6–9**, Videos 3 and 4).

Smaller specimens may require the knowledge of laterality (right, left, midline) and orientation by sutures or ink (**Fig. 10**).

MARGIN SHRINKAGE

Immediately after resection, the tissue shrinks by 20% to 40% due to unopposed muscle contraction, especially for lower stage (pT1-2) tumors.[25,26] The extent of tissue shrinkage and of artifactual changes (eg, up to 0.15 cm of cautery) depend on resection technique: cold steel, electrocautery, laser.[27] Formalin fixation adds additional 10% of shrinkage. Most importantly, tissue shrinkage takes place in all resections and cannot be used as the only explanation of margin status.[1] Shrinkage of a mucosal floor of mouth margin is illustrated in Video 2. Video 4 shows shrinkage and curling of the deep/midline oral tongue margin.

NONMARGIN CUT AND TEARS AND EXTENSION OF RESECTION

While performing resection, a surgeon may decide that the plane of section should be adjusted and additional cuff of tissue is needed. Such additional tissue should be re-approximated to the initial defect on resection specimen (Video 3).

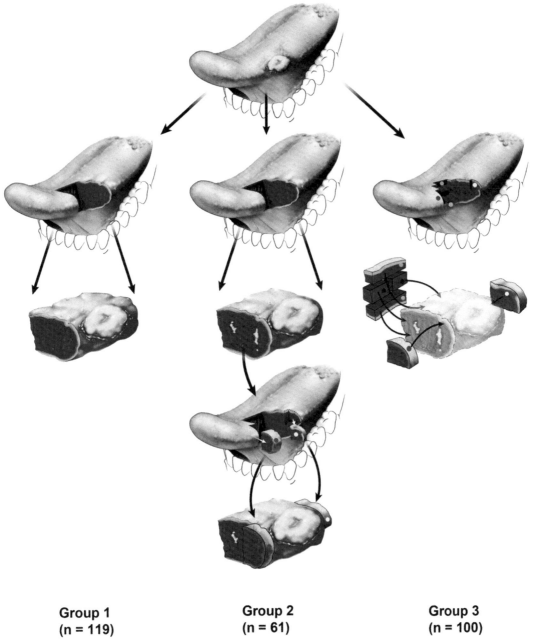

Group 1
(n = 119)

Group 2
(n = 61)

Group 3
(n = 100)

Fig. 1. Schematic representation of the glossectomy workflow. The baseline characteristics of patients and their tumors were similar. For simplicity, a predominantly exophytic tumor at the lateral edge of the oral tongue is illustrated, with each row representing the next step in the operative workflow. In group 1 (*left column*), tumor bed margins were not sampled. In group 2 (*middle column*), margins were examined from the glossectomy specimen and found to be positive or otherwise suboptimal. The surgeon revised margins by obtaining additional tissue from the tumor bed. White irregular areas in the anterior aspect of glossectomy specimen represent residual carcinoma at the initial anterior margin (*third row*). Red (erythematous) mucosa behind the tumor at the posterior aspect of the glossectomy illustrates the second positive margin (*third row*). The surgeon revised anterior and posterior margins by obtaining additional tissue form the tumor bed: new anterior margin (*red dot*) and new posterior margin (*yellow dot*) (*fourth row*). To imagine the relationship between the actual glossectomy margins and additional tissue, the 2 types of margins are superimposed in the fifth row. Due to the challenges of relocating the exact aspect of the relevant anterior margin in the tumor bed, size discrepancy, and uncertain orientation of the additional tissue, it is conceivable that in some cases the revised margin may not actually cover the entire residual tumor at the anterior glossectomy margin. In group 3 (*right column*), 5 margins are primarily sampled from the tumor bed (*red, green, yellow, blue, and black dots*), without preceding examination of the glossectomy specimen (*displayed in lighter colors in the third row*) by the pathologist. (Reproduced with permission from Maxwell JH, Thompson LD, Brandwein-Gensler MS, et al. Early oral tongue squamous cell carcinoma: sampling of margins from tumor bed and worse local control. JAMA Otolaryngol Head Neck Surg 2015;141(12):1104–10. Copyright©2015 American Medical Association. All rights reserved.)

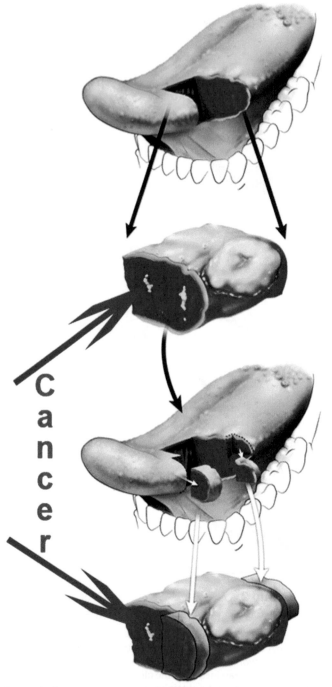

**Pathology Report:
Part 1: ...carcinoma
extends to margin.**

What is the
final margin status?

**Pathology Report:
Part 2: ...re-excision:
No tumor seen.**

Fig. 2. Challenges of margin revision. Spatial relationship between resection specimen, tumor at the resection specimen margin, additional revision margin, and the structure of the pathology report. Tumor bed sampling not only affects pathologists' sampling and reporting of margins, it may influence oncologists in a yet unknown manner. How oncologists read multipart pathology reports and resolve the issue of discrepant margins: positive margin on resection specimen and negative tumor bed margin?

MARGINS: RADIAL OR SHAVE?

Tissue sections that allow examination of the relationship between the bulk of the tumor and margin are referred to as "radial" or "perpendicular" margins. Tissue sections taken parallel to the margin are referred to as "shave" margins. Radial and shaved margins are compared in **Table 1**. The method of margin sampling depends on gross findings. Based on results of visual inspection and

---

Box 1
Pitfalls, challenges, and limitations of upfront tumor bed margin sampling without prior evaluation of the resection specimen (see Fig. 1, group 3)

1. The status of tumor bed margins (ie, positive vs negative):
   a. Does not correlate with local recurrence.
   b. Does not correlate with the status of margins obtained from the resection specimen. Tumor bed margins are characterized by a very low sensitivity for identifying positive margins from resection specimen (approximately 24%) rendering tumor bed margins inadequate for "mapping out" the tumor.[21]

2. Piecemeal removal/specimen fragmentation precludes confident and independent margin assessment by pathologists, as the spatial relationship between tissue fragments is difficult to reconstruct.

3. Tumor bed sampling results in complex multipart surgical pathology reports (see Fig. 2) rendering the overall margin status unclear to cancer registrars and oncologists.

4. Tumor bed margins discourage reporting of margins from the resection specimen and lead to equivocal terminology (ie, tissue edge) and misleading comments (eg, see other parts for "true" margins).

5. Most tumor bed margins are benign. This false reassurance may explain the narrower margin clearance (as measured on resection specimen) when surgeons routinely prefer to rely on tumor bed margins.

---

palpation, closest margins can be radially sectioned to better appreciate the distance to the tumor (see Figs. 4, 7, and 8, Video 1). If the gross distance between the tumor and margin is 0.3 to 1.0 cm, then microscopic examination of the closest section may be of help. Gross examination (with serial radial sections of most concerning margins) allows rapid detection of the closest margin. It may help to discuss gross findings (ie, close margins, <3 mm) with surgeons before microscopic examination. Such preliminary discussions allow for deciding whether more precise microscopic measurements are clinically meaningful. If microscopic examination of the margin is needed, such conversations allow pathologists to prioritize most clinically relevant margins (ie,

---

Box 2
An adequate study design to address the issue of margin clearance would satisfy the following requirements:

1. Local recurrence (rather than locoregional recurrence or survival) as a primary outcome endpoint.

2. Statement on how local recurrence is distinguished from regional recurrence in neck level I.[23]

3. Clear distinction of local recurrence from second primary squamous cell carcinoma.[12]

4. Actual measurement of the distance from the tumor to closest margin (margin clearance) and analysis of this distance as a continuous variable, rather than arbitrary grouping of cases into "close" and "negative" based on historically purported cutoffs (eg, 5 mm).

5. Margin clearance best correlates with relatively early, up to 24 months, local recurrences. Time-dependent receiver operating characteristic analysis is best suited for studies of discriminatory ability of margin clearance.[24]

6. Cases with positive margins should be excluded when attempting to determine the best cutoff between close and negative margins.[12,13]

7. Unequivocal definition of margins' source: resected specimen or additional tissue obtained from the tumor bed.

8. Statement on how discrepancies between the status of resection specimen margin and tumor bed margin are resolved.

9. Margin studies based on review of surgical pathology reports or cancer registry databases are suboptimal, due to potentially inadequate documentation of margin sampling in surgical pathology reports (ie, tissue section summary, inking code, radial or shave nature of the margin). Pathology material has to be re-reviewed.

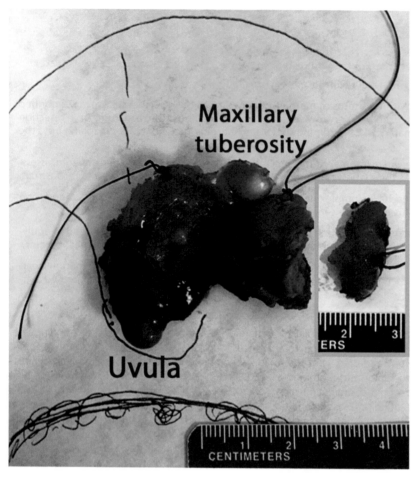

Fig. 3. Partial maxillectomy and adequate margin revision. Anatomic landmarks are indicated. The mucosa at the left buccal margin was inadvertently stripped and surgeon revised left buccal margin (double stitch). Single stitch indicates midline superior (as in "superior to uvula, toward the palate"). This is an example of adequate margin revision: the additional tissue obtained from the defect (*green rectangle*) "fits" the corresponding aspect of the resected specimen both in terms of shape and size and the new true margin was indicated by double stitch on the smaller fragment of tissue (green rectangle).

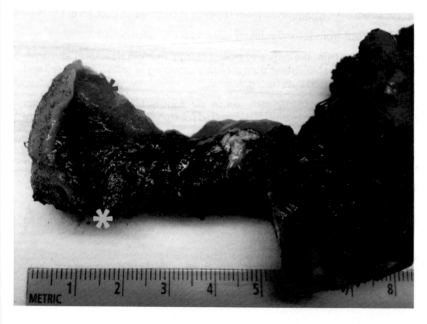

Fig. 4. Representative cross-section of the posterior tongue margin from anterior composite resection with segmental mandibulectomy shown in Video 1. Red asterisk indicates tumor and green asterisk indicates posterior tongue margin. The posterior tongue margin is wide and benign.

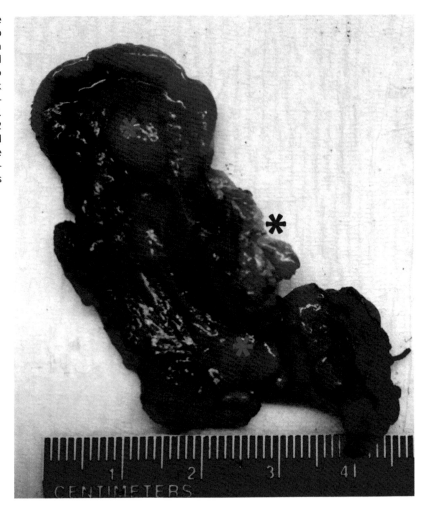

Fig. 5. The deep/midline tongue margin and deep floor of mouth margin were inked and sectioned (frontal plane, radial to deep margin). Black asterisk indicates exophytic part of the tumor. Red asterisks indicate 2 deep well-circumscribed tumor foci, shown to be vascular invasion microscopically. Deep margins are free of tumor.

the order in which margins are frozen, interpreted, and reported).

Radial sections are preferred in cases with close margins. Shave mucosal margins are preferred by some in cases with wider (>1 cm) margins. However, in most cases with such wide margins one could advocate for gross examination only. Of note, prior surgery, radiation, or chemotherapy render gross examination less reliable.

Both types of margin sampling are least reliable in tumors with discontinuous growth pattern (extratumoral vascular or perineural invasion) (see **Fig. 5**).

Neither radial nor shave margin sections allow *microscopic* examination of the *entire* margin. A greater margin area can be examined microscopically on one slide when margin is shaved off. However, processing (embedding, sectioning) of irregular or curved specimens results in significant tissue loss (ie, "shavings" lost in cryostat while attempting to get a section with profile

corresponding to the examined aspect of the resection specimen, see **Fig. 10B**).

RESOLVING SAMPLING DISCREPANCIES

Benign versus malignant sampling discrepancies (ie, no tumor on frozen section and tumor on permanent section of the frozen section remnant) for radial margins are exceedingly rare, because radial margins include the tumor. On deeper permanent sections of radial margins, usually, only subtle variations in the distance to margins are noticed. In contrast, 3% to 5% of shaved margins will reveal frozen versus permanent sampling discrepancy. Determining the actual margin status when such a discrepancy occurs is impossible unless true new margin surface was indicated (**Figs. 11** and **12**). Without such orientation, it is unclear whether "deeper" sections are away from or toward the true margin; that is, when the frozen section is

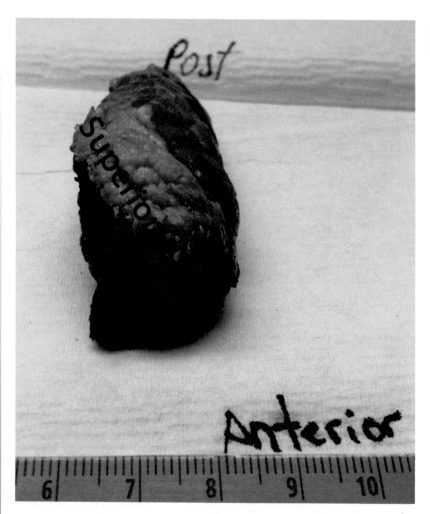

Fig. *6.* Left partial glossectomy specimen orientation.

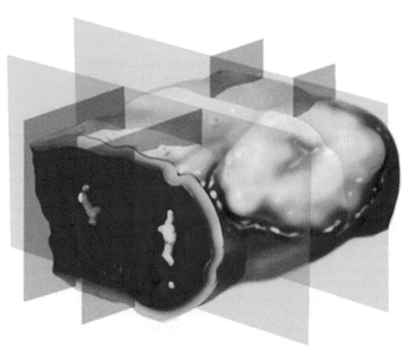

Fig. *7.* Schematic summary of preferred sectioning of partial glossectomies. Planes of radial sectioning are shown.

Fig. 8. Left partial glossectomy specimen from Figs. 6 and 9 is sectioned according to the schema in Fig. 7 after all mucosal and deep margins were differentially inked. Mid part with superior (*), inferior, & deep (ˆ) margins.

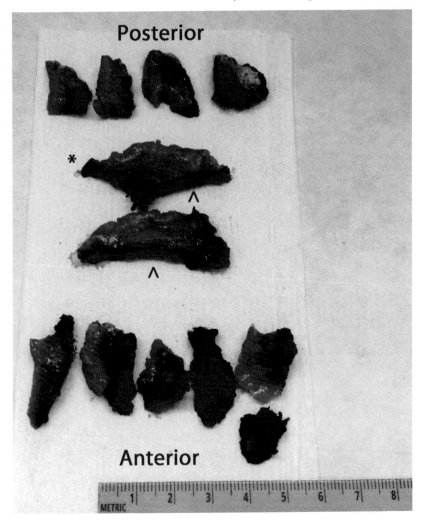

Fig. 9. Photograph of the frozen block. The deep margin (*black ink*) is several millimeters away from the tumor (*white-pink*).

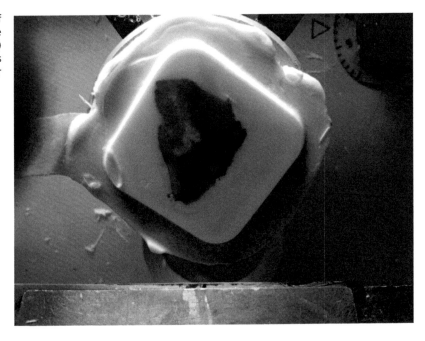

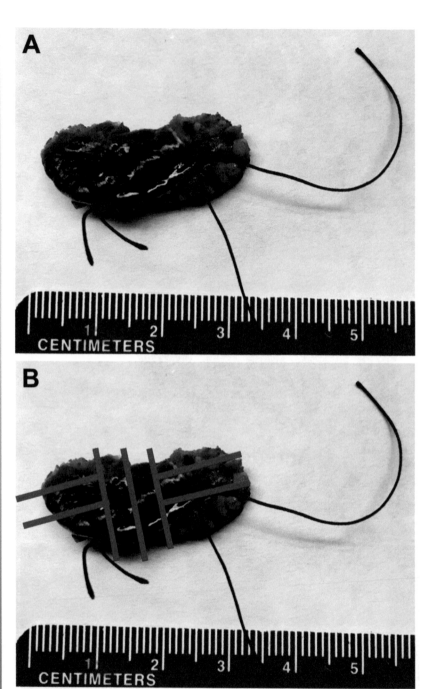

Fig. 10. (A) Small excision of the anterior floor of mouth for a superficially invasive squamous cell carcinoma that is unrecognizable grossly. Short stitch indicates anterior midline and long stitch indicates left (double stitch). In the left aspect of the specimen, note the difference in the amount of soft tissue/submucosa (abundant) and mucosa (scant). Processing this margin as a shave would require a very oblique section. Furthermore, attempts to get a section with adequate representation of squamous mucosa will result in the loss of some submucosal soft tissue. (B) The entire specimen was examined microscopically and the preferred way of sectioning this specimen is shown.

benign but deeper permanent tissue section reveals tumor, if true margin is not indicated, one cannot just assume that frozen section (or permanent section for that matter) reflects the true status of the margin.

Most tumor bed margins are represented by rather thin piece(s) of tissue (<5 mm), usually strips of mucosa with little to no underlying submucosa. Technically, such fragments of tissue have to be processed as shaved margins.

PROCESSING, REPORTING, AND SIGNIFICANCE OF REVISED MARGINS

When intraoperative examination of the resected specimen identifies a suboptimal margin (ie, close, positive, torn, ulcerated, stripped of mucosa), additional tissue is obtained from the tumor bed. Attempts to revise margins, as performed currently, do not improve clinical outcome and

Table 1
Comparison of shave and radial margins

Margin Type	Advantages	Disadvantages
Radial	Allows measurement of the exact distance between the tumor and margin. Fewer frozen vs permanent sampling issues. Easier to interpret (representative tumor is available for direct comparison with other atypical foci). Smaller area to be scrutinized by microscopic examination: margin is limited to inked or cauterized area.	Smaller area of the margin is examined microscopically.
Shave	Greater margin area is examined microscopically.	Precludes microscopic measurement of the distance between the tumor and margin. Underestimates distance to margin, especially in irregular or curved specimens. 3%–5% chance of frozen vs permanent sampling issue. More challenging to interpret: small clusters of tumor cells could "appear" anywhere on the tissue section, because the location of the bulk of the tumor is unknown.

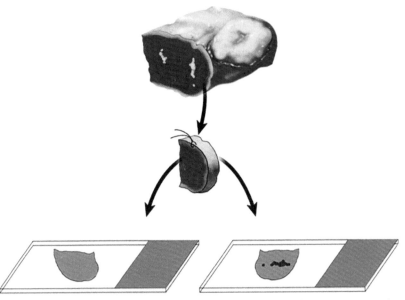

Fig. 11. Orientation of the revised (or tumor bed) margin. Stitch indicates the new true margin surface of the revised anterior margin from left partial glossectomy. The dark blue irregular area on the right glass slide represents tumor. Without orientation, the surface to be examined intraoperatively is picked randomly. The new margin surface will be examined first intraoperatively (see **Fig. 12**, Video 5). If frozen section is negative for tumor, but permanent section of the frozen remnant reveals tumor, the overall margin status is "close, but negative." Such determination is impossible if the tumor bed margin was fragmented or the new true margin surface was not indicated. Without such orientation, the assumption that frozen section represents true margin is wrong in half of the cases.

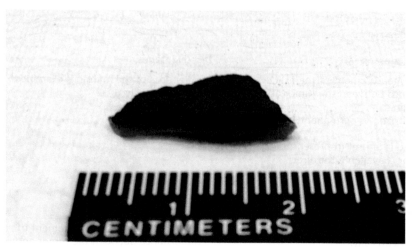

Fig. 12. Revised mucosal margin oriented by ink. Blue ink applied by surgeon indicates new true margin surface. Surgeon's ink indicates the surface to be examined first. There is no need to re-ink the surface of interest: it is thin and is best processed as shave margin.

the need for margin revision appears to be an adverse prognosticator.[12,17–20]

The challenges and limitations of margin revision are summarized in **Box 3**.

When the new true margin is indicated, it is best examined as illustrated in Video 5. To save time and if the tumor bed margin is processed as shave, there is no real need to re-ink the new true margin surface. "Ink on true margin" indicates which aspect of the tumor bed margin should be examined first. If the tumor bed margin is thick enough to be processed as a radial margin, re-inking true margin surface is needed (followed by sectioning radially to the new margin and embedding "on edge").

FINAL MARGIN: RECONCILING MARGINS OBTAINED FROM THE RESECTION SPECIMEN AND THOSE FROM THE TUMOR BED

Tumor bed margins discourage sampling and reporting of margins from the resection specimen by pathologists, lead to interdisciplinary friction, equivocal terminology (tissue edge, rather than margin), and misleading comments (eg, see other parts for "true margins").[6,7] Occasionally, resected specimens are even labeled by surgeons as "nonmarginal tissue" to further discourage margin reporting from resected specimens by pathologists. To optimize and encourage conveying of margin status from resection specimens, the updated College of American Pathologist oral cancer checklist recommends separate reporting of *both* resection specimen margins and tumor bed margins (when tumor bed margins are sampled).

The determination of the "final" margin status (for case synopsis) requires resolution of conflicting tumor bed and resection specimen margins. In at least half of cases when margin revision was attempted, the new margin is negative while the initial resection specimen margin is positive. To reconcile such a discrepancy and to assist oncologists in the scenario illustrated in **Fig. 2**, pathologists have to consider the size, shape, tissue type, and orientation of the tumor

---

Box 3
Pitfalls and limitations of margin revision

1. Suboptimal relocalization of the area of concern in the tumor bed: relocation of the site of interest in the tumor bed might be off target by approximately 1 cm in one-third of cases.[28] Up to 78% of the revised margins do not contain residual tumor, further implying that the revised margin is taken from a nonrepresentative area.[20]

2. The unclear spatial relationship between the main resection specimen and revised margin (see **Fig. 2**).

3. Even when tumor bed margin is taken from the correct site, the new true surface/margin may not always be designated (see **Figs. 11** and **12**).

4. If revised margin is thin (eg, <3 mm), positive margin may actually be revised to "close," rather than "negative" margin.

bed. Overall, pathologists have the following options:

1. Acknowledge adequate revision and state that the final margin is negative (see **Fig. 3**).
2. State that due to fragmentation, the final margin status cannot be determined (especially if the revision margin itself is small, fragmented, or unoriented as to the new margin).
3. State the inadequacy of revision margin and report margin status based on the resection specimen only. The latter scenario is most appropriate if revised margin is small, unoriented, fragmented, and, histologically, does not correspond to the positive resection specimen margin. For instance, if the tumor extends to the deeper part of the anterior glossectomy specimen margin (eg, tumor is several millimeters under the mucosa and is surrounded by intrinsic tongue musculature), but the revised margin consists of a strip of squamous mucosa, such a revision is inadequate.

SUMMARY

Margin status is one of the quality measures for head and neck cancer care.[29,30] However, the controversial coexistence of 2 types of margins,[6,7] those from the tumor bed and the ones from the resected specimen, only recently was addressed.[10,12–14] In approximately a quarter of cases, the status of the 2 types of margins is discordant. When the tumor bed margin is negative, but the resection specimen margin is positive, planning of patients' postoperative care should primarily rely on the status of resection specimen margins. In this review, deficiencies of margin revision were highlighted. In the margin revision literature, there seems to be a consensus that margin revision, as performed currently, is of little clinical value.[9,12,17–20] There appear to be no studies on perceived merits of upfront tumor bed sampling. Upfront tumor bed sampling without preceding examination of the resection specimen (see **Fig. 1**, group 3) appears to be a matter of surgeon preference and is unguided by formal intraoperative assessment of the resection specimen. The "merits" of such approach are subjective and appear to include the following:

1. Surgeon control over tumor bed margin labeling.
2. "Streamlining" the intraoperative consultation with pathologists by avoiding the need for specimen orientation (as in "margins are submitted separately anyway"?!).
3. Pathologists' inability to contest margin status due to specimen fragmentation.

The surgical method of margin sampling affects local control, pathologists' approach to margin sampling, and clarity of pathology reports. Studies have shown that exclusive reliance on tumor bed margins is associated with worse local control and should be avoided.[10–14] En bloc resections and margins obtained from the resection specimen remain the "gold standard." Successful surgical treatment of early carcinomas of oral cavity relies on close cooperation between surgeons and pathologists on issues of specimen orientation and margin sampling.

ACKNOWLEDGMENTS

The author thanks Robyn Roche for outstanding administrative assistance, Laura Pliego for medical illustrations, and Rochelle DiCianno, PA (ASCP) for assistance with preparation of videos of gross examination.

SUPPLEMENTARY DATA

Supplementary data related to this article can be found online at 10.1016/j.path.2016.10.002.

REFERENCES

1. Weinstock YE, Alava I 3rd, Dierks EJ. Pitfalls in determining head and neck surgical margins. Oral Maxillofac Surg Clin North Am 2014;26(2):151–62.
2. Gerber S, Gengler C, Gratz KW, et al. The impact of frozen sections on final surgical margins in squamous cell carcinoma of the oral cavity and lips: a retrospective analysis over an 11 years period. Head Neck Oncol 2011;3:56.
3. Gokavarapu S, Chandrasekhara Rao LM, Patnaik SC, et al. Prognostic value of frozen section in t1, t2 carcinoma of oral cavity. Indian J Otolaryngol Head Neck Surg 2015;67(Suppl 1):86–90.
4. Chaturvedi P, Datta S, Nair S, et al. Gross examination by the surgeon as an alternative to frozen section for assessment of adequacy of surgical margin in head and neck squamous cell carcinoma. Head Neck 2014;36(4):557–63.
5. DiNardo LJ, Lin J, Karageorge LS, et al. Accuracy, utility, and cost of frozen section margins in head and neck cancer surgery. Laryngoscope 2000; 110(10 Pt 1):1773–6.
6. Black C, Marotti J, Zarovnaya E, et al. Critical evaluation of frozen section margins in head and neck cancer resections. Cancer 2006;107(12): 2792–800.
7. Meier JD, Oliver DA, Varvares MA. Surgical margin determination in head and neck oncology: current

clinical practice. The results of an International American Head and Neck Society Member Survey. Head Neck 2005;27(11):952–8.

8. Hinni ML, Ferlito A, Brandwein-Gensler MS, et al. Surgical margins in head and neck cancer: a contemporary review. Head Neck 2013;35(9):1362–70.

9. Patel RS, Goldstein DP, Guillemaud J, et al. Impact of positive frozen section microscopic tumor cut-through revised to negative on oral carcinoma control and survival rates. Head Neck 2010;32(11):1444–51.

10. Yahalom R, Dobriyan A, Vered M, et al. A prospective study of surgical margin status in oral squamous cell carcinoma: a preliminary report. J Surg Oncol 2008;98(8):572–8.

11. Amit M, Na'ara S, Leider-Trejo L, et al. Improving the rate of negative margins after surgery for oral cavity squamous cell carcinoma: a prospective randomized controlled study. Head Neck 2016;38(Suppl 1):E1803–9.

12. Chang AM, Kim SW, Duvvuri U, et al. Early squamous cell carcinoma of the oral tongue: comparing margins obtained from the glossectomy specimen to margins from the tumor bed. Oral Oncol 2013; 49(11):1077–82.

13. Maxwell JH, Thompson LD, Brandwein-Gensler MS, et al. Early oral tongue squamous cell carcinoma: sampling of margins from tumor bed and worse local control. JAMA Otolaryngol Head Neck Surg 2015;141(12):1104–10.

14. Varvares MA, Poti S, Kenyon B, et al. Surgical margins and primary site resection in achieving local control in oral cancer resections. Laryngoscope 2015;125(10):2298–307.

15. Baddour HM Jr, Magliocca KR, Chen AY. The importance of margins in head and neck cancer. J Surg Oncol 2016;113(3):248–55.

16. Ettl T, El-Gindi A, Hautmann M, et al. Positive frozen section margins predict local recurrence in R0-resected squamous cell carcinoma of the head and neck. Oral Oncol 2016;55:17–23.

17. Guillemaud JP, Patel RS, Goldstein DP, et al. Prognostic impact of intraoperative microscopic cut-through on frozen section in oral cavity squamous cell carcinoma. J Otolaryngol Head Neck Surg 2010;39(4):370–7.

18. Jackel MC, Ambrosch P, Martin A, et al. Impact of re-resection for inadequate margins on the prognosis of upper aerodigestive tract cancer treated by laser microsurgery. Laryngoscope 2007;117(2):350–6.

19. Kwok P, Gleich O, Hubner G, et al. Prognostic importance of "clear versus revised margins" in oral and pharyngeal cancer. Head Neck 2010;32(11): 1479–84.

20. Scholl P, Byers RM, Batsakis JG, et al. Microscopic cut-through of cancer in the surgical treatment of squamous carcinoma of the tongue. Prognostic and therapeutic implications. Am J Surg 1986; 152(4):354–60.

21. Hinni ML, Zarka MA, Hoxworth JM. Margin mapping in transoral surgery for head and neck cancer. Laryngoscope 2013;123(5):1190–8.

22. Anderson CR, Sisson K, Moncrieff M. A meta-analysis of margin size and local recurrence in oral squamous cell carcinoma. Oral Oncol 2015;51(5):464–9.

23. Duvvuri U, Seethala RR, Chiosea S. Margin assessment in oral squamous cell carcinoma. Cancer 2014;120(3):452–3.

24. Heagerty PJ, Lumley T, Pepe MS. Time-dependent ROC curves for censored survival data and a diagnostic marker. Biometrics 2000;56(2):337–44.

25. Johnson RE, Sigman JD, Funk GF, et al. Quantification of surgical margin shrinkage in the oral cavity. Head Neck 1997;19(4):281–6.

26. Mistry RC, Qureshi SS, Kumaran C. Post-resection mucosal margin shrinkage in oral cancer: quantification and significance. J Surg Oncol 2005;91(2): 131–3.

27. George KS, Hyde NC, Wilson P, et al. Does the method of resection affect the margins of tumours in the oral cavity? Prospective controlled study in pigs. Br J Oral Maxillofac Surg 2013;51(7):600–3.

28. Kerawala CJ, Ong TK. Relocating the site of frozen sections–is there room for improvement? Head Neck 2001;23(3):230–2.

29. Hessel AC, Moreno MA, Hanna EY, et al. Compliance with quality assurance measures in patients treated for early oral tongue cancer. Cancer 2010; 116(14):3408–16.

30. Chen AY. Quality initiatives in head and neck cancer. Curr Oncol Rep 2010;12(2):109–14.

Laryngeal Dysplasia, Squamous Cell Carcinoma, and Variants

Lester D.R. Thompson, MD

KEYWORDS

- Carcinoma, squamous cell • Carcinoma, adenosquamous • Carcinoma, verrucous • Larynx
- Dysplasia

Key points

- Dysplasia is now separated into 2 categories: low and high grade.
- Verrucous squamous cell carcinoma is usually a clinicopathologic correlation.
- Basaloid squamous cell carcinoma shows abrupt keratinization and comedonecrosis.
- Up to 30% of Spindle cell squamous cell carcinoma lacks epithelial differentiation by immunohistochemistry.
- Exophytic and papillary squamous cell carcinoma usually have a better prognosis than conventional squamous cell carcinoma.

ABSTRACT

Squamous cell carcinoma (SCC) is a malignant epithelial tumor showing evidence of squamous differentiation. It is the most common malignancy of the larynx, with several variants (verrucous, exophytic or papillary, spindle-cell, basaloid, acantholytic, adenosquamous) recognized, with well-established precursor lesions. Dysplasia is now separated into only low-grade and high-grade categories. Each SCC variant has unique cytomorphologic features and histologic differential diagnoses that are important to consider, as management and outcomes are different.

OVERVIEW

Squamous cell carcinoma (SCC) is a malignant epithelial tumor showing evidence of squamous differentiation and is the single most important and most common malignant neoplasm of the larynx. Although not always present, precursor dysplasia is usually seen.[1] In general, men are affected much more frequently than women, usually in the middle to later decades of life, although any age can be affected.[2,3] Symptoms are nonspecific, with hoarseness, dyspnea, stridor, and dysphagia most common.[4] Independently and synergistically, tobacco (cigarette, cigar, pipe) and alcohol use are the most important risk factors,[5–7] whereas transcriptionally active human papillomavirus (HPV) is less common in laryngeal tumors, detected in up to 15% of cases.[8–10] Genetic predisposition (such as with Lynch syndrome, Bloom syndrome, and Li-Fraumeni, among others), susceptibility (immunologic factors and age), and other environmental and occupational factors probably interact in this multifactorial and multistep process.[11,12] Variants of SCC account for up to 4% of tumors,[13–19] and are separated primarily because they show a different clinical presentation and outcome, as well as frequently raising different differential diagnoses. In the United States, most tumors develop in the glottis, followed by the supraglottis and rarely subglottis, although geographic variation is common. Direct

Disclosure Statement: No disclosures.
Department of Pathology, Southern California Permanente Medical Group, Woodland Hills Medical Center, 5601 De Soto Avenue, Woodland Hills, CA 91367, USA
E-mail address: Lester.D.Thompson@kp.org

Surgical Pathology 10 (2017) 15–33
http://dx.doi.org/10.1016/j.path.2016.10.003
1875-9181/17/Published by Elsevier Inc.

surgpath.theclinics.com

extension into contiguous structures or lympho-vascular invasion is common, the latter resulting in a high incidence of regional lymph node metastases. Surgery, laser therapy, and radiation continue to be the mainstays of therapy, with changes in protocols for the specific histologic variants.[20] Outcomes are heavily influenced by tumor stage, localization (glottic), and age,[20–22] whereas differentiation, invasive pattern, vascular and/or perineural invasion, margin status, and extranodal extension play a significant role.[23–33]

DYSPLASIA (PRECURSOR LESIONS)

Dysplasia is defined by a morphologic spectrum of architectural and cytologic changes in the squamous mucosal epithelium that is associated with an increased likelihood of progression to SCC. Gastroesophageal reflux disease is considered a risk factor in addition to tobacco and alcohol use,[34,35] whereas transcriptionally active HPV seems to be of minor importance.[36–38] There are frequent chromosomal changes and loss of heterozygosity, with CDKN2A gene alterations most frequently identified, associated with TP53 and cyclin-D1 overexpression and activated telomerase activity, but these are not yet clinically useful.[39–41] The vocal cords are affected most frequently, with rare involvement of the commisures.[42]

Leukoplakia, erythroplakia, or mixed leukoerythroplakia appear in the larynx as localized or diffuse patches or flat to exophytic or papillary lesions that mimic SCC. Therefore, histologic evaluation is mandatory for diagnosis.

Over the years, many different grading schemes have been proposed,[43–45] often subject to significant interobserver variability. With a trend in other organs to a 2-grade system,[46,47] generally lesions that are traditionally considered mild dysplasia would be categorized as "low grade" whereas lesions classified as moderate to severe dysplasia/carcinoma in situ can be categorized as "high grade." **Table 1** highlights the architectural and cytomorphological features used to distinguish between low-grade and high-grade dysplasia (as modified from the World Health Organization Classification of Tumours of the Head and Neck). In general, it is a qualitative and quantitative

---

Table 1
Dysplasia criteria

Low-grade dysplasia (previously mild dysplasia)	Architecture	• Overall stratification is preserved, whereas basal-parabasal layer is abnormal • Basal-parabasal layer is increased, up to lower half of the epithelium • Spinous layer may be increased, with prickle cells usually seen only in upper half of the epithelium
	Cytology	• Limited pleomorphism • Enlarged nuclei with increased nuclear-to-cytoplasmic ratio, but evenly distributed chromatin; vague cytoplasmic pinking with limited intercellular spinous processes • Isolated dyskeratosis cells • Mitoses (typical forms) limited to lower third of epithelium
High-grade dysplasia (previously moderate and severe dysplasia, and carcinoma in situ)	Architecture	• Keratinizing or nonkeratinizing (basal cell) types • Loss of maturation, with disordered stratification and loss of polarity up to full thickness • Cellular pleomorphism from one-half up to full thickness, frequently severe • Basement membrane remains intact (no stromal changes) around irregular-shaped rete (bulbous, downwardly extending)
	Cytology	• Often conspicuous pleomorphism with marked variation in cell and nuclear size and shape, marked variation in staining intensity (often hyperchromatic), and increased size and number of nucleoli • High nuclear-to-cytoplasmic ratio • Dyskeratotic cells increased throughout the epithelium • Increased mitoses anywhere in the epithelial, to include atypical forms (the latter qualifies as high-grade by itself)

Modified from Gale N, Hille J, Jordan R, et al. Tumours of the hypopharynx, larynx, trachea, and parapharyngeal space: precursor lesions. In: El-Naggar AK, Chan JKC, Grandis JR, et al, editors. Pathology and genetics of head and neck tumours. 4th edition. World Health Organization Classification of Tumours. Lyon, France: IARC Press, 2017, in press.

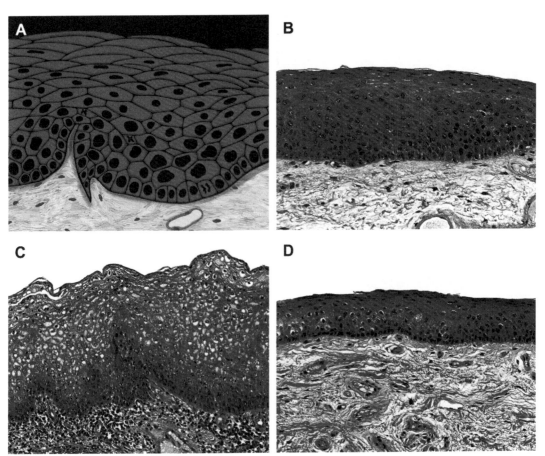

Fig. 1. Low-grade keratinizing dysplasia. (*A*) Schematic showing expanded basal-parabasal zone, nuclear hyperchromasia and irregularities, with increased normal mitoses. (*B*) Disorganized basal zone (lower one-third) with nuclear crowding and increased nuclear-to-cytoplasmic ratio, with maturation. (*C*) Expanded parabasal zone with maturation toward the surface, with nuclear irregularities and cytoplasmic pinking and spinous zone expansion. (*D*) Subtle increased cellularity with nuclear atypia limited to the lower half, showing surface maturation.

accumulation of features that moves a particular lesion into a dysplasia grade. It is important to note, however, that the traditional use of "thirds" in the uterine cervix does not apply to upper aerodigestive tract lesions. Particularly if there is profound pleomorphism and atypical mitoses confined to the lower third, it still represents high-grade dysplasia in the larynx. The vast majority of dysplasia in the larynx is keratinizing, with only a small number non-keratinizing. Loss of maturation, disordered polarity, and expansion of the basal layer (**Fig. 1**) is an architectural feature of dysplasia, whereas increased cell size, increase in nuclear-to-cytoplasmic ratio, nuclear contour irregularities, nuclear chromatin distribution changes, cytoplasmic pinking, prominent intercellular borders, and increased mitoses are some of the cytologic features seen in dysplasia (see **Fig. 1**). Sometimes, the low-power appearance is more innocuous because the dysplasia is often associated with surface maturation and multiple layers of epithelial cells, but careful examination on high power will help reveal the histologic features of dysplasia. Importantly, significant keratosis and parakeratosis only may behave similarly to low-grade dysplasia, showing a similar progression risk. No one feature in isolation is diagnostic, but in general, the presence of atypical mitoses is seen only in high-grade dysplasia (**Fig. 2**). By definition, the process is confined to the surface epithelium or showing gland-duct extension, but without stromal alterations or breach of the basement membrane. There are inconsistent findings with p53 (increased), p21, p27 (decreased), cyclin D1, bcl-2, p16, Ki-67 (increased), β-catenin, and epidermal growth factor receptor (EGFR) when used to separate between dysplasia grading, partly due to immunohistochemistry overexpression not necessarily correlating to molecular alterations or progression of disease.[48–52]

Distinction from epithelial hyperplasia, pseudoepitheliomatous hyperplasia, necrotizing sialometaplasia, verrucous changes, and invasive

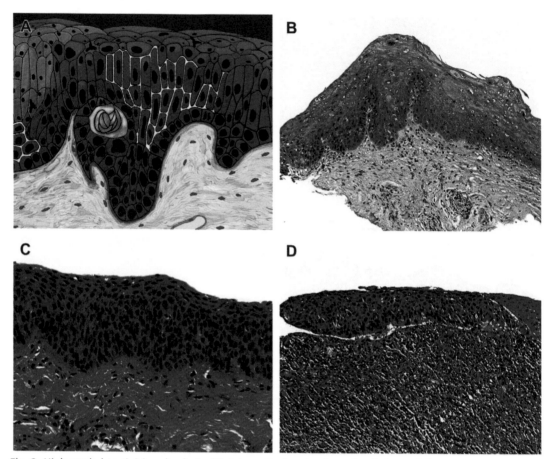

Fig. 2. High-grade keratinizing dysplasia. (*A*) Schematic showing loss of polarity and disorganization of upper half, with dyskeratosis, keratin pearl formation, and atypical mitoses. (*B*) Dyskeratosis at the surface, loss of maturation, and cellular pleomorphism. (*C*) Almost full-thickness atypia, perpendicular nuclear arrangement, increased mitoses, and very high nuclear-to-cytoplasmic ratio. (*D*) Full-thickness disorganization, loss of maturation, increased nuclear-to-cytoplasmic ratio, and pleomorphism. Note right side has uninvolved epithelium.

carcinoma are necessary to assess appropriate risk of progression, modify etiologic contributing risk factors, or to treat adequately, particularly when present intraoperatively at margins (Table 2). The sometimes very subtle findings in low-grade dysplasia may make separation of small or tangentially sectioned biopsies very challenging. Keeping in mind what the clinical consequences of each diagnosis will be, may help to apply the criteria more uniformly and reproducibly. High-grade dysplasia is associated with invasive carcinoma development in up to 40% of cases, whereas low-grade dysplasia shows malignant progression in only approximately 2% of cases.[45,53,54]

SQUAMOUS CELL CARCINOMA

SCC may be ulcerated, endophytic, flat, exophytic, polypoid, or verrucous, ranging from minute mucosal thickenings to occlusive masses. The tumors are erythematous to tan-white, frequently firm.

SCC is composed of variable degrees of squamous differentiation associated with invasion (Fig. 3). SCC is generally divided into 3 histologic grades (well, or moderately or poorly differentiated), with or without keratinization (see Fig. 3). SCC shows a desmoplastic stromal reaction, frequently perineural or lymphovascular invasion, and disruption of the basement membrane by cords, nests, islands, or individual cells (different invading fronts; see Fig. 3A). There is a loss of polarity, disorganization, dyskeratosis, and keratin pearl formation. Intercellular bridges are noted between cells that have an increased nuclear-to-cytoplasmic ratio, cytoplasmic opacification, and irregular, polygonal shapes. There are nuclear chromatin irregularities, prominent eosinophilic nucleoli, and increased mitoses, including atypical forms. Well-developed keratinization is not seen in poorly differentiated tumors (see **Fig. 3**). In poorly differentiated or high-grade tumors, immunohistochemistry studies for CK5/6, p63, p40, and epithelial membrane antigen (EMA) may help confirm the epithelial nature of the proliferation.[55]

Generally, hyperplasia, papilloma, dysplasia, and select SCC variants, mainly verrucous carcinoma (VC) are the major differential diagnostic considerations for a well-differentiated tumor (**Table 2**). Hyperplasia lacks individual cell infiltration and severe pleomorphism, usually showing the infectious agent or perhaps a granular cell tumor in the background. A squamous papilloma lacks significant pleomorphism and is noninvasive. Dysplasia by definition lacks breach of the basement membrane. SCC may develop in the absence of surface dysplasia. VC shows a specific architecture (bulbous rete, no atypia, limited mitoses, parakeratotic crypting, church-spire keratosis) that is not seen in SCC. The differential diagnosis for

differentiation and selected, pertinent, and focused immunohistochemistry studies (S100 protein, SOX10, CD45RB, synaptophysin, chromogranin) will help with this distinction.

Prognosis is separated by anatomic site, stage, and other factors, such as age, comorbidities, and the patient's performance status, with overall 5-year survival rate of 80% to 85% for glottic, 65% to 75% for supraglottic, and 40% for subglottic SCCs.[20–22] Stage, including regional and/or distant metastases, depth of invasion, pattern of invasive front (single cells), perineural and lymphovascular invasion, extranodal extension in lymph node metastases, and positive resection margins are all prognostic factors that correlate with increased risk of recurrence, lymph node metastases, and decreased survival.[23–33]

VERRUCOUS CARCINOMA

Table 2
Pitfalls

Tumor Type	Pitfall
Dysplasia	• Pseudoepitheliomatous hyperplasia has bulbous rete, but etiologic agent frequently present • Tangential sections must be carefully reviewed • Gland-duct extension is not invasion • Parakeratosis and keratosis in the larynx are abnormal
SCC	• Basement membrane must be breached • Invasive tumor may develop without surface dysplasia • Poorly differentiated tumors must be evaluated for neuroendocrine carcinoma and mucosa melanoma
Verrucous carcinoma	• Inadequate biopsy precludes definitive diagnosis • Tangential sectioning may overestimate thickness • Do not diagnose verrucous hyperplasia on a biopsy because more extensive sampling may reveal carcinoma
Papillary/Exophytic SCC	• Orientation is critical • Must make sure you have an adequate specimen (ie, stalk or base of lesion)
Spindle cell SCC	• Surface epithelium generally absent • 30% lack epithelial immuno markers • Hypocellular tumors still show atypia
Basaloid SCC	• Must find squamous differentiation • Mucohyaline material mimics adenoid cystic carcinoma • Superficial biopsy fails to show true tumor appearance
Adenosquamous carcinoma	• High-grade mucoepidermoid carcinoma still shows mucocytes • Two distinct populations are seen

Abbreviation: SCC, squamous cell carcinoma.

poorly differentiated SCC may include a variety of different tumor types. Melanoma, lymphoma, and neuroendocrine carcinomas are uncommon in the larynx, but the presence of squamous

Comprising approximately 3% of laryngeal SCC,[14,56] VC is not associated with transcriptionally active HPV, with most developing in older men.[57,58] A clinicopathologic correlation with the

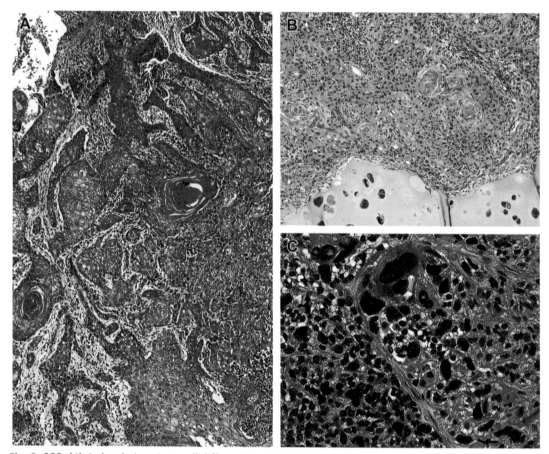

Fig. 3. SCC. (*A*) A deeply invasive, well-differentiated, keratinizing SCC with keratin pearls. (*B*) A moderately differentiated keratinizing SCC shows cartilage invasion. (*C*) Poorly differentiated SCC with marked pleomorphism.

gross or endoscopic appearance of a large, broad-based, warty, exophytic or fungating bulky, firm to hard, tan or white mass, is required in many cases to yield a diagnosis, especially if biopsies are superficial, small, and/or lack a good stromal interface (Table 3).[59–62] VCs are important to recognize because they are only locally aggressive without metastatic capacity unless there is a conventional SCC component.

VC is a highly differentiated, slow-growing, locally invasive SCC lacking cytologic features of malignancy, usually affecting the true vocal cord, but any site may be affected. Thickened, club-shaped, broad to bulbous rete pushing into the stroma below the level of the neighboring normal basal cell layer is one of the histologic hallmarks (Fig. 4). Desmoplasia is usually absent, but a lymphoplasmacytic infiltrate is common. The extraordinarily well-differentiated epithelium is greatly expanded, showing "church-spire" keratosis, parakeratosis, and parakeratotic crypting between the exophytic-warty tumor projections. There is absent atypia, orderly maturation toward the surface, and isolated to absent mitoses that are confined to the basal-parabasal zone (Fig. 5). In some cases, foci of conventional SCC are seen, diagnosed as a hybrid or mixed tumor, and showing the outcome of conventional SCC.[59,61,62]

The differential diagnosis of VC includes verrucous hyperplasia, squamous papilloma, conventional SCC, papillary and exophytic SCC, and hybrid carcinomas (Table 2). The constant challenge is that VC is not cytologically malignant and requires invasion for a definitive diagnosis. If a biopsy is small or superficial, this becomes almost impossible to determine. In fact, it has been argued that the difference between verrucous hyperplasia and VC is only in stage and size, considered to be a developmental spectrum,[63–65] a bias shared by this author. Thus, a definitive diagnosis can be rendered only when the relationship of the lesion to the stroma can be adequately assessed, made more challenging

Table 3
Pathologic key features of SCC variants

Feature	Verrucous	Papillary/Exophytic	Variant Spindle Cell (Sarcomatoid)	Basaloid	Adenosquamous
Macroscopic	Broad-based, warty and fungating mass	Polypoid, exophytic, bulky, papillary, fungiform	Polypoid mass	Firm to hard with central necrosis	Indurated submucosal mass
Microscopic	Pushing border of infiltration; abrupt transition with normal; large, blunt club-shaped rete; no pleomorphism; nearly absent mitoses; abundant keratin, including parakeratin crypting and "church-spire" keratosis	>70% exophytic or papillary architecture; unequivocal cytomorphologic malignancy; surface keratinization; invasive by definition; koilocytic atypia	Biphasic; SCC present, but ulcerated; transition of epithelial to atypical spindled cells; hypercellular; variable patterns of spindle-cell growth; pleomorphism; opacified cytoplasm; increased mitoses	Deeply invasive; lobular; basaloid component most prominent; peripheral nuclear palisading; high N:C ratio; abrupt squamous differentiation (metaplasia, dysplasia, CIS or invasive); increased mitoses; central comedonecrosis; hyaline stroma material	Biphasic; SCC and adenocarcinoma; undifferentiated clear-cell component; separate or intermixed with areas of transition; infiltrative
Special studies	No transcriptionally active HPV identified	None	30% negative with epithelial immunohistochemistry markers	Keratin, EMA, CK7, and 34βE12; negative neuroendocrine markers	Mucin-positive glandular/goblet cells
Differential diagnosis	Hyperplasia; squamous papilloma; conventional SCC; hybrid carcinoma	In situ SCC; squamous papilloma; reactive hyperplasia	Inflammatory myofibroblastic tumor; mucosal melanoma; synovial sarcoma; other malignant mesenchymal tumors	Adenoid cystic carcinoma; neuroendocrine carcinoma (small cell carcinoma); adenosquamous carcinoma; mucoepidermoid carcinoma	Basaloid SCC; mucoepidermoid carcinoma; adenocarcinoma with squamous metaplasia; adenoid SCC

Abbreviations: CIS, carcinoma in situ; EMA, epithelial membrane antigen; HPV, human papillomavirus; N:C ratio, nuclear-to-cytoplasmic ratio; SCC, squamous cell carcinoma.

A

B

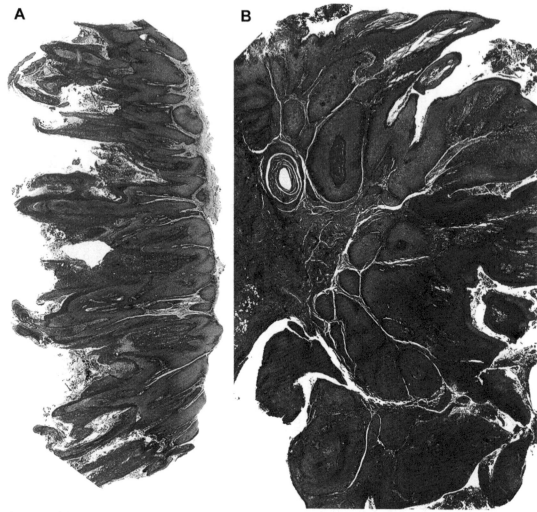

Fig. 4. VC. (*A*) Marked verruciform proliferation with church-spire–type keratosis and club-shaped rete pushing into the stroma. (*B*) Broad pushing border of infiltration by club-shaped rete lacking atypia and associated with keratosis.

with tangential sectioning, sample fragmentation, and frozen section artifacts. Using the term "verruciform squamous proliferation," followed by a comment will provide the necessary guidance to the treating physician and highlight the difficulties experienced. There is often an increased expression of p53 and EGFR in VC versus squamous epithelium alone,[66] but in daily practice almost impossible to apply. Squamous papilloma is usually an exophytic rather than an endophytic growth, often showing koilocytic changes and atypia of the basal-parabasal zones. When conventional SCC is noted within a VC, a hybrid diagnosis is rendered. The amount and extent of the conventional SCC component may determine extent of therapy (ie, managed as conventional SCC).[56]

Radiotherapy or surgery may be used, with an overall 5-year survival of 85% to 95%, with stage the most important prognostic factor.[14,56,62,67–69]

EXOPHYTIC AND PAPILLARY SQUAMOUS CELL CARCINOMA

Rare in the larynx, men are affected more often than women, usually in the seventh decade of life (**Table 3**). Macroscopically, exophytic SCC (ESCC) and papillary SCC (PSCC) are polypoid, exophytic, bulky, papillary, or fungiform tumors, soft to firm, arising from a broad base or from a narrow pedicle/stalk.[16,70–73]

By definition, ESCC and PSCC are de novo malignancies without a preexisting or coexisting

Fig. 5. The proliferation is cytologically bland without mitotic figures but demonstrating a broad, bulbous type infiltration into the stroma. Parakeratotic crypting is noted.

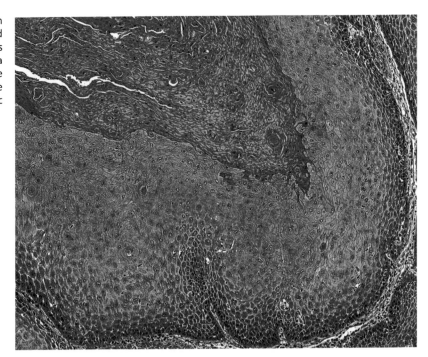

benign lesion, showing severely dysplastic epithelium lining the fronds, frequently lacking well-developed histologic invasion. The neoplasm must demonstrate a dominant (>70%) exophytic or papillary growth with frank cytomorphologic evidence of malignancy.[70] The exophytic pattern consists of broad-based, bulbous growths of rounded atypical epithelium, often with a rounded to lobular surface appearance (**Fig. 6**). The papillary pattern shows multiple, thin, delicate filiform, projections with delicate fibrovascular cores covered by the neoplastic epithelium, creating numerous surface fronds (**Fig. 7**). When both patterns are seen, ESCC is diagnosed. The lining squamous epithelium is frankly malignant, showing similar features to high-grade dysplasia or carcinoma in situ (see **Fig. 6**). Stromal invasion is difficult to document, but present by definition, along with a heavy inflammatory infiltrate.[16,70] "Koilocytic atypia" may be focally noted, correlated with transcriptionally active HPV in some cases.[74]

The cytomorphologic features of malignancy would help distinguish a squamous papilloma and VC from these variants. Reactive hyperplasia may show atypia, but does not have well-developed exophytic or papillary architecture (**Table 2**).

This variant of SCC has a better prognosis than conventional SCC, usually related to low-stage presentation and low metastatic potential because of the exophytic growth, with an approximately 85% 5-year survival.[16,70,71,74]

SPINDLE-CELL SQUAMOUS CELL CARCINOMA

Spindle-cell (sarcomatoid) squamous cell carcinoma (SCSCC) is a morphologically biphasic tumor with a carcinoma that has surface epithelial changes (dysplasia to invasive carcinoma) and an underlying malignant spindle and/or pleomorphic proliferation. This tumor shows a profound male-to-female ratio (11:1), generally presenting in the seventh decade of life, usually involving the glottis, and usually with low tumor stage (**Table 3**).[15,17,75–78]

Nearly all cases are polypoid masses (**Fig. 8**) with a mean size of approximately 2.0 cm. They are frequently ulcerated with a covering of fibrinoid necrosis. They have a firm and fibrous cut surface.[15,17,77]

As a consequence of ulceration, surface origin or transition is difficult to identify. Review of the base of the stalk, invaginated regions or noneroded areas may help highlight epithelial dysplasia, carcinoma in situ, or infiltrating SCC (see **Fig. 8**; **Fig. 9**). Frequently, limited stromal invasion beyond the stalk is noted, as the tumors are predominantly polypoid. There is an imperceptible blending and continuity of the epithelial to spindled morphology (see **Fig. 8**).[79,80] By definition, the spindled population dominates, arranged

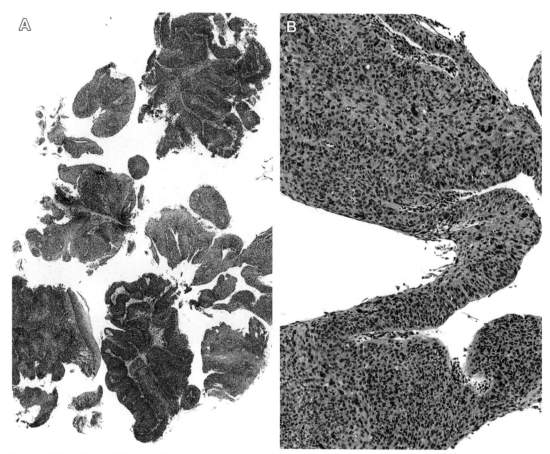

Fig. 6. ESCC. (*A*) An ESCC with fragments of tissue showing broad projections. (*B*) Marked pleomorphism and frank anaplasia.

in a storiform, cartwheel, whorled to intersecting fascicular architecture. Hypocellular areas with collagen deposition contain pleomorphic cells, but can be deceptively bland (see **Fig. 8**). Most tumors are hypercellular, lacking maturation, with easily identified but usually not profound pleomorphism. Tumor cells are fusiform to polygonal (see **Fig. 8**). Opacified, dense cytoplasm suggests squamous differentiation. Easily identified mitoses, including atypical forms, are common, but necrosis is rare.[15,17,77,81] Rarely, metaplastic or frankly neoplastic cartilage or bone or rhabdomyoblastic heterologous elements may be present.[77,82,83]

SCSCC is the most likely SCC variant to benefit from immunohistochemistry evaluation, in which approximately 70% show reactivity for AE1/AE3, EMA, p63, and/or p40.[77,84] p53 is usually overexpressed.[85] Tumors without epithelial reactivity must still be interpreted as SCSCC until proven otherwise. Importantly, focal reactivity for smooth muscle actin, muscle-specific actin, and, rarely, S-100 protein may be seen.[76,77,86,87] This degree

of lineage infidelity is expected in tumors that show significant epithelial-mesenchymal–type transition.[79,80]

Given a very limited stroma in the vocal cords, genuine mesenchymal lesions of the larynx are very rare. Thus, a spindled cell proliferation of the larynx must be considered an SCSCC until further evaluation proves otherwise. Inflammatory myofibroblastic tumor, mucosal melanoma, and synovial sarcoma are occasionally seen, whereas fibrosarcoma, pleomorphic sarcoma, leiomyosarcoma, rhabdomyosarcoma, malignant peripheral nerve sheath tumor, and angiosarcoma are vanishingly rare (**Table 2**). The presence of squamous differentiation usually makes distinction possible. The rich inflammatory infiltrate along with a myofibroblastic haphazard spindled cell proliferation with feathery cytoplasm, often with anaplastic lymphoma kinase (ALK) expression and a lack of epithelial features helps to diagnose an inflammatory myofibroblastic tumor.[88,89] A monophasic synovial sarcoma tends to occur in young patients, usually arises in the soft tissues

A
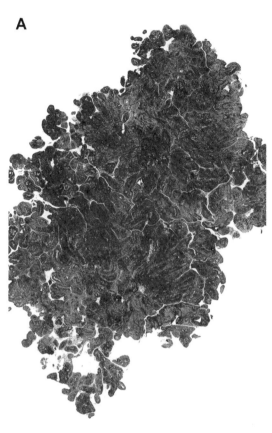

B
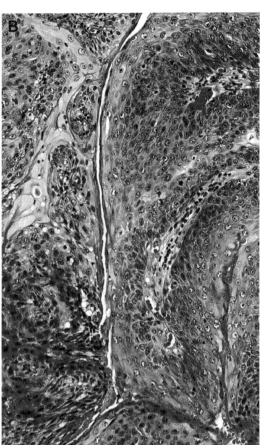

Fig. 7. PSCC. (*A*) A PSCC with numerous individual, delicate fingerlike projections with fibrovascular cores. (*B*) Marked pleomorphism is seen in the lining epithelium of the papillary projections.

of the neck, will show a marbled pattern, expresses TLE1, and will usually show the specific characteristic translocation (*SS18-SSX*).[90,91]

Although the terms "spindle cell" or "sarcomatoid," sound ominous, laryngeal SCSCC, irrespective of T-stage, actually shows a statistically significant better patient outcome when no epithelial marker immunoreactivity can be demonstrated (ie, patients with tumors that are keratin immunoreactive tend to have a worse prognosis), although patients generally show an excellent prognosis in comparison with conventional SCC.[15,17,77]

BASALOID SQUAMOUS CELL CARCINOMA

Basaloid SCC (BSCC) is a high-grade SCC variant showing a prominent basaloid component and evidence of squamous cell differentiation, showing a predilection for the supraglottis, frequently presenting with multifocality, primarily affecting men in the seventh decade of life with frequent advanced stage at presentation (**Table 3**).[18,92–95]

There is no significant transcriptionally active HPV association with laryngeal tumors.[94,96,97] Macroscopically, these tumors are usually firm to hard with associated central necrosis.

Histologically, the tumor invades in a submucosal distribution as smooth-bordered lobules, cords, and nests, frequently showing peripheral palisading (**Fig. 10**A). The depth of invasion may not be obvious on a superficial biopsy, and thus generous sampling is necessary for diagnosis. Lymphovascular invasion is common. The basaloid component is the most diagnostic feature, showing closely approximated cells with a high nuclear-to-cytoplasmic ratio and hyperchromatic chromatin. The cells are often separated by a prominent, hyalinized densely eosinophilic stroma that may form small droplets or cylinders within the tumor, creating a jigsaw puzzle appearance (**Fig. 10**B). Glandlike foci often with mucomyxoid material can mimic adenocarcinoma. Squamous differentiation may be in the form of abrupt keratinization, squamous pearls, individual cell

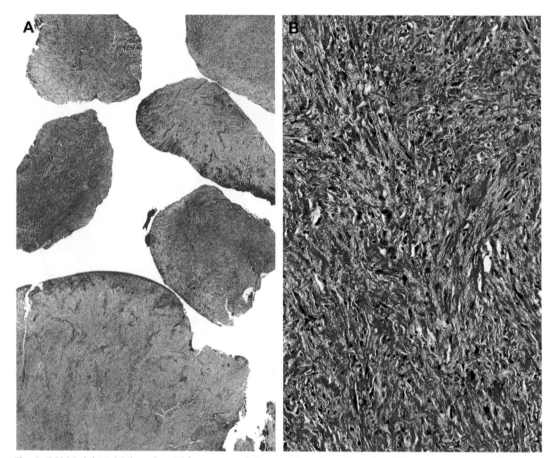

Fig. 8. SCSCC. (*A*) Multiple polypoid fragments of tissue with surface ulceration. (*B*) Hypocellular spindled tumor showing isolated pleomorphic cells with hyperchromatic nuclei.

keratinization, dysplasia, or SCC (in situ or invasive). Although both basaloid and squamous cell components can be seen in metastases, the basaloid features predominate. Epithelial markers (pancytokeratin, CAM5.2, EMA, CK7, 34ßE12) and p63 and p40 are consistently reactive, whereas neuroendocrine markers are negative; p53 is overexpressed.[98–100] A perinuclear "dot" of vimentin immunoreactivity is occasionally seen.[93,101]

The differential diagnosis includes neuroendocrine carcinoma (small cell and large cell types), SCC, adenoid cystic carcinoma (ACC), adenosquamous carcinoma (ASC), and high-grade mucoepidermoid carcinoma (MEC) (**Table 2**). All these diagnoses require sufficient sampling to demonstrate the heterogeneous components of the tumor.[18,99,102] ACC lacks squamous differentiation, usually shows limited mitoses and necrosis, and shows biphasic distribution of p63 and epithelial markers.[93,98,103] *MYB* is seen in ACC and not in BSCC.[104,105] Neuroendocrine carcinoma may show squamous differentiation, but demonstrates

nuclear molding, salt-and-pepper nuclear chromatin distribution, and demonstrates neuroendocrine markers.[103] Combined features of true mucinous differentiation with transitional cells would confirm an MEC, whereas two distinct tumors would define an ASC. True glandular elements would define ASC.

BSCC of the larynx has an overall worse prognosis compared with conventional SCC, especially in active smokers, but irrespective of stage, tumor location, or treatment received, and showing high rates of nodal metastases (50%–70%) and distant metastases.[18,94,106]

ADENOSQUAMOUS CARCINOMA

ASC shows an admixture of SCC and adenocarcinoma, often accompanied by an undifferentiated cellular component. The SCC can be in situ or invasive, showing intercellular bridges, keratin pearl formation, and dyskeratosis (**Fig. 11**). The adenocarcinoma shows glandular differentiation (see

Fig. 9. SCSCC. An SCSCC blending of the surface epithelium with the spindle-cell component. Abrupt transitions with conventional SCC is present (*left*), with focal profoundly pleomorphic cells.

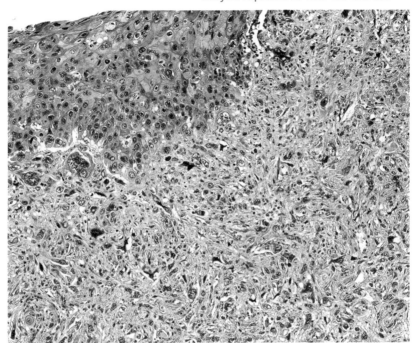

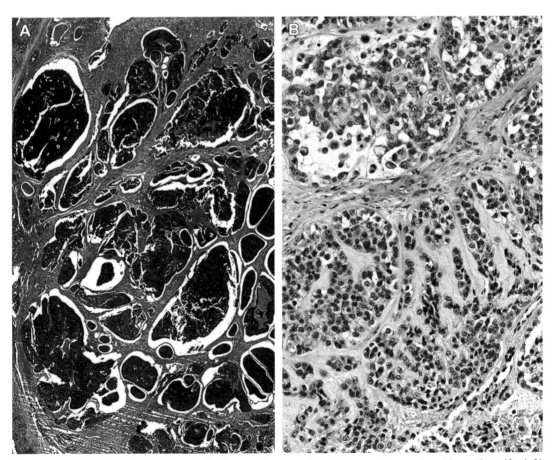

Fig. 10. BSCC. (*A*) There is a lobular architecture, with areas of central comedonecrosis, with cartilage (*far left*). The neoplastic proliferation is highly basaloid. (*B*) A prominent hyalinized material between tumor cells with associated myxoid material. Focal squamous differentiation is noted.

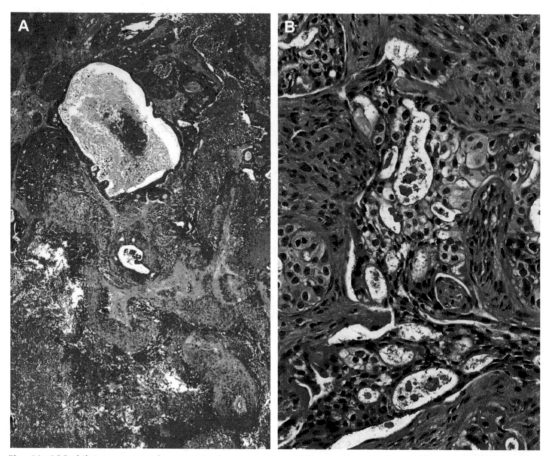

Fig. 11. ASC. (*A*) Low power shows a single tumor mass with an adenocarcinoma (*upper*) blending with a keratinizing SCC (*lower*). (*B*) High power demonstrates blending of an adenocarcinoma and SCC (*far left*) within a single tumor mass associated with desmoplasia.

Fig. 11), including mucocytes or goblet cells (**Table 3**). Basaloid cells in either the SCC or adenocarcinoma may make distinction from BSCC arbitrary. The two tumors may be separate or intermixed, with areas of commingling. The "undifferentiated" transition areas often show cytoplasmic clearing. Increased mitoses and necrosis may be seen.[107–112]

Although impossible to distinguish in some cases, MEC shows intermediate type cells and generally lacks true squamous cell differentiation (**Table 2**). Two distinct tumor populations are not seen in MEC. Further, *CRTC1-MAML2* translocation is not seen in ASC.[108] BSCC shows islands of basaloid cells, peripheral nuclear palisading, and lacks true glandular differentiation. An adenocarcinoma with surface squamous metaplasia lacks the malignant squamous cell component. An adenoid SCC (acantholytic SCC) shows acantholysis of the squamous cells, mimicking glandular differentiation, but lacking a positive mucicarmine reaction.[113] Synchronous collision tumors (SCC and adenocarcinoma) may affect the larynx, with the

bulk of the tumors temporally distinct. The overall outcome is historically poor, although recent data suggest no significant differences in outcome as compared with conventional SCC when matched for stage and other variables.[108,112]

RARE VARIANTS

NUT CARCINOMA

NUT carcinoma is exceedingly rare in the larynx and is a poorly differentiated carcinoma often with evidence of abrupt squamous differentiation, at least focally, and defined by the presence of *NUT* (*NUTM1*) gene rearrangement, detected by a strongly expressed NUT protein by immunohistochemistry.[114,115]

SMARCB1-DEFICIENT CARCINOMAS

SMARCB1-deficient carcinomas develop all over the body, although rare, frequently showing poorly differentiated cells with rhabdoid features and by definition lacking *SMARCB1* (INI-1) protein by immunohistochemistry. They are not yet reported in the larynx.[116]

LYMPHOEPITHELIAL CARCINOMA

Lymphoepithelial carcinoma is an SCC that is identical to nonkeratinizing undifferentiated nasopharyngeal carcinoma, although exceptional in the larynx. There is less of an association with Epstein-Barr virus in the larynx. The histologic features of large cells with high nuclear-to-cytoplasmic ratio, and prominent nucleoli within vesicular nuclei associated with lymphoid cells is characteristic.[117,118]

REFERENCES

1. Hu Y, Liu H. Diagnostic variability of laryngeal premalignant lesions: histological evaluation and carcinoma transformation. Otolaryngol Head Neck Surg 2014;150:401–6.
2. Cattaruzza MS, Maisonneuve P, Boyle P. Epidemiology of laryngeal cancer. Eur J Cancer B Oral Oncol 1996;32B:293–305.
3. Rafferty MA, Fenton JE, Jones AS. The history, aetiology and epidemiology of laryngeal carcinoma. Clin Otolaryngol Allied Sci 2001;26:442–6.
4. Raitiola H, Pukander J. Symptoms of laryngeal carcinoma and their prognostic significance. Acta Oncol 2000;39:213–6.
5. Bagnardi V, Rota M, Botteri E, et al. Alcohol consumption and site-specific cancer risk: a comprehensive dose-response meta-analysis. Br J Cancer 2015;112:580–93.
6. Paget-Bailly S, Cyr D, Luce D. Occupational exposures and cancer of the larynx-systematic review and meta-analysis. J Occup Environ Med 2012;54:71–84.
7. Hashibe M, Brennan P, Benhamou S, et al. Alcohol drinking in never users of tobacco, cigarette smoking in never drinkers, and the risk of head and neck cancer: pooled analysis in the International Head and Neck Cancer Epidemiology Consortium. J Natl Cancer Inst 2007;99:777–89.
8. Lewis JS Jr, Ukpo OC, Ma XJ, et al. Transcriptionally-active high-risk human papillomavirus is rare in oral cavity and laryngeal/hypopharyngeal squamous cell carcinomas–a tissue microarray study utilizing E6/E7 mRNA in situ hybridization. Histopathology 2012;60:982–91.
9. Chernock RD, Wang X, Gao G, et al. Detection and significance of human papillomavirus, CDKN2A(p16) and CDKN1A(p21) expression in squamous cell carcinoma of the larynx. Mod Pathol 2013;26:223–31.
10. Halec G, Holzinger D, Schmitt M, et al. Biological evidence for a causal role of HPV16 in a small fraction of laryngeal squamous cell carcinoma. Br J Cancer 2013;109:172–83.
11. Wagner M, Bolm-Audorff U, Hegewald J, et al. Occupational polycyclic aromatic hydrocarbon exposure and risk of larynx cancer: a systematic review and meta-analysis. Occup Environ Med 2015;72:226–33.
12. Brown T, Darnton A, Fortunato L, et al. Occupational cancer in Britain. Respiratory cancer sites: larynx, lung and mesothelioma. Br J Cancer 2012; 107(Suppl 1):S56–70.
13. Bice TC, Tran V, Merkley MA, et al. Disease-specific survival with spindle cell carcinoma of the head and neck. Otolaryngol Head Neck Surg 2015;153:973–80.
14. Dubal PM, Svider PF, Kam D, et al. Laryngeal verrucous carcinoma: a population-based analysis. Otolaryngol Head Neck Surg 2015;153:799–805.
15. Dubal PM, Marchiano E, Kam D, et al. Laryngeal spindle cell carcinoma: a population-based analysis of incidence and survival. Laryngoscope 2015;125:2709–14.
16. Dutta R, Husain Q, Kam D, et al. Laryngeal papillary squamous cell carcinoma: a population-based analysis of incidence and survival. Otolaryngol Head Neck Surg 2015;153:54–9.
17. Gerry D, Fritsch VA, Lentsch EJ. Spindle cell carcinoma of the upper aerodigestive tract: an analysis of 341 cases with comparison to conventional squamous cell carcinoma. Ann Otol Rhinol Laryngol 2014;123:576–83.
18. Fritsch VA, Lentsch EJ. Basaloid squamous cell carcinoma of the larynx: analysis of 145 cases with comparison to conventional squamous cell carcinoma. Head Neck 2014;36:164–70.
19. Hoffman HT, Porter K, Karnell LH, et al. Laryngeal cancer in the United States: changes in demographics, patterns of care, and survival. Laryngoscope 2006;116:1–13.
20. Zhu J, Fedewa S, Chen AY. The impact of comorbidity on treatment (chemoradiation and laryngectomy) of advanced, nondistant metastatic laryngeal cancer: a review of 16 849 cases from the national cancer database (2003-2008). Arch Otolaryngol Head Neck Surg 2012;138:1120–8.
21. Singh B, Alfonso A, Sabin S, et al. Outcome differences in younger and older patients with laryngeal cancer: a retrospective case-control study. Am J Otolaryngol 2000;21:92–7.
22. Chen AY, Matson LK, Roberts D, et al. The significance of comorbidity in advanced laryngeal cancer. Head Neck 2001;23:566–72.
23. Sethi S, Lu M, Kapke A, et al. Patient and tumor factors at diagnosis in a multi-ethnic primary head and neck squamous cell carcinoma cohort. J Surg Oncol 2009;99:104–8.

24. Yilmaz T, Hosal AS, Gedikoglu G, et al. Prognostic significance of histopathological parameters in cancer of the larynx. Eur Arch Otorhinolaryngol 1999;256:139–44.

25. Yilmaz T, Hosal AS, Gedikoglu G, et al. Prognostic significance of vascular and perineural invasion in cancer of the larynx. Am J Otolaryngol 1998;19:83–8.

26. Brandwein-Gensler M, Smith RV, Wang B, et al. Validation of the histologic risk model in a new cohort of patients with head and neck squamous cell carcinoma. Am J Surg Pathol 2010;34:676–88.

27. Suoglu Y, Erdamar B, Katircioglu OS, et al. Extracapsular spread in ipsilateral neck and contralateral neck metastases in laryngeal cancer. Ann Otol Rhinol Laryngol 2002;111:447–54.

28. Ferlito A, Rinaldo A, Devaney KO, et al. Prognostic significance of microscopic and macroscopic extracapsular spread from metastatic tumor in the cervical lymph nodes. Oral Oncol 2002;38:747–51.

29. Nakayama M, Holsinger C, Okamoto M, et al. Clinicopathological analyses of fifty supracricoid laryngectomized specimens: evidence base supporting minimal margins. ORL J Otorhinolaryngol Relat Spec 2009;71:305–11.

30. Hinni ML, Ferlito A, Brandwein-Gensler MS, et al. Surgical margins in head and neck cancer: a contemporary review. Head Neck 2013;35:1362–70.

31. Bryne M, Boysen M, Alfsen CG, et al. The invasive front of carcinomas. The most important area for tumour prognosis? Anticancer Res 1998;18:4757–64.

32. Bryne M, Jenssen N, Boysen M. Histological grading in the deep invasive front of T1 and T2 glottic squamous cell carcinomas has high prognostic value. Virchows Arch 1995;427:277–81.

33. Jones AS, Bin HZ, Nadapalan V, et al. Do positive resection margins after ablative surgery for head and neck cancer adversely affect prognosis? A study of 352 patients with recurrent carcinoma following radiotherapy treated by salvage surgery. Br J Cancer 1996;74:128–32.

34. Sereg-Bahar M, Jerin A, Hocevar-Boltezar I. Higher levels of total pepsin and bile acids in the saliva as a possible risk factor for early laryngeal cancer. Radiol Oncol 2015;49:59–64.

35. Sadri M, McMahon J, Parker A. Laryngeal dysplasia: aetiology and molecular biology. J Laryngol Otol 2006;120:170–7.

36. Pagliuca G, Martellucci S, Degener AM, et al. Role of human papillomavirus in the pathogenesis of laryngeal dysplasia. Otolaryngol Head Neck Surg 2014;150:1018–23.

37. Mooren JJ, Gultekin SE, Straetmans JM, et al. P16(INK4A) immunostaining is a strong indicator for high-risk-HPV-associated oropharyngeal carcinomas and dysplasias, but is unreliable to predict low-risk-HPV-infection in head and neck papillomas and laryngeal dysplasias. Int J Cancer 2014;134:2108–17.

38. Isayeva T, Li Y, Maswahu D, et al. Human papillomavirus in non-oropharyngeal head and neck cancers: a systematic literature review. Head Neck Pathol 2012;6(Suppl 1):S104–20.

39. Yoo WJ, Cho SH, Lee YS, et al. Loss of heterozygosity on chromosomes 3p,8p,9p and 17p in the progression of squamous cell carcinoma of the larynx. J Korean Med Sci 2004;19:345–51.

40. Nadal A, Campo E, Pinto J, et al. p53 expression in normal, dysplastic, and neoplastic laryngeal epithelium. Absence of a correlation with prognostic factors. J Pathol 1995;175:181–8.

41. Liu Y, Dong XL, Tian C, et al. Human telomerase RNA component (hTERC) gene amplification detected by FISH in precancerous lesions and carcinoma of the larynx. Diagn Pathol 2012;7:34.

42. Gale N, Zidar N, Poljak M, et al. Current views and perspectives on classification of squamous intraepithelial lesions of the head and neck. Head Neck Pathol 2014;8:16–23.

43. Fleskens S, Slootweg P. Grading systems in head and neck dysplasia: their prognostic value, weaknesses and utility. Head Neck Oncol 2009;1:11.

44. Fleskens SA, Bergshoeff VE, Voogd AC, et al. Interobserver variability of laryngeal mucosal premalignant lesions: a histopathological evaluation. Mod Pathol 2011;24:892–8.

45. Gale N, Blagus R, El-Mofty SK, et al. Evaluation of a new grading system for laryngeal squamous intraepithelial lesions–a proposed unified classification. Histopathology 2014;65:456–64.

46. Waxman AG, Chelmow D, Darragh TM, et al. Revised terminology for cervical histopathology and its implications for management of high-grade squamous intraepithelial lesions of the cervix. Obstet Gynecol 2012;120:1465–71.

47. Cheng L, MacLennan GT, Lopez-Beltran A. Histologic grading of urothelial carcinoma: a reappraisal. Hum Pathol 2012;43:2097–108.

48. Lopez F, varez-Marcos C, onso-Guervos M, et al. From laryngeal epithelial precursor lesions to squamous carcinoma of the larynx: the role of cell cycle proteins and beta-catenin. Eur Arch Otorhinolaryngol 2013;270:3153–62.

49. Hussein MR. Alterations of p53 and Bcl-2 protein expression in the laryngeal intraepithelial neoplasia. Cancer Biol Ther 2005;4:213–7.

50. Jeannon JP, Soames JV, Aston V, et al. Molecular markers in dysplasia of the larynx: expression of cyclin-dependent kinase inhibitors p21, p27 and p53 tumour suppressor gene in predicting cancer risk. Clin Otolaryngol Allied Sci 2004;29:698–704.

51. Ioachim E, Peschos D, Goussia A, et al. Expression patterns of cyclins D1, E in laryngeal epithelial

lesions: correlation with other cell cycle regulators (p53, pRb, Ki-67 and PCNA) and clinicopathological features. J Exp Clin Cancer Res 2004;23: 277–83.

52. Sengiz S, Pabuccuoglu U, Sarioglu S. Immunohistological comparison of the World Health Organization (WHO) and Ljubljana classifications on the grading of preneoplastic lesions of the larynx. Pathol Res Pract 2004;200:181–8.

53. Karatayli-Ozgursoy S, Pacheco-Lopez P, Hillel AT, et al. Laryngeal dysplasia, demographics, and treatment: a single-institution, 20-year review. JAMA Otolaryngol Head Neck Surg 2015;141:313–8.

54. Zhang HK, Liu HG. Is severe dysplasia the same lesion as carcinoma in situ? 10-Year follow-up of laryngeal precancerous lesions. Acta Otolaryngol 2012;132:325–8.

55. Mallofre C, Cardesa A, Campo E, et al. Expression of cytokeratins in squamous cell carcinomas of the larynx: immunohistochemical analysis and correlation with prognostic factors. Pathol Res Pract 1993; 189:275–82.

56. Orvidas LJ, Olsen KD, Lewis JE, et al. Verrucous carcinoma of the larynx: a review of 53 patients. Head Neck 1998;20:197–203.

57. Odar K, Kocjan BJ, Hosnjak L, et al. Verrucous carcinoma of the head and neck—not a human papillomavirus-related tumour? J Cell Mol Med 2014;18:635–45.

58. Patel KR, Chernock RD, Zhang TR, et al. Verrucous carcinomas of the head and neck, including those with associated squamous cell carcinoma, lack transcriptionally active high-risk human papillomavirus. Hum Pathol 2013;44:2385–92.

59. Batsakis JG, Hybels R, Crissman JD, et al. The pathology of head and neck tumors: verrucous carcinoma, Part 15. Head Neck Surg 1982;5:29–38.

60. Ferlito A. Histological classification of larynx and hypopharynx cancers and their clinical implications. Pathologic aspects of 2052 malignant neoplasms diagnosed at the ORL Department of Padua University from 1966 to 1976. Acta Otolaryngol Suppl 1976;342:1–88.

61. Ferlito A, Recher G. Ackerman's tumor (verrucous carcinoma) of the larynx: a clinicopathologic study of 77 cases. Cancer 1980;46:1617–30.

62. Koch BB, Trask DK, Hoffman HT, et al. National survey of head and neck verrucous carcinoma: patterns of presentation, care, and outcome. Cancer 2001;92:110–20.

63. Slootweg PJ, Muller H. Verrucous hyperplasia or verrucous carcinoma. An analysis of 27 patients. J Maxillofac Surg 1983;11:13–9.

64. Medina JE, Dichtel W, Luna MA. Verrucous-squamous carcinomas of the oral cavity. A clinicopathologic study of 104 cases. Arch Otolaryngol 1984; 110:437–40.

65. Shear M, Pindborg JJ. Verrucous hyperplasia of the oral mucosa. Cancer 1980;46:1855–62.

66. Wu M, Putti TC, Bhuiya TA. Comparative study in the expression of p53, EGFR, TGF-alpha, and cyclin D1 in verrucous carcinoma, verrucous hyperplasia, and squamous cell carcinoma of head and neck region. Appl Immunohistochem Mol Morphol 2002;10:351–6.

67. Huang SH, Lockwood G, Irish J, et al. Truths and myths about radiotherapy for verrucous carcinoma of larynx. Int J Radiat Oncol Biol Phys 2009;73: 1110–5.

68. McCaffrey TV, Witte M, Ferguson MT. Verrucous carcinoma of the larynx. Ann Otol Rhinol Laryngol 1998;107:391–5.

69. Ferlito A, Rinaldo A, Mannara GM. Is primary radiotherapy an appropriate option for the treatment of verrucous carcinoma of the head and neck? J Laryngol Otol 1998;112:132–9.

70. Thompson LD, Wenig BM, Heffner DK, et al. Exophytic and papillary squamous cell carcinomas of the larynx: a clinicopathologic series of 104 cases. Otolaryngol Head Neck Surg 1999;120:718–24.

71. Russell JO, Hoschar AP, Scharpf J. Papillary squamous cell carcinoma of the head and neck: a clinicopathologic series. Am J Otolaryngol 2011;32: 557–63.

72. Jo VY, Mills SE, Stoler MH, et al. Papillary squamous cell carcinoma of the head and neck: frequent association with human papillomavirus infection and invasive carcinoma. Am J Surg Pathol 2009;33:1720–4.

73. Suarez PA, Adler-Storthz K, Luna MA, et al. Papillary squamous cell carcinomas of the upper aerodigestive tract: a clinicopathologic and molecular study. Head Neck 2000;22:360–8.

74. Mehrad M, Carpenter DH, Chernock RD, et al. Papillary squamous cell carcinoma of the head and neck: clinicopathologic and molecular features with special reference to human papillomavirus. Am J Surg Pathol 2013;37:1349–56.

75. Nappi O, Wick MR. Sarcomatoid neoplasms of the respiratory tract. Semin Diagn Pathol 1993;10: 137–47.

76. Lewis JE, Olsen KD, Sebo TJ. Spindle cell carcinoma of the larynx: review of 26 cases including DNA content and immunohistochemistry. Hum Pathol 1997;28:664–73.

77. Thompson LD, Wieneke JA, Miettinen M, et al. Spindle cell (sarcomatoid) carcinomas of the larynx: a clinicopathologic study of 187 cases. Am J Surg Pathol 2002;26:153–70.

78. Batsakis JG, Suarez P. Sarcomatoid carcinomas of the upper aerodigestive tracts. Adv Anat Pathol 2000;7:282–93.

79. Choi HR, Sturgis EM, Rosenthal DI, et al. Sarcomatoid carcinoma of the head and neck: molecular

evidence for evolution and progression from conventional squamous cell carcinomas. Am J Surg Pathol 2003;27:1216–20.

80. Zidar N, Bostjancic E, Gale N, et al. Down-regulation of microRNAs of the miR-200 family and miR-205, and an altered expression of classic and desmosomal cadherins in spindle cell carcinoma of the head and neck–hallmark of epithelial-mesenchymal transition. Hum Pathol 2011;42:482–8.

81. Viswanathan S, Rahman K, Pallavi S, et al. Sarcomatoid (spindle cell) carcinoma of the head and neck mucosal region: a clinicopathologic review of 103 cases from a tertiary referral cancer centre. Head Neck Pathol 2010;4:265–75.

82. Roy S, Purgina B, Seethala RR. Spindle cell carcinoma of the larynx with rhabdomyoblastic heterologous element: a rare form of divergent differentiation. Head Neck Pathol 2013;7:263–7.

83. Bishop JA, Thompson LD, Cardesa A, et al. Rhabdomyoblastic differentiation in head and neck malignancies other than rhabdomyosarcoma. Head Neck Pathol 2015;9:507–18.

84. Lewis JS, Ritter JH, El-Mofty S. Alternative epithelial markers in sarcomatoid carcinomas of the head and neck, lung, and bladder-p63, MOC-31, and TTF-1. Mod Pathol 2005;18:1471–81.

85. Ansari-Lari MA, Hoque MO, Califano J, et al. Immunohistochemical p53 expression patterns in sarcomatoid carcinomas of the upper respiratory tract. Am J Surg Pathol 2002;26:1024–31.

86. Zarbo RJ, Crissman JD, Venkat H, et al. Spindle-cell carcinoma of the upper aerodigestive tract mucosa. An immunohistologic and ultrastructural study of 18 biphasic tumors and comparison with seven monophasic spindle-cell tumors. Am J Surg Pathol 1986;10:741–53.

87. Scully C, Porter SR, Speight PM, et al. Adenosquamous carcinoma of the mouth: a rare variant of squamous cell carcinoma. Int J Oral Maxillofac Surg 1999;28:125–8.

88. Wenig BM, Devaney K, Bisceglia M. Inflammatory myofibroblastic tumor of the larynx. A clinicopathologic study of eight cases simulating a malignant spindle cell neoplasm. Cancer 1995;76:2217–29.

89. Volker HU, Scheich M, Zettl A, et al. Laryngeal inflammatory myofibroblastic tumors: different clinical appearance and histomorphologic presentation of one entity. Head Neck 2010;32:1573–8.

90. Salcedo-Hernandez RA, Lino-Silva LS, Luna-Ortiz K. Synovial sarcomas of the head and neck: comparative analysis with synovial sarcoma of the extremities. Auris Nasus Larynx 2013;40:476–80.

91. Thway K, Fisher C. Synovial sarcoma: defining features and diagnostic evolution. Ann Diagn Pathol 2014;18:369–80.

92. Banks ER, Frierson HF, Mills SE, et al. Basaloid squamous cell carcinoma of the head and neck. A clinicopathologic and immunohistochemical study of 40 cases. Am J Surg Pathol 1992;16:939–46.

93. Barnes L, Ferlito A, Altavilla G, et al. Basaloid squamous cell carcinoma of the head and neck: clinicopathological features and differential diagnosis. Ann Otol Rhinol Laryngol 1996;105:75–82.

94. Fritsch VA, Lentsch EJ. Basaloid squamous cell carcinoma of the head and neck: location means everything. J Surg Oncol 2014;109:616–22.

95. Seidman JD, Berman JJ, Yost BA, et al. Basaloid squamous carcinoma of the hypopharynx and larynx associated with second primary tumors. Cancer 1991;68:1545–9.

96. Chernock RD, Lewis JS Jr, Zhang Q, et al. Human papillomavirus-positive basaloid squamous cell carcinomas of the upper aerodigestive tract: a distinct clinicopathologic and molecular subtype of basaloid squamous cell carcinoma. Hum Pathol 2010;41:1016–23.

97. Begum S, Westra WH. Basaloid squamous cell carcinoma of the head and neck is a mixed variant that can be further resolved by HPV status. Am J Surg Pathol 2008;32:1044–50.

98. Klijanienko J, el Naggar A, Ponzio-Prion A, et al. Basaloid squamous carcinoma of the head and neck. Immunohistochemical comparison with adenoid cystic carcinoma and squamous cell carcinoma. Arch Otolaryngol Head Neck Surg 1993;119:887–90.

99. Morice WG, Ferreiro JA. Distinction of basaloid squamous cell carcinoma from adenoid cystic and small cell undifferentiated carcinoma by immunohistochemistry. Hum Pathol 1998;29:609–12.

100. Calli C, Calli A, Pinar E, et al. Prognostic significance of p63, p53 and ki67 expression in laryngeal basaloid squamous cell carcinomas. B-ENT 2011;7:37–42.

101. Wieneke JA, Thompson LD, Wenig BM. Basaloid squamous cell carcinoma of the sinonasal tract. Cancer 1999;85:841–54.

102. Emanuel P, Wang B, Wu M, et al. p63 immunohistochemistry in the distinction of adenoid cystic carcinoma from basaloid squamous cell carcinoma. Mod Pathol 2005;18:645–50.

103. Serrano MF, El-Mofty SK, Gnepp DR, et al. Utility of high molecular weight cytokeratins, but not p63, in the differential diagnosis of neuroendocrine and basaloid carcinomas of the head and neck. Hum Pathol 2008;39:591–8.

104. Fonseca FP, Sena FM, Altemani A, et al. Molecular signature of salivary gland tumors: potential use as diagnostic and prognostic marker. J Oral Pathol Med 2016;45:101–10.

105. Ho AS, Kannan K, Roy DM, et al. The mutational landscape of adenoid cystic carcinoma. Nat Genet 2013;45:791–8.

106. Ereno C, Gaafar A, Garmendia M, et al. Basaloid squamous cell carcinoma of the head and neck: a clinicopathological and follow-up study of 40 cases and review of the literature. Head Neck Pathol 2008;2:83–91.

107. Keelawat S, Liu CZ, Roehm PC, et al. Adenosquamous carcinoma of the upper aerodigestive tract: a clinicopathologic study of 12 cases and review of the literature. Am J Otolaryngol 2002;23:160–8.

108. Kass JI, Lee SC, Abberbock S, et al. Adenosquamous carcinoma of the head and neck: molecular analysis using CRTC-MAML FISH and survival comparison with paired conventional squamous cell carcinoma. Laryngoscope 2015;125:E371–6.

109. Kusafuka K, Muramatsu K, Iida Y, et al. MUC expression in adenosquamous carcinoma of the head and neck regions of Japanese patients: immunohistochemical analysis. Pathol Int 2014;64:104–14.

110. Alos L, Castillo M, Nadal A, et al. Adenosquamous carcinoma of the head and neck: criteria for diagnosis in a study of 12 cases. Histopathology 2004;44:570–9.

111. Damiani JM, Damiani KK, Hauck K, et al. Mucoepidermoid-adenosquamous carcinoma of the larynx and hypopharynx: a report of 21 cases and a review of the literature. Otolaryngol Head Neck Surg 1981;89:235–43.

112. Schick U, Pusztaszeri M, Betz M, et al. Adenosquamous carcinoma of the head and neck: report of 20 cases and review of the literature. Oral Surg Oral Med Oral Pathol Oral Radiol 2013;116:313–20.

113. Ferlito A, Devaney KO, Rinaldo A, et al. Mucosal adenoid squamous cell carcinoma of the head and neck. Ann Otol Rhinol Laryngol 1996;105: 409–13.

114. French CA. The importance of diagnosing NUT midline carcinoma. Head Neck Pathol 2013;7: 11–6.

115. Stelow EB. A review of NUT midline carcinoma. Head Neck Pathol 2011;5:31–5.

116. Bishop JA, Antonescu CR, Westra WH. SMARCB1 (INI-1)-deficient carcinomas of the sinonasal tract. Am J Surg Pathol 2014;38:1282–9.

117. Wenig BM. Lymphoepithelial-like carcinomas of the head and neck. Semin Diagn Pathol 2015;32: 74–86.

118. Chan JY, Wong EW, Ng SK, et al. Non-nasopharyngeal head and neck lymphoepithelioma-like carcinoma in the United States: a population-based study. Head Neck 2016;38(Suppl 1):E1294–300.

Human Papillomavirus–Associated Neoplasms of the Head and Neck

Aaron M. Udager, MD, PhD[a], Jonathan B. McHugh, MD[b],*

KEYWORDS

- Oropharynx • Squamous cell carcinoma • Nasopharyngeal carcinoma
- Carcinoma with adenoid cystic-like features • Sinonasal (Schneiderian) papilloma

Key points

- Human papillomavirus (HPV)–associated head and neck squamous cell carcinoma occurs most commonly in the oropharynx, typically shows a nonkeratinizing morphology, and is associated with a better clinical outcome.

- A subset of Epstein-Barr virus (EBV)–negative nasopharyngeal carcinoma is associated with high-risk HPV infection, particularly in countries where EBV is not endemic.

- Carcinoma with adenoid cystic-like features is a recently described HPV-associated tumor of the sinonasal cavities that has morphologic and immunophenotypic overlap with adenoid cystic carcinoma.

- A subset of sinonasal (Schneiderian) papillomas are associated with HPV infection, in particular those with epithelial dysplasia and/or associated sinonasal carcinoma.

ABSTRACT

Human papillomavirus (HPV) is an essential causal factor in a subset of head and neck neoplasms, most notably oropharyngeal squamous cell carcinoma, for which HPV infection has important diagnostic, prognostic, and therapeutic implications. This article summarizes the current understanding of HPV-associated neoplasms of the head and neck, including the recently described carcinoma with adenoid cystic-like features. Salient clinical, gross, and microscopic features are discussed, and the utility of specific ancillary studies is highlighted.

OVERVIEW

Over the past 2 decades, human papillomavirus (HPV) infection has emerged as an important causal factor in a subset of head and neck neoplasms.[1,2] HPV is a double-stranded DNA virus with more than 200 unique subtypes, which can be broadly categorized into low-risk (eg, subtypes 6 and 11) and high-risk (eg, subtypes 16 and 18) groups.[3] HPV-associated oncogenesis is mediated predominantly by the E6 and E7 oncoproteins,[3] although the E5 oncoprotein may also play a role in some tumors.[4] Similar to high-risk HPV-associated neoplasms at other anatomic sites (eg, cervix, anus), viral integration and overexpression of high-risk E6 and E7 oncoproteins in head and neck malignancies drives cellular transformation via disruption of p53 and retinoblastoma (RB) pathway activity, respectively, whereas low-risk E6 and E7 oncoproteins do not significantly affect p53 and RB pathway activity.[3] These distinct pathogenetic pathways have important implications for tumor biology and histopathologic diagnosis.

Disclosures: The authors have nothing to disclose.
Funding: None.
[a] Department of Pathology, University of Michigan Health System, 2G309 UH, 1500 East Medical Center Drive, Ann Arbor, MI 48109-5054, USA; [b] Department of Pathology, University of Michigan Health System, 2G332 UH, 1500 East Medical Center Drive, Ann Arbor, MI 48109-5054, USA
* Corresponding author.
E-mail address: jonamch@umich.edu

surgpath.theclinics.com

SQUAMOUS CELL CARCINOMA AND VARIANTS

INTRODUCTION

Squamous cell carcinoma (SCC) is the most common malignant tumor of the head and neck and may arise in the oral cavity, pharynx, larynx, or sinonasal cavities.[5] Although most head and neck SCCs (HNSCCs) are related to alcohol and/or tobacco use, the incidence of HPV-associated HNSCC is increasing worldwide.[6] High-risk HPV subtype 16 is the most common HPV subtype detected in HPV-associated HNSCC, although other high-risk subtypes have also been identified.[7] In contrast with alcohol-associated and tobacco-associated HNSCC, which typically occur in older male patients, HPV-associated HNSCC is more common in younger patients.[6] HPV-associated HNSCC most commonly involves the oropharynx, and more than 70% of oropharyngeal SCCs are HPV-associated. Tonsillar crypt epithelium is a hotspot for HPV infection in the head and neck, and therefore the lingual and palatine tonsil are particularly common sites for HPV-associated HNSCC.[2] Although less common than the oropharynx, HPV-associated HNSCC also occurs in the sinonasal cavities[8,9]; it is rare in the oral cavity and larynx.[2] Patients with HPV-associated HNSCC may be clinically asymptomatic or may present with dysphagia and/or tonsillar asymmetry. HPV-associated HNSCC often metastasizes to lateral cervical lymph nodes; for a subset of patients, the primary tumor is clinically occult, and the first indication of disease is an enlarging lateral neck mass.

GROSS FEATURES

There are no specific gross features of primary HPV-associated HNSCC, which may be erythroplakic, exophytic, ulcerative, infiltrative, or clinically occult. Lymph node metastases may have a cystic gross appearance.

MICROSCOPIC FEATURES

HPV-associated HNSCC shows a diverse morphologic spectrum with varied architectural patterns.[2,10,11] Most commonly, HPV-associated HNSCC presents as nonkeratinizing SCC, which has an immature squamous (basaloid) appearance.[12] These tumors are composed of polygonal to spindled cells with minimal cytoplasm, hyperchromatic nuclei, and inconspicuous nucleoli, arranged in variably sized solid expansile nests with abundant associated inflammatory cells,

frequent mitotic activity and apoptosis, and occasional comedonecrosis (**Fig. 1**). Overall, these features recapitulate the appearance of tonsillar crypts. As such, the term poorly differentiated is a misnomer. Similarly, although technically true, the term basaloid is discouraged to avoid confusion with true basaloid SCC (discussed later). Squamous maturation and keratinization are typically minimal (<10% of overall tumor volume), and overlying squamous epithelial dysplasia is rarely present because these are mainly tumors of tonsillar crypt rather than surface mucosa. Metastatic nonkeratinizing SCC in lateral cervical lymph nodes may undergo degeneration, imparting a cystic gross and/or microscopic appearance (**Fig. 2**). Occasionally, HPV-associated nonkeratinizing SCC shows more extensive squamous maturation and keratinization, but only rarely is HPV infection associated with true keratinizing SCC (**Fig. 3**).[13]

Other morphologic variants of SCC that may be associated with HPV infection include papillary, basaloid, adenosquamous, lymphoepithelial-like/undifferentiated, and spindle cell (sarcomatoid). In general, these SCC variants are uncommon, and although they may occur at essentially any site in the head and neck, they are most commonly HPV-associated when occurring in the oropharynx (similar to HNSCC overall). Papillary SCC shares many morphologic features with nonkeratinizing SCC but has a characteristic exophytic/papillary growth pattern with fibrovascular cores (**Fig. 4**).[14,15] Basaloid SCC is a unique tumor with a biphasic appearance; it is composed predominantly of basaloid cells, arranged in nests, cords, and cribriform structures with abundant basement membrane–type material, characteristic myxoid stroma, and admixed foci of abrupt squamous maturation and keratinization (**Fig. 5**).[16,17] Adenosquamous carcinoma also has a biphasic appearance, with intimately admixed areas of squamous and glandular differentiation (**Fig. 6**).[18] In general, oropharyngeal adenosquamous carcinoma is a cytologically malignant tumor composed of tumor cells resembling both nonkeratinizing SCC and adenocarcinoma; however, 2 recent studies have reported morphologically bland forms of HPV-associated adenosquamous carcinoma with ciliated glandular epithelial cells.[19,20] Lymphoepithelial-like/undifferentiated carcinoma has a similar morphology to nonkeratinizing undifferentiated type nasopharyngeal carcinoma (NPC; discussed later for details).[21,22] Spindle cell (sarcomatoid) SCC is often a biphasic tumor and is composed of a malignant spindle cell population with admixed or overlying foci of morphologically identifiable SCC (**Fig. 7**).[23,24]

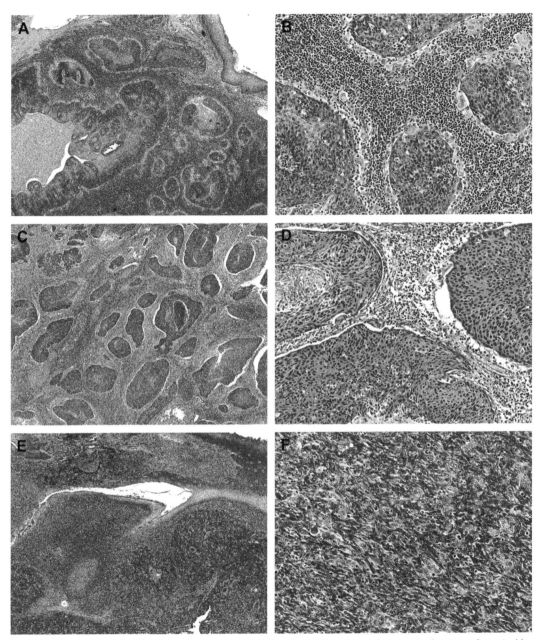

Fig. 1. Nonkeratinizing SCC. (*A–F*) Nonkeratinizing SCC showing infiltrative and/or expansile nests of atypical basaloid squamous cells (hematoxylin-eosin, original magnification ×4 [*A, C, E*] and ×20 [*B, D, F*]).

Although not strictly a variant of SCC, HPV-associated small cell carcinoma of the head and neck is often associated with concurrent SCC and, therefore, may represent a form of divergent differentiation.[25,26] In these cases, the small cell component shows the typical morphology of small cell carcinomas at other sites: small to intermediate cells with scant cytoplasm, salt-and-pepper chromatin, and inconspicuous nucleoli, arranged in discohesive cords, nests, and sheets with frequent mitotic activity and apoptosis and admixed comedonecrosis (**Fig. 8**). Rare HPV-associated large cell neuroendocrine carcinomas (LCNEC) of the head and neck have also been described and show similar morphologic features to LCNEC of the lung and other sites: large cells with abundant cytoplasm and prominent nucleoli, arranged in nests and trabeculae with frequent

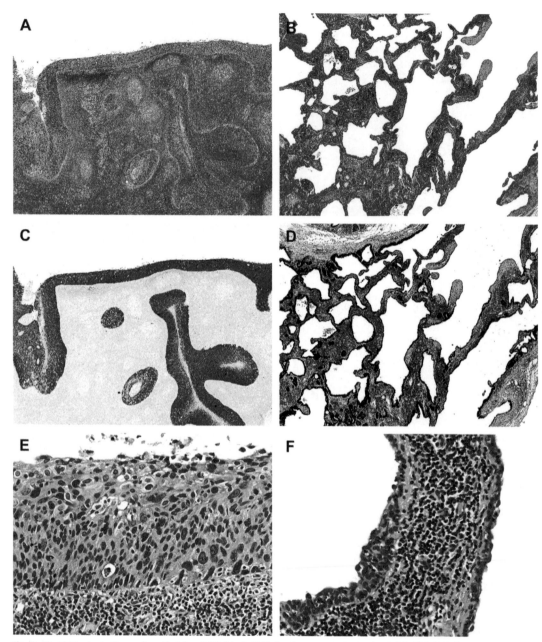

Fig. 2. Cystic metastatic nonkeratinizing SCC. (*A, B, E, F*) Cystic metastatic nonkeratinizing SCC showing a unicystic (*A, E*) or multicystic (*B, F*) tumor lined by atypical basaloid squamous cells. (*C, D*) p16 immunohistochemistry (IHC) shows diffuse cytoplasmic and nuclear staining, consistent with an HPV-associated tumor (hematoxylin-eosin [*A, B, E, F*], original magnification ×4 [*A–D*] and ×40 [*E, F*]).

necrosis, peripheral palisading, and rosette forma-tion.[27] Similarly, HPV-associated pure adenocarci-nomas without a squamous component have been described.[28,29] These are most commonly solid to cribriform and may show moderate to severe cyto-logic atypia, although 1 case with nuclear stratifi-cation and a papillary growth pattern has been

reported.[29] The main pitfalls include metastatic adenocarcinomas from other sites, particularly the gastrointestinal tract, and primary salivary gland carcinomas. Site-selective markers (ie, CDX2 and TTF-1) are negative in HPV-associated adenocarcinomas. Because they do not have the distinctive morphology of described salivary gland

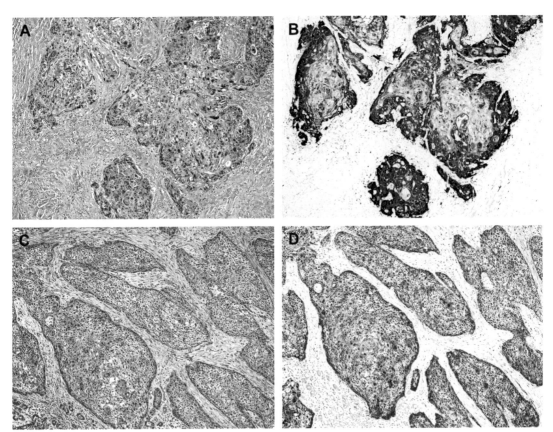

Fig. 3. Keratinizing SCC. (*A, C*) Keratinizing SCC showing infiltrative nests of atypical squamous cells with conspicuous maturation and keratinization. (*B, D*) p16 IHC shows diffuse cytoplasmic and nuclear staining, consistent with an HPV-associated tumor (hematoxylin-eosin [*A, C*], original magnification ×20).

tumor types, HPV-associated adenocarcinoma should be considered when encountering any intermediate-grade to high-grade adenocarcinoma without defining features for a specific salivary gland tumor.

DIFFERENTIAL DIAGNOSIS

The primary differential diagnosis for HPV-associated nonkeratinizing SCC is normal tonsillar tissue and/or tonsillitis. In particular, hyperplastic and/or reactive tonsillar crypt epithelium may be confused with HPV-associated nonkeratinizing SCC; however, identification of areas of significant squamous atypia and/or expansile growth supports a diagnosis of carcinoma. Cystic metastatic HPV-associated nonkeratinizing SCC may present a diagnostic challenge on fine-needle aspiration or primary surgical excision, because these tumors may be confused with benign cystic squamous lesions (ie, branchial cleft cyst) or primary salivary gland tumors (ie, mucoepidermoid

carcinoma [MEC]; discussed later). The presence of conspicuous squamous atypia in a cystic lesion of the lateral neck should prompt consideration of HPV-associated nonkeratinizing SCC, especially in older patients with a new enlarging lateral neck mass.

Additional differential considerations include melanoma and large cell lymphoma; however, HPV-associated nonkeratinizing SCC typically shows more cellular cohesion and architecture, and, even if only focal, squamous maturation and/or keratinization is often present. In diagnostically challenging cases, immunohistochemistry (IHC) for broad-spectrum pan-cytokeratins, p63, S100, CD45, and/or CD20, may be useful. In addition, depending on the anatomic site, nonkeratinizing NPC, lymphoepithelial carcinoma, sinonasal undifferentiated carcinoma (SNUC), SMARCB1 (INI-1)-deficient sinonasal carcinoma, NUT midline carcinoma, and synovial sarcoma may enter the differential diagnosis of nonkeratinizing HPV-associated SCC. In these rare cases, additional

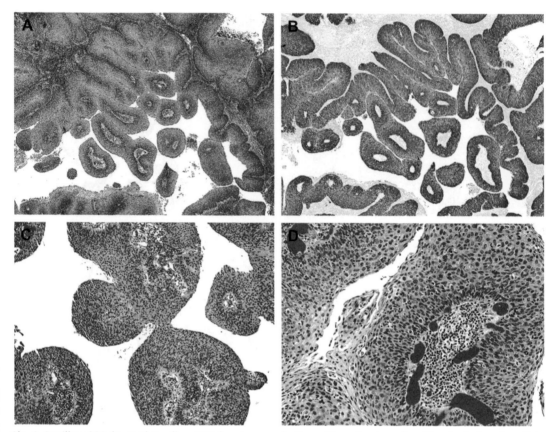

Fig. 4. Papillary SCC. (*A, C, D*) Papillary SCC showing exophytic papillary structures lined by atypical nonkeratinizing squamous epithelium. (*B*) p16 IHC shows diffuse cytoplasmic and nuclear staining, consistent with an HPV-associated tumor (hematoxylin-eosin [*A, C, D*], original magnification ×4 [*A, B*], ×10 [*C*], ×20 [*D*]).

clinical information and ancillary studies for HPV infection (discussed later; HPV-associated non-keratinizing SCC), specific cytokeratins (eg, CK5/6, CK7; SNUC), EBV infection (Epstein-Barr virus-encoded small RNA [EBER] in situ hybridization [ISH]; nonkeratinizing NPC and lymphoepithelial carcinoma), INI-1 expression (SMARCB1 [INI-1]-deficient sinonasal carcinoma), *NUT* gene rearrangement (NUT IHC or *NUT* fluorescent ISH [FISH]; NUT midline carcinoma), and/or TLE-1 expression or *SYT-SSX* gene rearrangements (synovial sarcoma) may be helpful.

In addition, specific morphologic variants of HPV-associated HNSCC, including basaloid SCC and adenosquamous carcinoma, may have unique differential diagnoses. Because of its prominent basaloid cell population, adenoid cystic carcinoma (ACC), as well as carcinoma with adenoid cystic-like features (discussed later), may enter the differential diagnosis for HPV-associated basaloid SCC; however, ACC typically shows true ductal and myoepithelial

differentiation and does not show overt squamous differentiation. In diagnostically challenging cases (eg, the solid variant of ACC), IHC for myoepithelial markers (eg, p63, calponin) may be useful to highlight the biphasic nature of ACC, whereas FISH to detect the *MYB-NFIB* gene fusion may help exclude ACC. Similarly, because of its mixed squamous and glandular morphology, MEC may enter the differential diagnosis for HPV-associated adenosquamous carcinoma (in particular, the recently described bland form with ciliated glandular epithelial cells), although MEC is uncommon outside of parotid gland and palatal/buccal mucosa. This differential diagnosis is further compounded by conflicting evidence for HPV infection in MEC, with at least 1 study reporting the presence of high-risk HPV subtypes in approximately one-third of tumors.[30] The role of HPV in true MEC is now considered dubious in light of the inability to duplicate these findings in other studies.[31] In these rare cases, FISH to detect *MAML2* gene

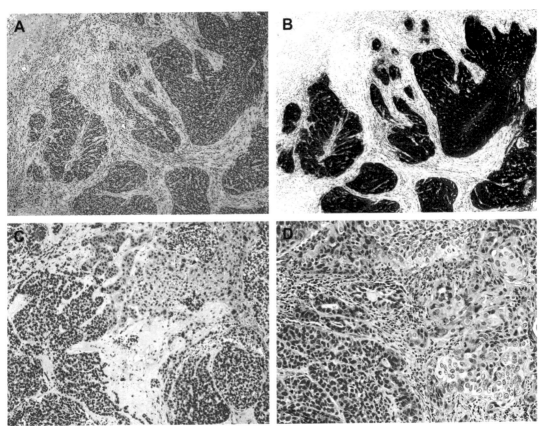

Fig. 5. Basaloid SCC. (*A, C, D*) Basaloid SCC showing a biphasic population of basaloid cells arranged in variably sized nests and cords with admixed areas of abrupt squamous maturation and keratinization. (*B*) p16 IHC shows diffuse cytoplasmic and nuclear staining, consistent with an HPV-associated tumor (hematoxylin-eosin [*A, C, D*], original magnification ×10 [*A, B*], ×20 [*C, D*]).

rearrangements may be helpful, because this genomic alteration is present in most MEC and has not been reported in HPV-associated adenosquamous carcinoma.[19,20]

DIAGNOSIS

In general, the diagnosis of HPV-associated HNSCC can be made on morphologic grounds, although consideration should be given to the clinicopathologic context (eg, anatomic site), and, if necessary, robust confirmatory ancillary studies are available for routine clinical use (**Fig. 9**).[32] These confirmatory assays include p16 IHC and DNA ISH for high-risk HPV subtypes.[33] As discussed earlier, malignant transformation by high-risk HPV subtypes involves viral integration and overexpression of high-risk E6 and E7 oncoproteins. The E7 oncoprotein, in particular, suppresses RB pathway activity, which eliminates negative feedback on p16 gene expression and

results in p16 protein overexpression.[3] Thus, in the appropriate clinical context (ie, oropharyngeal nonkeratinizing SCC), strong, diffuse nuclear and cytoplasmic p16 staining by IHC is a surrogate biomarker for high-risk HPV infection.[33] In the oropharynx, p16 IHC alone has high sensitivity and specificity for HPV-associated HNSCC. Similarly, for metastatic nonkeratinizing SCC in lateral cervical lymph nodes, p16 IHC alone has high sensitivity and specificity for HPV-associated HNSCC. However, it is important to remember that p16 is also a tumor suppressor protein and may be overexpressed in cancer cells independent of HPV status. Accordingly, at other anatomic sites in the head and neck (as well as for rare HPV-associated SCC variants), the specificity of p16 IHC alone decreases, and, if confirmation of HPV infection is needed, a second method is strongly recommended.[32] For this purpose, high-risk HPV DNA ISH is often used, and although the specificity is high, the sensitivity of this assay may be limited

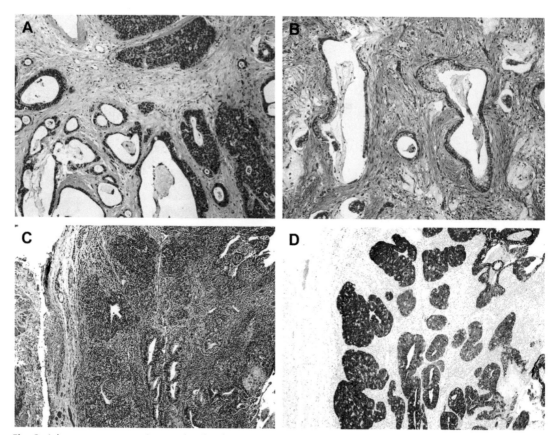

Fig. 6. Adenosquamous carcinoma. (*A–C*) Adenosquamous carcinoma showing infiltrating glands lined by atypical epithelium with admixed atypical squamous cells (atypical squamous component not present in [*B*]). (*D*) p16 IHC shows diffuse cytoplasmic and nuclear staining, consistent with an HPV-associated tumor (hematoxylin-eosin [*A–C*], original magnification ×20).

by the number of subtypes probed. Therefore, in the appropriate clinical context (ie, oropharyngeal nonkeratinizing SCC), a negative HPV DNA ISH result may be a false-negative and does not exclude HPV-associated HNSCC. Other assays, including HPV DNA PCR and RNA ISH for high-risk E6 and E7 messenger RNA expression, are increasingly used in the research setting but have not yet found widespread utility in routine clinical practice.[7,34,35]

PROGNOSIS

In general, despite often presenting with locally advanced disease (ie, lateral cervical lymph node metastases), patients with HPV-associated HNSCC have a better overall clinical outcome than those with non–HPV-associated HNSCC, although this effect is mitigated by a history of heavy tobacco use.[2,36] This favorable prognosis applies particularly to patients with

oropharyngeal tumors, and there are emerging data to suggest that patients with HPV-associated HNSCC of the sinonasal cavity may also have better clinical outcome than those with non–HPV-associated tumors.[37] Many of the HNSCC variants, including basaloid SCC, sarcomatoid SCC, and small cell carcinoma, are associated with aggressive disease and poor clinical outcome.[16,17,23–26] Given the small numbers of HPV-associated SCC variants reported in the literature, there is currently insufficient evidence to determine whether HPV infection in these rare tumor subtypes portends a better overall clinical outcome (relative to their non–HPV-associated counterparts). Regardless, HPV-associated HNSCC is particularly sensitive to treatment with radiation therapy, and therefore, if possible, patients with HPV-associated HNSCC typically undergo primary surgical excision and then receive adjuvant radiation therapy with or without platinum-based chemotherapy.[38]

Pathologic Key Features
SQUAMOUS CELL CARCINOMA AND VARIANTS

- Relative to alcohol-related and tobacco-related tumors, HPV-associated HNSCC occurs in younger patients, has a predilection for the oropharynx, frequently metastasizes to lateral cervical lymph nodes, and is associated with better clinical outcome

- Nonkeratinizing morphology is the most common type of HPV-associated HNSCC and shows an immature (basaloid) squamous appearance with minimal squamous maturation and/or keratinization

- SCC variants, including papillary SCC, basaloid SCC, adenosquamous carcinoma, lymphoepithelial-like/undifferentiated carcinoma, spindle cell (sarcomatoid) SCC, and small cell carcinoma, may also be HPV-associated, particularly when occurring in the oropharynx

- p16 IHC is a reliable surrogate biomarker for high-risk HPV infection in nonkeratinizing oropharyngeal SCC; however, in non-oropharyngeal tumors or rare SCC variants, p16 IHC should be paired with another HPV detection method (ie, HPV DNA ISH)

Differential Diagnosis
SQUAMOUS CELL CARCINOMA AND VARIANTS

Differential Diagnosis	Diagnostic Pathologic Features and/or Ancillary Studies
Benign or reactive tonsillar tissue	• Absence of cytologic atypia and expansile growth of tonsillar crypts; p16 IHC and high-risk HPV DNA ISH negative
Benign cystic squamous lesions of the lateral neck (ie, branchial cleft cyst)	• Unilocular and absence of cytologic atypia; p16 IHC and high-risk HPV DNA ISH negative
MEC	• CRTC1-MAML2 or CRTC3-MAML2 FISH positive
Melanoma	• Melanin pigment; absence of squamous maturation and/or keratinization; melanocytic markers (S100, HMB-45, melan-A) positive; pan-cytokeratin negative
Large cell lymphoma	• Absence of squamous maturation and/or keratinization; lymphoid markers (CD45, CD20) positive; pan-cytokeratin negative
Nonkeratinizing NPC	• Clinicoradiographic correlation; EBER RNA ISH positive
Lymphoepithelial carcinoma	• EBER RNA ISH positive
SNUC	• Absence of squamous maturation and/or keratinization; CK7 positive and CK5/6 negative
SMARCB1 (INI-1)-deficient sinonasal carcinoma	• Absence of squamous maturation and/or keratinization; INI-1 negative
NUT midline carcinoma	• NUT IHC or NUT FISH positive
Synovial sarcoma	• Absence of squamous maturation and/or keratinization; TLE-1 and SYT-SSX FISH positive

Pitfalls
SQUAMOUS CELL
CARCINOMA AND VARIANTS

! HPV-associated nonkeratinizing oropharyngeal SCC may be difficult to distinguish from hyperplastic or reactive tonsillar crypt epithelium; look for conspicuous cytologic atypia and/or expansile growth

! Maintain a low threshold of suspicion for HPV-associated cystic metastatic nonkeratinizing SCC in older patients with a new enlarging lateral neck mass

! When used as a surrogate of high-risk HPV infection in oropharyngeal SCC, p16 IHC should show strong and diffuse nuclear and cytoplasmic staining; weak and/or patchy cytoplasmic staining in less than half of tumor cells should be reported as negative

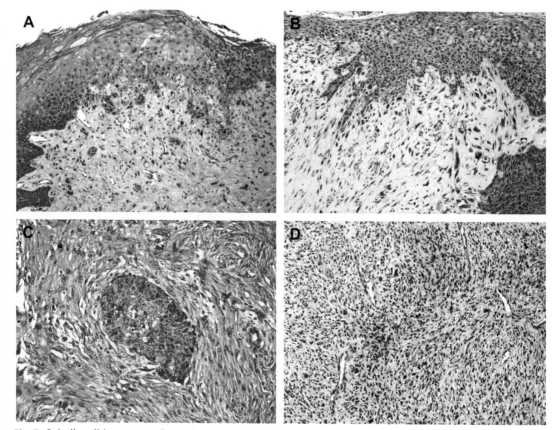

Fig. 7. Spindle cell (sarcomatoid) SCC. (*A–D*) Sarcomatoid SCC showing atypical spindled cells with (*A, B*) overlying or (*C*) admixed atypical squamous epithelium (atypical squamous component not present in [*D*]) (hematoxylin-eosin, original magnification ×20).

NASOPHARYNGEAL CARCINOMA

INTRODUCTION

NPC is the most common malignant neoplasm of the nasopharynx, and although rare in the United States, it is one of the most common tumors overall in countries where EBV is endemic (eg, China).[39] In addition to a presumed pathogenetic role for EBV, the development of NPC has been linked to a variety of environmental exposures; prior radiation exposure; and, occasionally, HPV

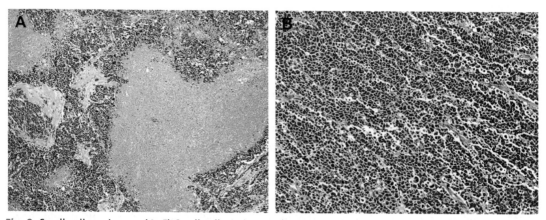

Fig. 8. Small cell carcinoma. (*A, B*) Small cell carcinoma showing markedly atypical basaloid cells with nuclear molding and increased mitotic activity and apoptosis, arranged in diffuse sheets with admixed comedonecrosis (hematoxylin-eosin, original magnification, ×10 [*A*], ×20 [*B*]).

Fig. 9. Ancillary studies in HPV-associated nonkeratinizing SCC. (*A*) HPV-associated nonkeratinizing SCC. (*B*) p16 IHC shows diffuse cytoplasmic and nuclear staining in tumor cells, and (*C*) high-risk HPV DNA ISH shows punctate nuclear staining. The overlying benign squamous mucosa (*right*) shows focal, patchy p16 IHC staining and is negative for high-risk HPV DNA (hematoxylin-eosin [*A*], original magnification ×20 [*A–C*], ×60 [inset in *C*]).

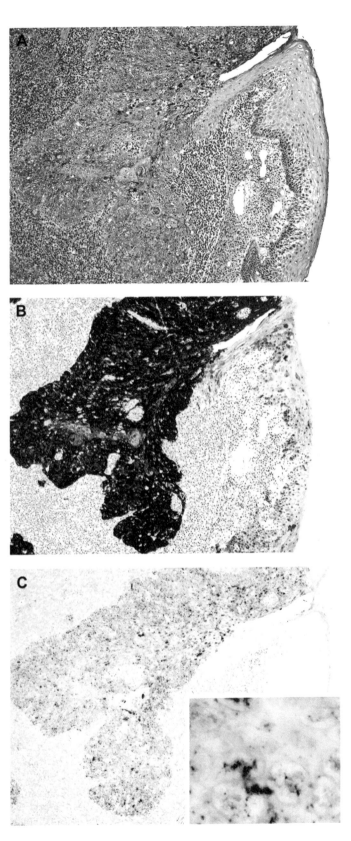

infection. In countries where EBV is endemic, almost all NPCs are associated with the presence of EBV, whereas in nonendemic countries, a subset of EBV-negative tumors seem to be associated with high-risk HPV infection.[40] NPC occurs predominantly in adult patients and shows a moderate male predilection.[39] Patients with NPC typically present with nasopharyngeal obstruction, eustachian tube dysfunction, and/or cranial nerve impingement. NPC often metastasizes to regional lymph nodes, and most patients present with locally advanced disease; similar to HPV-associated HNSCC, for a subset of patients with NPC, the first indication of disease is an enlarging lateral neck mass.

GROSS FEATURES

There are no specific gross features of NPC, and tumors may be exophytic, ulcerative, infiltrative, or clinically occult.

MICROSCOPIC FEATURES

NPC is classified into 3 morphologic subtypes: keratinizing, nonkeratinizing differentiated, and nonkeratinizing undifferentiated.[39] Keratinizing NPC is morphologically identical to keratinizing SCC and is composed of irregular nests of atypical epithelial cells with squamous maturation and keratinization. Nonkeratinizing differentiated NPC is morphologically similar to nonkeratinizing SCC and is composed of pleomorphic, immature cells with minimal basophilic cytoplasm, hyperchromatic nuclei, and inconspicuous nucleoli, arranged in infiltrative nests and interconnecting cords and trabeculae with minimal squamous maturation and keratinization and frequent mitotic activity, apoptosis, and comedonecrosis (Fig. 10A, B). Nonkeratinizing undifferentiated NPC is morphologically similar to lymphoepithelial carcinoma and is composed of large cells with amphophilic cytoplasm, vesicular chromatin, and conspicuous nucleoli, arranged singly and in

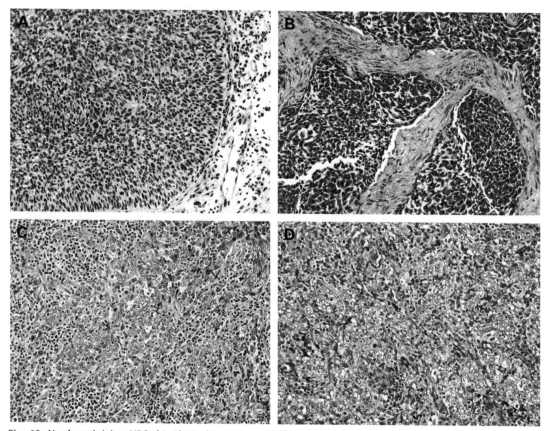

Fig. 10. Nonkeratinizing NPC. (*A, B*) Nonkeratinizing differentiated NPC showing infiltrative and/or expansile nests of atypical basaloid squamous cells. (*C, D*) Nonkeratinizing undifferentiated NPC showing large atypical cells with abundant syncytial cytoplasm, large vesicular nuclei, prominent nucleoli, and conspicuous admixed lymphocytic inflammation (hematoxylin-eosin, original magnification ×20).

small syncytial clusters with prominent associated lymphoplasmacytic inflammation (Fig. 10C, D). HPV infection has been documented in all 3 morphologic subtypes but is most commonly observed in nonkeratinizing differentiated NPC, which, as described earlier, is morphologically similar to HPV-associated nonkeratinizing SCC.[40,41]

DIFFERENTIAL DIAGNOSIS

The main differential diagnosis for keratinizing NPC is extension or metastasis of a keratinizing SCC from another anatomic site (eg, sinus cavity), which can typically be resolved on clinicoradiographic grounds. The primary differential diagnosis for nonkeratinizing differentiated NPC is melanoma, although secondary involvement by a nonkeratinizing SCC should also be excluded clinicoradiographically. Similar to nonkeratinizing SCC, nonkeratinizing differentiated NPC usually shows more defined cellular architecture, and focal squamous maturation and/or keratinization may be present; these morphologic features, as well as the lack of intracellular melanin pigment, may be helpful for excluding melanoma, however in some cases, IHC for broad-spectrum pan-cytokeratins, high-molecular-weight cytokeratins, and S100 are necessary. SNUC, SMARCB1 (INI-1)-deficient sinonasal carcinoma, and NUT midline carcinoma is also occasionally a differential diagnostic consideration for nonkeratinizing differentiated NPC, and, in these rare cases, additional clinical information and ancillary studies for specific cytokeratins (ie, CK7), INI-1 expression, and/or NUT gene rearrangement may be useful. Finally, the major differential diagnosis for nonkeratinizing undifferentiated NPC is large cell lymphoma, although secondary involvement by a lymphoepithelial carcinoma or lymphoepithelial-like SCC should be excluded on clinicoradiographic grounds. Although the presence of focal squamous maturation and/or keratinization helps exclude large cell lymphoma, it may be difficult to reliably distinguish it from nonkeratinizing undifferentiated NPC based on morphology alone. In these cases, IHC for broad-spectrum pan-cytokeratins, CD45, and CD20 should be helpful.

DIAGNOSIS

The diagnosis of HPV-associated NPC involves integration of available clinicoradiographic information, morphologic features, and focused ancillary study results. Given the high frequency of EBV-associated tumors even in nonendemic countries, all newly diagnosed NPC should be interrogated by EBER RNA ISH to evaluate for the presence of EBV.[39] In those cases that are negative for EBV, both p16 IHC and high-risk HPV DNA ISH should be performed, and only if both assays are unequivocally positive should a diagnosis of HPV-associated NPC be rendered (Fig. 11).[40]

PROGNOSIS

Similar to HPV-associated HNSCC, despite often presenting with locally advanced disease, patients with NPC typically have a moderate clinical outcome.[39] The overall 5-year survival rate is approximately 75% and is markedly better for patients with clinically localized disease. Given the small numbers of HPV-associated NPC reported in the literature, it is currently unclear whether HPV infection is associated with a better or worse overall clinical outcome, although at least 1 study has reported decreased overall and progression-free survival.[42] Regardless, similar to HPV-associated HNSCC, NPC is sensitive to treatment with radiation, which most patients receive as primary treatment.[39]

Pathologic Key Features
NASOPHARYNGEAL CARCINOMA

- NPC is the most common malignant neoplasm of the nasopharynx; it often presents with locally advanced disease and/or regional lymph node metastases

- Most tumors are associated with EBV infection; however, in countries where EBV is not endemic, a subset of EBV-negative NPCs are HPV-associated

- Of the 3 morphologic subtypes (keratinizing, nonkeratinizing differentiated, and nonkeratinizing undifferentiated), HPV-associated NPC are most commonly nonkeratinizing differentiated tumors

- All NPCs should be evaluated for EBV infection with EBER RNA ISH; in those cases that are EBV negative, p16 IHC and HPV DNA ISH should be used to assess for possible high-risk HPV infection, because this may portend a worse clinical outcome

Differential Diagnosis
NASOPHARYNGEAL CARCINOMA

Differential Diagnosis	Diagnostic Pathologic Features and/or Ancillary Studies
Nonkeratinizing SCC	• Clinicoradiographic correlation; EBER RNA ISH negative
Melanoma	• Melanin pigment; melanocytic markers (S100, HMB-45, melan-A) positive; pan-cytokeratin negative
Large cell lymphoma	• Lymphoid markers (CD45, CD20) positive; pan-cytokeratin negative
SNUC	• CK7 positive and CK5/6 negative
SMARCB1 (INI-1)-deficient sinonasal carcinoma	• INI-1 negative
NUT midline carcinoma	• NUT IHC or NUT FISH positive

Pitfalls
NASOPHARYNGEAL CARCINOMA

! The nasopharynx may be secondarily involved by sinonasal or oropharyngeal tumors, and thus clinicoradiographic correlation and focused ancillary studies (ie, EBER RNA ISH) are necessary in the work-up of presumptive NPC

! Always consider the possibility of melanoma and large cell lymphoma in the work-up of a nonkeratinizing undifferentiated tumor of the nasopharynx

! When evaluating EBV-negative NPC for possible high-risk HPV infection, p16 IHC alone is insufficient and should paired with another more specific method (ie, HPV DNA ISH)

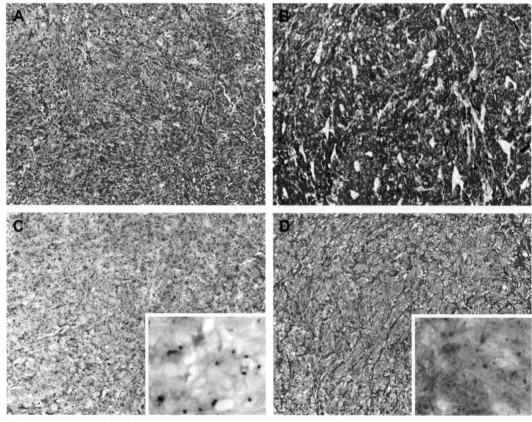

Fig. 11. HPV-associated nonkeratinizing NPC. (*A*) Nonkeratinizing undifferentiated NPC. (*B*) p16 IHC shows diffuse cytoplasmic and nuclear staining in tumor cells, and (*C*) high-risk HPV DNA ISH shows punctate nuclear staining; (*D*) EBER RNA ISH is negative (hematoxylin-eosin [*A*], original magnification ×20 [*A–D*], ×60 [insets in *C, D*]).

HUMAN PAPILLOMAVIRUS VIRUS–RELATED CARCINOMA WITH ADENOID CYSTIC-LIKE FEATURES

INTRODUCTION

HPV-related carcinoma with ACC-like features is a unique, recently described tumor of the head and neck, which, to date, has only been reported to occur in the sinonasal cavities[8,43] (See Lisa M. Rooper and Justin A. Bishop's article, "Sinonasal Small Round Blue Cell Tumors: An Immunohistochemical Approach," in this issue). Although only a few cases have been described, patients with HPV-related carcinoma with ACC-like features were typically older adults and presented with symptoms of nasal obstruction; approximately half of the patients presented with locally advanced disease, but no regional lymph node metastases have been reported. In contrast with HPV-associated nonkeratinizing SCC, carcinoma with ACC-like features is associated with high-risk HPV subtype 33, not high-risk HPV subtype 16.

GROSS FEATURES

No specific gross features of carcinoma with ACC-like features have been described.

MICROSCOPIC FEATURES

Carcinoma with ACC-like features is a biphasic tumor composed of basaloid myoepithelial-type cells with scant cytoplasm and hyperchromatic nuclei surrounding cuboidal ductal-type cells with moderate pale to eosinophilic cytoplasm, vesicular nuclei, and variably prominent nucleoli; tumor cells are arranged in variably sized expansile solid nests with occasional microcystic cribriform architecture (Fig. 12A, B). Squamous dysplasia of the overlying sinonasal epithelium is often present.

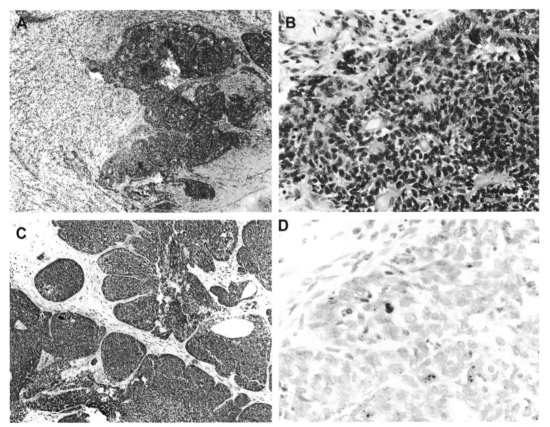

Fig. 12. HPV-related carcinoma with adenoid cystic-like features. (*A, B*) H&E images of carcinoma with adenoid cystic-like features showing basaloid tumor cells in expansile solid nests with a cribriform appearance generated by microcystic spaces filled by eosinophilic basement membrane–like material. (*C*) p16 IHC shows diffuse cytoplasmic and nuclear staining in tumor cells, and (*D*) high-risk HPV DNA ISH shows punctate nuclear staining (hematoxylin-eosin [*A, B*], original magnification ×4 [*A, C*], ×20 [*B*], ×40 [*D*]). (*Courtesy of* Dr Raja R. Seethala, University of Pittsburgh Medical Center, Pittsburgh, PA.)

DIFFERENTIAL DIAGNOSIS

The differential diagnosis for carcinoma with ACC-like features includes ACC and basaloid SCC. In contrast with basaloid SCC, carcinoma with ACC-like features typically shows true ductal differentiation and does not show overt squamous differentiation. In diagnostically challenging cases, IHC for myoepithelial markers (eg, calponin) may be useful to highlight the biphasic nature of carcinoma with ACC-like features. Given the substantial morphologic and immunophenotypic overlap, the distinction between carcinoma with ACC-like features and ACC may be challenging. In these cases, the presence of overlying squamous dysplasia, evidence of high-risk HPV infection (particularly high-risk HPV subtype 33), and lack of *MYB-NFIB* gene fusion by FISH support the diagnosis of carcinoma with ACC-like features. CD117 IHC is not helpful in this differential diagnosis, because it is expressed by both ACC and carcinoma with ACC-like features.

DIAGNOSIS

The diagnosis of carcinoma with ACC-like features requires recognition of the unique clinicopathologic characteristics of this rare HPV-associated tumor, including its predilection for the sinonasal cavities and striking resemblance to ACC (in particular, the solid variant). Given its strong association with high-risk HPV subtype 33, both p16 IHC and HPV DNA ISH should be used to evaluate for HPV infection (**Fig. 12**C, D).

PROGNOSIS

To date, only a few cases have been described with short clinical follow-up. Patients were treated with various combinations of surgical excision, radiation therapy, and chemotherapy, and a subset of patients showed local recurrence. No deaths caused by disease have yet been reported.

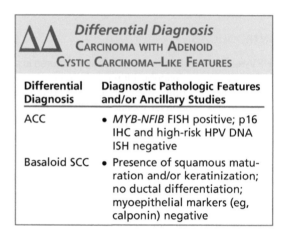

Differential Diagnosis	Diagnostic Pathologic Features and/or Ancillary Studies
ACC	• *MYB-NFIB* FISH positive; p16 IHC and high-risk HPV DNA ISH negative
Basaloid SCC	• Presence of squamous maturation and/or keratinization; no ductal differentiation; myoepithelial markers (eg, calponin) negative

Differential Diagnosis CARCINOMA WITH ADENOID CYSTIC CARCINOMA–LIKE FEATURES

Pitfalls CARCINOMA WITH ADENOID CYSTIC CARCINOMA–LIKE FEATURES

! Remember to consider carcinoma with ACC-like features in the work-up of basaloid and biphasic tumors of the sinonasal cavities

! The presence of overlying squamous dysplasia may be a helpful clue to the diagnosis of carcinoma with ACC-like features

! CD117 IHC is not helpful in differentiating carcinoma with ACC-like features from ACC

! When evaluating for possible high-risk HPV infection, p16 IHC should be paired with another more specific method (ie, HPV DNA ISH) to detect HPV subtype 33

Pathologic Key Features CARCINOMA WITH ADENOID CYSTIC CARCINOMA–LIKE FEATURES

• Carcinoma with ACC-like features is a rare HPV-associated sinonasal tumor that morphologically mimics ACC

• It shows a biphasic morphology with myoepithelial and ductal differentiation and does not show overt squamous differentiation

• Carcinoma with ACC-like features is strongly associated with infection by high-risk HPV subtype 33 and does not show *MYB-NFIB* gene fusions that are characteristic of ACC

SINONASAL (SCHNEIDERIAN) PAPILLOMAS

INTRODUCTION

Sinonasal (Schneiderian) papillomas are benign epithelial tumors of the sinonasal cavities.[44] Three types of sinonasal papillomas have been described: exophytic sinonasal papilloma (ESP), inverted sinonasal papilloma (ISP), and oncocytic sinonasal papilloma (OSP). ESPs typically occur on the nasal septum and are not associated with sinonasal carcinoma. In contrast, ISP and OSP usually occur on the lateral wall of the nasal cavity and/or paranasal sinuses and are associated with a synchronous or metachronous sinonasal carcinoma in a minority of cases (up to 15%). Patients with sinonasal papillomas are typically older adults

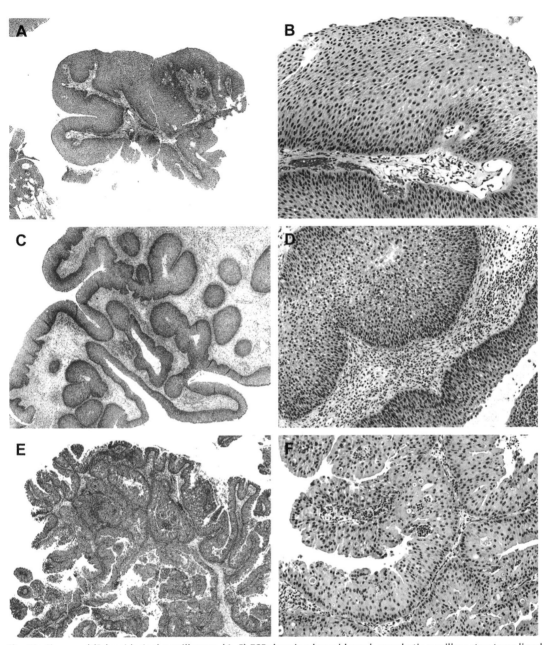

Fig. 13. Sinonasal (Schneiderian) papillomas. (*A, B*) ESP showing broad-based, exophytic papillary structures lined by benign nonkeratinizing squamous epithelium. (*C, D*) ISP showing predominantly inverted nests of benign nonkeratinizing squamous epithelium with conspicuous transmigrating neutrophilic inflammation. (*E, F*) OSP showing mixed exophytic papillary structures and endophytic (inverted) nests lined by benign multilayered columnar epithelium composed of cells with abundant eosinophilic (oncocytic) cytoplasm and conspicuous admixed neutrophilic abscesses (hematoxylin-eosin, original magnification ×4 [*A, C, E*], ×20 [*B, D, F*]).

and present with symptoms of nasal obstruction; associated sinonasal carcinomas may be locally aggressive and metastasize to regional lymph nodes.

The relationship between HPV infection and sinonasal papillomas is an area of ongoing investigation. No significant association between HPV infection and OSP has been established, and recent molecular profiling identified somatic *KRAS* mutations in 100% of tumors.[45] In contrast, ESP is almost exclusively associated with low-risk HPV subtypes (ie, subtypes 6 and 11), whereas a recent large meta-analysis of the published literature indicates that up to one-third of ISPs may be associated with HPV infection- either low-risk or high-risk HPV subtypes.[44,46] Recent molecular interrogation, however, has identified somatic *EGFR* mutations in approximately 90% of ISPs, and these mutations appear to be mutually exclusive of HPV infection.[47–49] The presence of high-risk HPV subtypes has been linked to epithelial dysplasia in ISP, as well as the development of associated sinonasal carcinoma, suggesting that high-risk HPV infection may play a role in malignant transformation of a subset of ISP-associated sinonasal carcinoma.[37,50–52]

GROSS FEATURES

ESPs are typically small, discrete, broad-based exophytic lesions arising from the mucosa, whereas ISP and OSP are often bulky, friable, papillary and polypoid tumors without clear delineation from the mucosa.[44]

MICROSCOPIC FEATURES

ESPs are exophytic, papillary tumors composed of hyperplastic nonkeratinizing squamous-type epithelium with scattered mucocytes (**Fig. 13**A, B). ISPs are predominantly endophytic tumors composed of hyperplastic nonkeratinizing squamous-type epithelium with scattered mucocytes and characteristic transmigrating neutrophils (**Fig. 13**C, D). OSPs are exophytic and endophytic tumors composed of hyperplastic columnar-type epithelium with abundant eosinophilic (oncocytic) cytoplasm and conspicuous intraepithelial mucin cysts with neutrophilic microabscesses (**Fig. 13**E, F). Epithelial dysplasia in ISP or OSP involves nuclear enlargement and hyperchromasia, architectural (intraepithelial) disorder, and increased mitotic activity. Sinonasal carcinomas associated with sinonasal papillomas are overwhelmingly SCC, which may be either keratinizing or nonkeratinizing.

DIFFERENTIAL DIAGNOSIS

Aside from distinguishing among the 3 subtypes, the major differential diagnoses for sinonasal papillomas are nonkeratinizing and/or papillary SCC. These entities can usually be readily distinguished on morphologic grounds alone because papillomas typically lack significant cytologic atypia; however, for some cases of ISP and OSP with high-grade epithelial dysplasia, this differential diagnosis is more difficult, and it is important to closely evaluate for evidence of invasive carcinoma (eg, stromal desmoplasia, infiltrative growth). Respiratory epithelial adenomatoid hamartoma (REAH), a circumscribed endophytic proliferation

of benign respiratory-type epithelium, may also enter the differential diagnosis for ISP; however, in contrast with REAH, ISP is composed predominantly of hyperplastic squamous epithelium and contains a prominent neutrophilic infiltrate.

DIAGNOSIS

The diagnosis of sinonasal papilloma is typically straightforward based on characteristic morphologic features but requires recognition of all 3 subtypes- most notably OSP, which is the least common papilloma subtype. More importantly, all specimens containing sinonasal papilloma should be extensively sampled to evaluate for the possibility of epithelial dysplasia and/or synchronous sinonasal carcinoma. In the event of a synchronous sinonasal carcinoma, several features are important for the diagnostic report, including the presence of invasion, the type of carcinoma (eg, keratinizing SCC), and the relative proportion of the specimen involved by carcinoma. In general, given the uncertain clinical significance of HPV infection in sinonasal carcinoma, p16 IHC and HPV DNA ISH are not recommended for routine clinical evaluation of sinonasal papilloma-associated carcinomas.[37]

PROGNOSIS

ESP is typically adequately treated with local surgical excision and usually does not recur.[44] ISP

Pathologic Key Features
SINONASAL (SCHNEIDERIAN)
PAPILLOMAS

- Sinonasal (Schneiderian) papillomas are group of benign epithelial tumors with 3 distinct morphologic subtypes: ESP, ISP, and OSP

- ESPs arise on the nasal septum, are associated with low-risk HPV infection, and typically do not progress to sinonasal carcinoma

- ISPs usually occur on lateral nasal wall and/or paranasal sinuses, are associated with somatic *EGFR* mutations or HPV infection, and progress to sinonasal carcinoma in a subset of cases; tumors with epithelial dysplasia and/or associated carcinoma may be associated with high-risk HPV infection

- OSPs typically occur on the lateral nasal wall and/or paranasal sinuses, are associated with somatic *KRAS* mutations, and progress to sinonasal carcinoma in a subset of cases; these tumors are not associated with HPV infection and OSP often require more extensive surgical debulking of the sinonasal mucosa and may recur and/or progress to sinonasal carcinoma. For patients who develop sinonasal carcinoma, treatment options include surgical excision, radiation therapy, and chemotherapy; the prognosis for sinonasal papilloma-associated sinonasal carcinoma may be similar to de novo sinonasal carcinoma, with a 5-year mortality approaching 40%.[53,54] As indicated earlier, there are recent data to indicate that patients with HPV-associated sinonasal SCC may have a better clinical outcome than those with non–HPV-associated tumors[44]; however, this has not been specifically examined in the context of sinonasal papilloma-associated sinonasal carcinoma.

△△ **Differential Diagnosis**
SINONASAL (SCHNEIDERIAN) PAPILLOMAS

Differential Diagnosis	Diagnostic Pathologic Features and/or Ancillary Studies
REAH	• Circumscribed growth; respiratory-type epithelium with abundant mucocytes and no squamous hyperplasia or transmigrating neutrophils
Nonkeratinizing or papillary SCC	• Infiltrative growth and/or stromal desmoplasia; presence of significant cytologic atypia; absence of transmigrating neutrophils

Pitfalls
SINONASAL (SCHNEIDERIAN) PAPILLOMAS

! The presence of significant cytologic atypia, infiltrative growth, and/or stromal desmoplasia should warrant consideration of nonkeratinizing or papillary SCC

! Although ISP may have a minor exophytic component, conspicuous endophytic (inverted) growth is a helpful clue for differentiating these tumors from ESP

! In contrast with ISP, REAH is a circumscribed proliferation of benign respiratory-type epithelium without significant squamous hyperplasia

REFERENCES

1. Gillison ML, Koch WM, Capone RB, et al. Evidence for a causal association between human papillomavirus and a subset of head and neck cancers. J Natl Cancer Inst 2000;92(9):709–20.
2. Westra WH. The pathology of HPV-related head and neck cancer: implications for the diagnostic pathologist. Semin Diagn Pathol 2015;32(1):42–53.
3. Galloway DA, Laimins LA. Human papillomaviruses: shared and distinct pathways for pathogenesis. Curr Opin Virol 2015;14:87–92.
4. Venuti A, Paolini F, Nasir L, et al. Papillomavirus E5: the smallest oncoprotein with many functions. Mol Cancer 2011;10:140.
5. Barnes L, Eveson JW, Reichart P, et al. Pathology and genetics of head and neck tumours. 3rd edition. Lyon (France): IARC; 2005.
6. Gillison ML, Chaturvedi AK, Anderson WF, et al. Epidemiology of human papillomavirus-positive head and neck squamous cell carcinoma. J Clin Oncol 2015;33(29):3235–42.
7. Walline HM, Komarck C, McHugh JB, et al. High-risk human papillomavirus detection in oropharyngeal, nasopharyngeal, and oral cavity cancers: comparison of multiple methods. JAMA Otolaryngol Head Neck Surg 2013;139(12):1320–7.
8. Bishop JA, Guo TW, Smith DF, et al. Human papillomavirus-related carcinomas of the sinonasal tract. Am J Surg Pathol 2013;37(2):185–92.
9. Larque AB, Hakim S, Ordi J, et al. High-risk human papillomavirus is transcriptionally active in a subset of sinonasal squamous cell carcinomas. Mod Pathol 2014;27(3):343–51.
10. El-Mofty SK. HPV-related squamous cell carcinoma variants in the head and neck. Head Neck Pathol 2012;6(Suppl 1):S55–62.
11. El-Mofty SK. Human papillomavirus-related head and neck squamous cell carcinoma variants. Semin Diagn Pathol 2015;32(1):23–31.
12. El-Mofty SK, Lu DW. Prevalence of human papillomavirus type 16 DNA in squamous cell carcinoma of the palatine tonsil, and not the oral cavity, in young patients: a distinct clinicopathologic and molecular disease entity. Am J Surg Pathol 2003;27(11):1463–70.
13. Cai C, Chernock RD, Pittman ME, et al. Keratinizing-type squamous cell carcinoma of the oropharynx: p16 overexpression is associated with positive high-risk HPV status and improved survival. Am J Surg Pathol 2014;38(6):809–15.
14. Jo VY, Mills SE, Stoler MH, et al. Papillary squamous cell carcinoma of the head and neck: frequent association with human papillomavirus infection and invasive carcinoma. Am J Surg Pathol 2009;33(11):1720–4.

15. Mehrad M, Carpenter DH, Chernock RD, et al. Papillary squamous cell carcinoma of the head and neck: clinicopathologic and molecular features with special reference to human papillomavirus. Am J Surg Pathol 2013;37(9):1349–56.

16. Begum S, Westra WH. Basaloid squamous cell carcinoma of the head and neck is a mixed variant that can be further resolved by HPV status. Am J Surg Pathol 2008;32(7):1044–50.

17. Chernock RD, Lewis JS Jr, Zhang Q, et al. Human papillomavirus-positive basaloid squamous cell carcinomas of the upper aerodigestive tract: a distinct clinicopathologic and molecular subtype of basaloid squamous cell carcinoma. Hum Pathol 2010;41(7):1016–23.

18. Masand RP, El-Mofty SK, Ma XJ, et al. Adenosquamous carcinoma of the head and neck: relationship to human papillomavirus and review of the literature. Head Neck Pathol 2011;5(2):108–16.

19. Radkay-Gonzalez L, Faquin W, McHugh JB, et al. Ciliated adenosquamous carcinoma: expanding the phenotypic diversity of human papillomavirus-associated tumors. Head Neck Pathol 2016;10(2):167–75.

20. Bishop JA, Westra WH. Ciliated HPV-related carcinoma: a well-differentiated form of head and neck carcinoma that can be mistaken for a benign cyst. Am J Surg Pathol 2015;39(11):1591–5.

21. Singhi AD, Stelow EB, Mills SE, et al. Lymphoepithelial-like carcinoma of the oropharynx: a morphologic variant of HPV-related head and neck carcinoma. Am J Surg Pathol 2010;34(6):800–5.

22. Carpenter DH, El-Mofty SK, Lewis JS Jr. Undifferentiated carcinoma of the oropharynx: a human papillomavirus-associated tumor with a favorable prognosis. Mod Pathol 2011;24(10):1306–12.

23. Bishop JA, Montgomery EA, Westra WH. Use of p40 and p63 immunohistochemistry and human papillomavirus testing as ancillary tools for the recognition of head and neck sarcomatoid carcinoma and its distinction from benign and malignant mesenchymal processes. Am J Surg Pathol 2014;38(2):257–64.

24. Watson RF, Chernock RD, Wang X, et al. Spindle cell carcinomas of the head and neck rarely harbor transcriptionally-active human papillomavirus. Head Neck Pathol 2013;7(3):250–7.

25. Kraft S, Faquin WC, Krane JF. HPV-associated neuroendocrine carcinoma of the oropharynx: a rare new entity with potentially aggressive clinical behavior. Am J Surg Pathol 2012;36(3):321–30.

26. Bishop JA, Westra WH. Human papillomavirus-related small cell carcinoma of the oropharynx. Am J Surg Pathol 2011;35(11):1679–84.

27. Thompson ED, Stelow EB, Mills SE, et al. Large cell neuroendocrine carcinoma of the head and neck: a clinicopathologic series of 10 cases with an emphasis on HPV status. Am J Surg Pathol 2016;40(4):471–8.

28. Chang AM, Nikiforova MN, Johnson JT, et al. Human papillomavirus-associated adenocarcinoma of the base of tongue: potentially actionable genetic changes. Head Neck Pathol 2014;8(2):151–6.

29. Hanna J, Reimann JD, Haddad RI, et al. Human papillomavirus-associated adenocarcinoma of the base of the tongue. Hum Pathol 2013;44(8):1516–23.

30. Isayeva T, Said-Al-Naief N, Ren Z, et al. Salivary mucoepidermoid carcinoma: demonstration of transcriptionally active human papillomavirus 16/18. Head Neck Pathol 2013;7(2):135–48.

31. Bishop JA, Yonescu R, Batista D, et al. Mucoepidermoid carcinoma does not harbor transcriptionally active high risk human papillomavirus even in the absence of the MAML2 translocation. Head Neck Pathol 2014;8(3):298–302.

32. Bishop JA, Lewis JS Jr, Rocco JW, et al. HPV-related squamous cell carcinoma of the head and neck: An update on testing in routine pathology practice. Semin Diagn Pathol 2015;32(5):344–51.

33. Jordan RC, Lingen MW, Perez-Ordonez B, et al. Validation of methods for oropharyngeal cancer HPV status determination in US cooperative group trials. Am J Surg Pathol 2012;36(7):945–54.

34. Bishop JA, Ma XJ, Wang H, et al. Detection of transcriptionally active high-risk HPV in patients with head and neck squamous cell carcinoma as visualized by a novel E6/E7 mRNA in situ hybridization method. Am J Surg Pathol 2012;36(12):1874–82.

35. Ukpo OC, Flanagan JJ, Ma XJ, et al. High-risk human papillomavirus E6/E7 mRNA detection by a novel in situ hybridization assay strongly correlates with p16 expression and patient outcomes in oropharyngeal squamous cell carcinoma. Am J Surg Pathol 2011;35(9):1343–50.

36. Chung CH, Gillison ML. Human papillomavirus in head and neck cancer: its role in pathogenesis and clinical implications. Clin Cancer Res 2009;15(22):6758–62.

37. Lewis JS Jr. Sinonasal squamous cell carcinoma: a review with emphasis on emerging histologic subtypes and the role of human papillomavirus. Head Neck Pathol 2016;10(1):60–7.

38. Gillison ML, Restighini C. Anticipation of the impact of human papillomavirus on clinical decision making for the head and neck cancer patient. Hematol Oncol Clin North Am 2015;29(6):1045–60.

39. Petersson F. Nasopharyngeal carcinoma: a review. Semin Diagn Pathol 2015;32(1):54–73.

40. Maxwell JH, Kumar B, Feng FY, et al. HPV-positive/p16-positive/EBV-negative nasopharyngeal carcinoma in white North Americans. Head Neck 2010;32(5):562–7.

41. Lo EJ, Bell D, Woo JS, et al. Human papillomavirus and WHO type I nasopharyngeal carcinoma. Laryngoscope 2010;120(10):1990–7.

42. Stenmark MH, McHugh JB, Schipper M, et al. Nonendemic HPV-positive nasopharyngeal carcinoma: association with poor prognosis. Int J Radiat Oncol Biol Phys 2014;88(3):580–8.

43. Bishop JA, Ogawa T, Stelow EB, et al. Human papillomavirus-related carcinoma with adenoid cystic-like features: a peculiar variant of head and neck cancer restricted to the sinonasal tract. Am J Surg Pathol 2013;37(6):836–44.

44. Barnes L. Schneiderian papillomas and nonsalivary glandular neoplasms of the head and neck. Mod Pathol 2002;15(3):279–97.

45. Udager AM, McHugh JB, Betz BL, et al. Activating KRAS mutations are characteristic of oncocytic sinonasal papilloma and associated sinonasal squamous cell carcinoma. J Pathol 2016;239(4):394–8.

46. Syrjanen K, Syrjanen S. Detection of human papillomavirus in sinonasal papillomas: systematic review and meta-analysis. Laryngoscope 2013;123(1):181–92.

47. Udager AM, Rolland DC, McHugh JB, et al. High-frequency targetable EGFR mutations in sinonasal squamous cell carcinomas arising from inverted sinonasal papilloma. Cancer Res 2015;75(13):2600–6.

48. Brown N, Udager A, McHugh J, et al. Human papillomavirus and activating EGFR mutations: alternative oncogenic mechanisms in inverted sinonasal papilloma. Mod Pathol 2016;29:319A.

49. Udager AM, McHugh JB, Elenitoba-Johnson KS, et al. EGFR mutations in sinonasal squamous tumors: oncogenic and therapeutic implications. Oncoscience 2015;2(11):908–9.

50. Strojan P, Ferlito A, Lund VJ, et al. Sinonasal inverted papilloma associated with malignancy: the role of human papillomavirus infection and its implications for radiotherapy. Oral Oncol 2012;48(3):216–8.

51. Lewis JS Jr, Westra WH, Thompson LD, et al. The sinonasal tract: another potential "hot spot" for carcinomas with transcriptionally-active human papillomavirus. Head Neck Pathol 2014;8(3):241–9.

52. Syrjanen K, Syrjanen S. Detection of human papillomavirus in sinonasal carcinoma: systematic review and meta-analysis. Hum Pathol 2013;44(6):983–91.

53. Tanvetyanon T, Qin D, Padhya T, et al. Survival outcomes of squamous cell carcinoma arising from sinonasal inverted papilloma: report of 6 cases with systematic review and pooled analysis. Am J Otolaryngol 2009;30(1):38–43.

54. Nudell J, Chiosea S, Thompson LD. Carcinoma ex-Schneiderian papilloma (malignant transformation): a clinicopathologic and immunophenotypic study of 20 cases combined with a comprehensive review of the literature. Head Neck Pathol 2014;8(3):269–86.

Autoimmune Disease Manifestations in the Oral Cavity

Kelly R. Magliocca, DDS, MPH[a],*, Sarah G. Fitzpatrick, DDS[b]

KEYWORDS

• Pemphigus • Pemphigoid • Pyostomatitis vegetans • Geographic tongue • Lichen planus

---

Key points

- Autoimmune diseases affecting the oral cavity may demonstrate clinical, histologic, and in some cases similar immunopathologic patterns.

- Infectious, reactive, and neoplastic entities may arise in the microscopic differential diagnosis of oral autoimmune disease.

- Identifying tissue reaction patterns, such as lichenoid, psoriasiform, spongiotic, and vesiculobullous, may form a component of the diagnostic algorithm for oral mucosal disease.

ABSTRACT

Immune-related disorders of the oral cavity may occur as primary disease process, secondary to systemic disease or neoplasm, or as a reaction to medications and other agents. The entities represented within this group may vary significantly by severity, clinical presentation, microscopic presentation, and special testing results. The selected immune-related conditions of the oral cavity in this article are categorized and presented by their prototypical tissue reaction patterns: vesiculobullous, including acantholytic and subepithelial separation; psoriasiform; spongiotic; and lichenoid reaction patterns.

OVERVIEW: IMMUNOPATHOLOGIC TESTING

Ancillary testing methods, such as special stains, immunohistochemical (IHC) testing, and immunopathologic and serologic testing, may be helpful in distinguishing between similar-appearing lesions. A brief overview of immunopathologic testing is provided: in direct immunofluorescence (DIF) testing, frozen perilesional tissue biopsy specimens are treated with fluorescein-labeled antibodies and evaluated under a fluorescence microscope.[1] Specimens for DIF must be transported to the laboratory in special medium, most commonly Michel solution, but other options include Zeus media, liquid nitrogen, or rarely saline (short-term storage only).[2] Fibrinogen, C3, IgA, IgM, and IgG represent the antibodies evaluated during the examination. In contrast, indirect immunofluorescence testing (IIF) uses patient serum applied to a secondary substrate tested for antibody presence with fluorescein labels.[1] The salt split technique can be performed either directly on patient tissue or indirectly using serum and is used to differentiate between certain entities with similar-appearing histology and DIF results.[3]

VESICULOBULLOUS REACTION PATTERN — ACANTHOLYSIS

PEMPHIGUS

Pemphigus is a group of autoimmune blistering diseases that may involve the skin and/or oral

---

Disclosure Statement: We the authors have no commercial or financial conflicts of interest or funding sources to disclose.
[a] Department of Pathology and Laboratory Medicine, Emory University, 500 Peachtree Street Northeast, Atlanta, GA 30308, USA; [b] Department of Oral and Maxillofacial Diagnostic Sciences, University of Florida, 1395 Center Drive, Gainesville, FL 32610, USA
* Corresponding author.
E-mail address: kmagliocca@emory.edu

mucosa. Four major categories of pemphigus have been described: pemphigus vulgaris (PV), pemphigus foliaceus, IgA pemphigus (IgAP), and paraneoplastic pemphigus (PNP).[4] This article focuses on the 2 forms of pemphigus with almost invariable involvement of oral mucosal surfaces: PV and PNP.

PV is a potentially life-threatening chronic bullous disease affecting patients worldwide, and although possible in the pediatric population, a majority of cases affect adults in the fourth to sixth decades of life.[5] The best known mechanism for blister formation in PV involves the autoantibody attack against the intercellular keratinocyte adhesion molecules, or desmosomes. Desmoglein-3 (Dsg3), a 130-kDa cadherin component of the desmosome is the main target of attack in mucosal predominant PV, with desmoglein-1 (Dsg1), a 160-kDa protein, additionally targeted in mucocutaneous PV.[6] The antibody-antigen attack results in loss of intercellular adhesion, resultant epithelial acantholysis, and development of blisters and bullae.[4] The process or event(s) precipitating autoantibody formation are unknown.[7]

PNP was first described in 1990 and most often occurs in association with an underlying neoplastic disorder.[8,9] Chronic lymphocytic lymphoma and other forms of non-Hodgkin lymphoma are often linked to PNP, but carcinoma and sarcoma, in addition to benign neoplasms, such as thymoma and Castleman disease, are reported.[9–11] The onset of PNP in relation to the identification of an underlying neoplasm is variable but in most cases the clinical history of neoplasm is known prior to the development of PNP.[12] In one-third of patients, oral mucosal lesions may be the first sign of any disease, with subsequent identification of a neoplasm during the diagnostic evaluation of the orocutaneous symptoms or within the ensuing months in approximately half of patients.[12,13] The average age of onset is 57 years with overall equal gender distribution.[10,13,14] The pathogenesis of PNP is complex and thought to occur as a result of the combined humoral autoimmune response and cellular immune response.[8,15] Antibody attack against a spectrum of targets, such as intercellular proteins (Dsg1 and Dsg3), plakin family proteins (envoplakin, periplakin, desmoplakin, plectin, and Bullous pemphigoid antigen 1 [BP230]), and the protease inhibitor alpha-2-macroglobulin-like antigen 1 (A2ML1), may be detected.[16] Of these, envoplakin and periplakin are most specific for PNP.[17]

Gross/Clinical Features

In PV, mucosal lesions tend to precede the development of cutaneous manifestations and in some cases may be the only site affected. Delicate, superficial blisters and erosions affect any oral site but the palate, tongue, and labial/buccal mucosa are often involved.[5,12,18] Erosion of the lower lip vermillion is not uncommon. Nonoral mucosal sites, such as pharyngeal, laryngeal, nasal, conjunctival, and genital mucosa, can be affected.[4] Localized or generalized cutaneous lesions exhibit a symmetric predilection for the trunk, groin, axilla, scalp, and face[12,18] and present as flaccid vesicles or bullae on uninflamed skin reported to rupture easily and appear as erythematous erosions.

For PNP, the earliest and most striking clinical features of PNP are painful, florid oral mucosal erosions and ulcers.[17] Oral mucosal involvement can be identified in nearly all patients, but extraoral mucosal sites, such as conjunctiva, genital, pharyngeal, esophageal, nasopharyngeal, and laryngeal mucosa, may also occur[13,15] as well as cutaneous lesions (often sparing the face)[15,17] or viscera, justifying designation of paraneoplastic autoimmune multiorgan syndrome.[19] Pulmonary involvement is devastating and typically manifests as bronchiolitis obliterans.[10]

Microscopic Features

A developing lesion of PV may demonstrate eosinophilic spongiosis, whereas the center of a deeply entrenched mucosal ulceration may show a nonspecific ulceration on microscopic examination. Clinicians carefully sampling the edge of the blister should include lesion and perilesional mucosa to confirm the level of the separation and demonstrate the presence of the characteristic suprabasilar acantholysis in PV.[18] Rounded acantholytic cells with eosinophilic cytoplasm and pyknotic nuclei are present within intraepithelial cleft spaces and lack overtly atypical features, despite their detachment (**Fig. 1**A). A mild to moderate mixed inflammatory infiltrate may be present in the subjacent connective tissue. The suprabasalar epithelial separation results in retention of only basal cells, an appearance that corresponds to the so-called tombstone effect.[4] Preservation of undulating connective tissue papillae lined by basal cells and devoid of suprabasal epithelium imparts a villous silhouette (**Fig. 1**B).

PNP shows variable morphologic features. The key and most frequent features include a combination of humoral mediated phenomena: suprabasal epithelial acantholysis, dyskeratosis, and cellular autoimmune phenomena: vacuolar interface change and lichenoid infiltrates. Dyskeratosis in the setting of suprabasal acantholysis may be an important clue to PNP.[8] In developing lesions,

Fig. 1. Histologic and DIF appearance of mucosal PV. (*A*) Characteristic suprabasal separation, rounded acantholytic cells with eosinophilic cytoplasm within intraepithelial cleft spaces (×100, H&E stain). (*B*) Suprabasal detachment and retention of basal cells results in a tombstone appearance to the retained basal cells (*arrows*). Undulating appearance of connective tissue papillae lined by basal cells and devoid of suprabasal epithelium imparts a villous tissue silhouette (×200, H&E stain). (*C*) DIF demonstrating intercellular deposition of IgG autoantibody (×200). (*Courtesy of* [*C*] University of Florida Oral Pathology Image Archive, Gaineville, FL; with permission.)

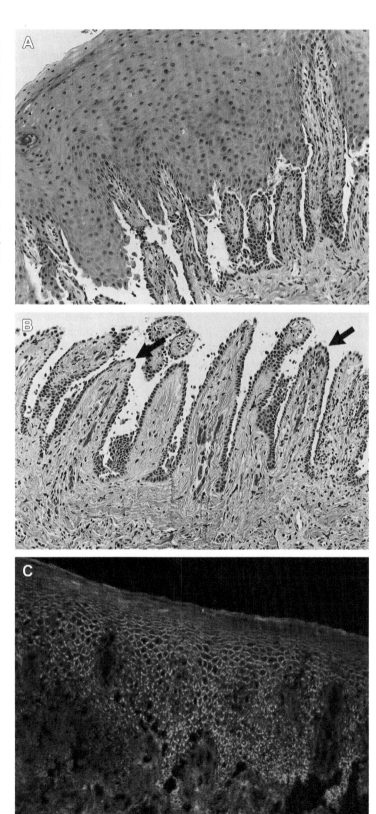

epithelial spongiosis (ES) with eosinophilic exocytosis may be identified prior to frank acantholysis.[20] In some cases, only dyskeratosis and lichenoid changes may be identified, without convincing acantholytic alterations.[15,19]

Differential Diagnosis

Based on light microscopy, PV may be indistinguishable from PNP and other forms of pemphigus. PNP is more likely to exhibit dyskeratotic cells within the epithelium than PV, and the 2 can be further distinguished by immunopathologic testing. Nonblistering PNP without acantholysis may mimic lichenoid reactions (discussed later). Warty dyskeratoma/Darier disease demonstrate acantholysis, but the presence of an endophytic epithelial proliferation with elongated narrow test-tube rete ridges, a central keratin-filled crater, and peculiar keratinocyte dyskeratosis (corp ronds and corp grains formation within the stratum spinosum and stratum corneum, respectively) are not features of pemphigus (Fig. 2). In immunocompromised patients, an atypical clinical presentation of herpes simplex virus (HSV) can mimic a vesiculobullous disease and lead to biopsy sampling. Identification of multinucleated epithelial cells, margination of chromatin, and molding of affected cells is supportive of viral cytopathic effect. A marked stromal inflammatory response is expected to accompany mucosal HSV (Fig. 3A–C). Pseudoacantholytic or pseudoadenoid epithelial alterations have been described in keratinizing oral squamous epithelial dysplasia.[21] Epithelial hyperplasia with budding or drop-shaped rete ridges, aberrant paradoxic keratinization, cellular and nuclear pleomorphism, and abnormal variation in cell size are some of the cytomorphologic and architectural disturbances that favor keratinizing epithelial dysplasia over true vesiculobullous disease (Fig. 4). Unintentional immersion of a fresh mucosal biopsy sample into a specimen cup filled with tap water instead of formalin fixative is known to result in marked epithelial acantholysis, an artifactual tissue distortion.[22] Clues to detecting an artifactual acantholytic pattern include the complete eosinophilic homogenization of the tissue tinctorial qualities on hematoxylin-eosin stain (H&E). In addition, artifactual vertical elongation or spiking of the retained basal layer is a helpful clue to the presence of artifact (Fig. 5). Although light microscopic evidence may be sufficient for accurate diagnostic classification of many of the entities discussed previously, others require clinical correlation and additional tissue for immunofluorescence and/or serologic confirmation.

Diagnosis

Definitive diagnosis of PV and PNP is secured based on combined clinical, histologic, immunopathologic, and serologic data.[4] In PV, the sample submitted for DIF should demonstrate intercellular IgG and C3 deposition in a netlike, or lattice-like pattern within the stratified squamous epithelium (Fig. 1C).[23] Detection of circulating IgG autoantibodies to epithelial intercellular antigens using serologic testing, such as IIF or ELISA, is an important component in arriving at a final diagnosis. Using IIF, autoantibodies directed against the epithelial cell surface can be detected on monkey or rat esophagus, and the test result is reported as a titer.[23] In addition to the diagnostic value, these tests allow for assessment of circulating autoantibody titers as a useful surrogate of disease severity against which to adjust treatment and monitor response.[12] At present, ELISA is considered the most sensitive test for the detection of circulating antibodies in PV.[4,23] IHC staining for Dsg3 is not widely used or widely available in the evaluation for pemphigus and does not obviate additional serologic testing.[24] When the light microscopic differential diagnosis includes epithelial acantholysis secondary to viral cytopathic effect of herpetic lesions, IHC staining to detect HSV-1/HSV-2 may prove useful in some cases (Fig. 3D).

In PNP, deposition of IgG and/or C3 at the intercellular epithelial cell surface is present alone or in combination with a granular-linear deposition of IgG or complement at the basement membrane zone (BMZ).[12,15] Although DIF lacks sensitivity as a test for PNP, the specificity is high and approaches 90%.[16,17] IIF has a higher sensitivity and specificity than DIF, 86% and 98%, respectively.[17] Using IIF, circulating IgG antibodies against intercellular surfaces and, in most cases, the BMZ can be detected in the serum of patients with PNP. Although stratified squamous epithelial substrate facilitates detection of some targets, plakin proteins are an important target of PNP and present in substrates, such as rat urothelium.[12,15,16] If PNP is still clinically suspected in the setting of negative IIF, additional testing for autoantibodies with immunoassays, such as ELISA, immunoblotting (IB), and immunoprecipitation (IP), is suggested.[12,15] Through use of 1 or more of these specific detection immunoassays, evidence of serum IgG/IgA autoantibodies against envoplakin, periplakin, Dsg3, Dsg1, desmoplakin, BP230, plectin, and/or A2ML1 provides additional support for the diagnosis of PNP.[14,25] Although IP is the most sensitive and specific test for antiplakin antibodies commonly associated with PNP, the

Fig. 2. Histologic appearance of mucosal Warty dyskeratoma/Darier disease. (*A*) Epithelial proliferation with surface keratosis (H&E, ×20). (*B*) Elongated narrow test-tube rete ridges (*arrows*) (H&E, ×200). (*C*) Dyskeratosis with corp ronds and corp grains formation within the stratum spinosum and stratum corneum respectively (*arrows*) (H&E, ×400).

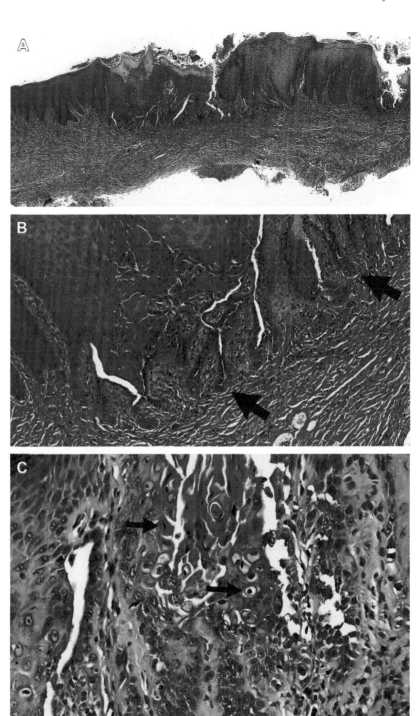

availability of IP testing is limited.[8,14] Recently, a European group viewed the combination of 2 of 3 serologic techniques (IIF on rat bladder, IB, and IP) as sufficient for establishing a diagnosis of PNP with sensitivity approaching approximately 100%.[12] PNP without a concurrent tumor should necessitate investigation for an occult malignancy. In some cases no malignancy is discovered and

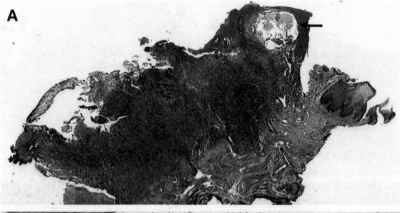

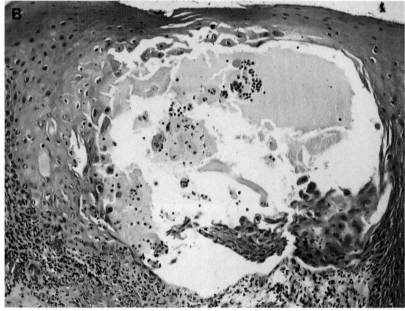

Fig. 3. Histologic and IHC appearance of HSV. (*A*) Intraepithelial vesicle formation within squamous epithelium (*arrow*), and marked stromal inflammation (H&E, ×27). (*B, C*) Acantholysis with multinucleated epithelial cells, margination of chromatin, and molding of affected cells (*arrows*), supportive of viral cytopathic effect (H&E, ×200 and H&E, ×400, respectively). (*D*) IHC reactivity to HSV I in affected cells (H&E, ×200).

classification of this latter group of patients is problematic. Such patients must be followed closely to exclude development of a tumor. If no tumor ever develops, this suggests other unidentified factors may induce a PNP-like profile.[10]

Prognosis

For PV, once diagnosis is confirmed, the goals of therapy with systemic immunosuppressive (steroidal agents) and/or immunomodulating agents, such as azathioprine, mycophenolate, rituximab, and even plasmapheresis in refractory cases, include a reduction in disease burden, quality-of-life improvement, and minimizing therapy-related complications.[26] Prior to the development or use of systemic corticosteroids, PV was associated with a mortality rate of approximately 90%[4] but

is now estimated at 5% to 10%, attributable to therapy-related complications in most cases.[4] High doses and/or prolonged steroid therapy can be associated with significant adverse events, such as heart disease, immunosuppression, sepsis, and even death.

PNP, on the other hand, has a high mortality rate, ranging between 68% and 90%, with a mean survival of less than 1 year.[9,10,13] Mortality is less when PNP occurs in association with benign neoplasms, such as thymoma and Castleman disease.[19] Commonly reported causes of mortality in PNP include the underlying neoplasm, respiratory failure, and septicemia. Treatment goals of PNP include balancing management of a neoplasm and the associated autoimmune and inflammatory response yet limiting morbidity

Fig. 3. (continued).

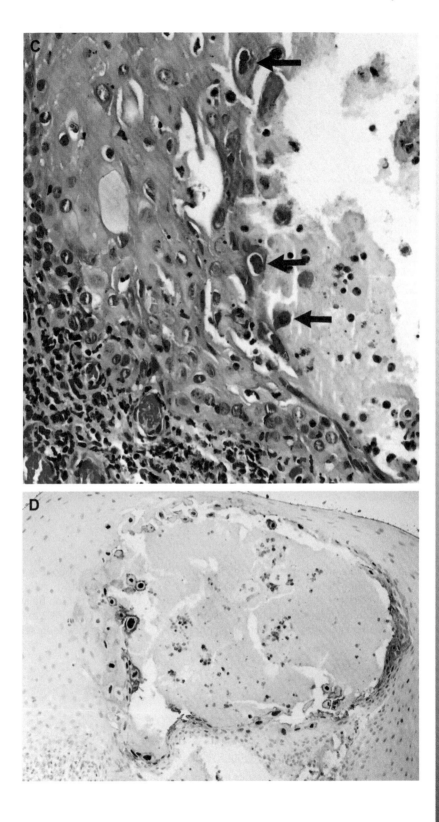

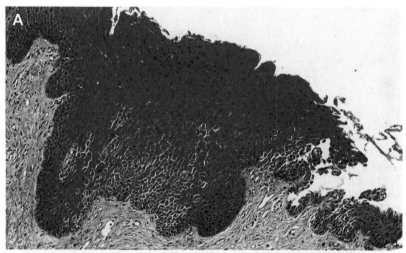

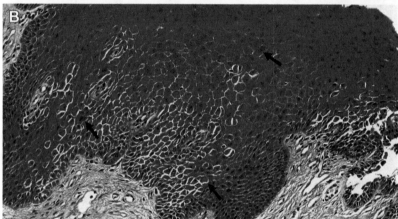

Fig. 4. Histologic appearance of keratinizing dysplasia exhibiting pseudoacantholysis. (*A*) Epithelial hyperplasia focal orthokeratosis, dyskeratosis and cellular pleomorphism (H&E, ×100). (*B*) Higher magnification of aberrant/paradoxic keratinization, pseudoacantholytic squamous epithelium, and cellular and nuclear pleomorphism (*arrows*) (H&E, ×180).

and complications of treatment and improving quality of life.[8] Removing the associated tumor if nonhematologic demonstrates variable clinical and symptomatic improvement.[15,27] Use of high-dose corticosteroids and immunosuppressive medication to control the immune phenomena in a patient with a history of malignancy increases morbidity, but, on balance, the reported high rate of mortality of PNP may be required and in some instances may represent a palliative approach.

Pathologic Key Features
ACANTHOLYTIC VESICULOBULLOUS REACTION PATTERN OF ORAL MUCOSA

- PV is the most common pemphigus variant to affect the oral mucosa.
- Intraepithelial separation results in retained basal layer, imparting a tombstone appearance.
- Intraepithelial separation with dyskeratosis and vacuolar interface should prompt a request for additional testing with DIF and IIF to evaluate for PNP.
- Multiple supportive parameters (clinical, light microscopic, DIF, IIF, and/or immunoassay) are essential to secure a diagnosis of PV or PNP.

Differential Diagnosis
ACANTHOLYTIC VESICULOBULLOUS REACTION PATTERN OF ORAL MUCOSA

Differential Diagnosis of Oral Mucosal Pemphigus Vulgaris

	Distinguishing Features
PNP	• Clinically recalcitrant oral ulcerations
	• Acantholysis, dyskeratosis, and vacuolar interface change
	• DIF intercellular deposition of IgG alone and/or with a granular-linear deposition of IgG or complement BMZ
	• IIF using rat bladder to detect plakins
Warty dyskeratoma/oral manifestation of Darier disease	• Warty dyskeratoma, isolated lesion, usually hard palate. Darier disease diffuses keratotic lesions, favoring palate.
	• Epithelial proliferation present with acantholysis, dyskeratosis, often keratotic central plug
	• Corps ronds and corp grains present
HSV	• Acantholysis, spongiosis, ulceration, and marked epithelial and stroma inflammation
	• Viral cytopathic effect present
Keratinizing acantholytic dysplasia	• Dyskeratosis, multinucleate keratinocytes, abnormal maturation of epithelium
	• No evidence of intracellular antigen-antibody reaction on DIF
Fixation artifact	• Low magnification washed-out eosinophilic appearance.
	• Stromal tissues poorly preserved
	• Spiked appearance to basal cell layer
	• May exhibit subepithelial separation in addition to suprabasal separation

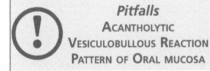

Pitfalls
ACANTHOLYTIC VESICULOBULLOUS REACTION PATTERN OF ORAL MUCOSA

! Definitive diagnosis of PV or PNP should not be established with H&E alone.

! Acantholytic pattern can be artifactual, can be seen in premalignant lesions in association with benign and malignant tumors, and can show syndromic association with Darier disease, autoimmune diseases, and virally mediated diseases.

! DIF and IIF or immunoassays are supportive for autoimmune disease and distinguishing from microscopic mimics.

VESICULOBULLOUS REACTION PATTERN — SUBEPITHELIAL SEPARATION

MUCOUS MEMBRANE PEMPHIGOID

Diseases associated with subepithelial separation affect the oral cavity with a wide range of clinical and microscopic features. Mucous membrane pemphigoid (MMP) is the most common of these to affect the oral mucosa. Related and rare disorders, such as linear IgA (LIGA) disease and epidermolysis bullosa acquisita (EBA), may have significant clinical and histologic overlap with MMP. Lichen planus pemphigoides (LPP) is an exceptionally rare disorder exhibiting a combined lichenoid and vesiculobullous reaction pattern.[28]

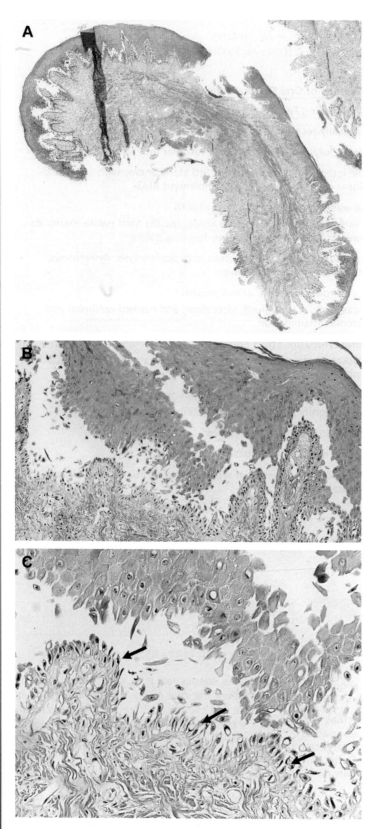

Fig. 5. Histologic appearance of artifactual acantholytic changes as a result of unintentional immersion/transport of an oral mucosal irritation fibroma (bite fibroma) in tap water. (*A*) Scanning magnification demonstrating pale eosinophilic tissue tinctorial qualities on H&E (H&E, ×20). (*B*) Suprabasal acantholysis with tombstone appearance (H&E, ×100). (*C*) Vertical elongation or spiking of the retained basal layer is a helpful clue to the presence of artifact (*arrows*) (H&E, ×380).

Fig. 6. Histologic and DIF appearance of MMP. (*A*) Subepithelial separation of epithelium from underlying connective tissue (H&E, ×40). (*B*) Zone of separation appears well defined, without suggestion of artifactual tissue tears, such as the presence of suprabasal and subepithelial separation (H&E, ×200). DIF demonstrates (*C*) IgG and (*D*) C3 linear deposition along BMZ in MMP (×200). (*Courtesy of [B and C] University of Florida Oral Pathology Image Archive, Gaineville, FL; with permission.*)

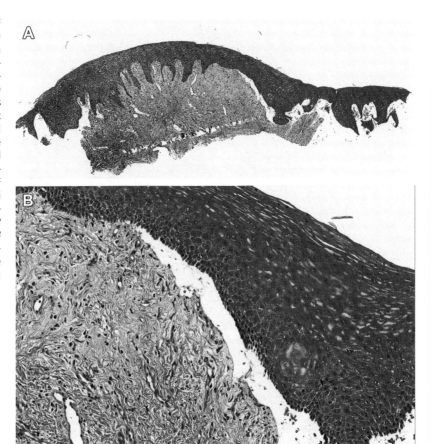

Gross/Clinical Features

MMP occurs mainly in middle-aged patients, with a female predominance. Although multiple areas of the oral cavity may be involved, the gingiva is most commonly affected and may be the only affected site in many cases. Lesions occur as relapsing and recurring chronic blood-filled blister formation that ruptures quickly, leaving painful ulcerations.[29] LIGA and EBA are rare bullous skin disorders skin that may exhibit oral lesions similar to MMP.[30,31] In the absence of skin findings, some pathologists are hesitant to provide a diagnosis of LIGA or EBA because these lesions may instead represent MMP.[32] In LPP, bullous lesions occur in an area of preexisting lichenoid patterned lesions.[28]

Microscopic Features

MMP is the prototypical subepithelial separation disease, showing separation epithelium from underlying inflamed connective tissue.[32] This zone of separation generally appears well defined, without suggestion of artifactual tearing (**Fig. 6**A,

B). LIGA and EBA appear similar to MMP with subepithelial bulla formation with or without inflammatory infiltrate, which may include neutrophils and eosinophils in addition to a nonspecific chronic inflammatory infiltrate.[30,31] LPP shows MMP-like histologic features with other areas compatible with lichenoid reaction patterned changes.[28]

Differential Diagnosis

In addition to differentiation of MMP from other closely related disorders, such as LIGA, EBA, and LPP, MMP with regenerative epithelial hyperplasia along the basal layer may suggest intraepithelial separation and should be distinguished from PV or variants of pemphigus. Artifactual epithelial separation, and trauma-related bullae may enter the differential diagnosis in some cases. Artifactual separation between the epithelium and connective tissue may occur for a variety of reasons, including intralesional injection of local anesthetic during biopsy.[33] This may mimic MMP but clinical history, histologic appearance, and negative DIF results may assist in identifying artifact

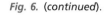

Fig. 6. (*continued*).

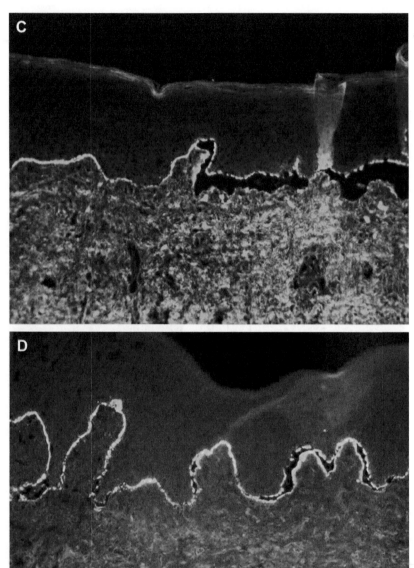

as etiology. Angina bullosa hemorrhagica is a lesion most likely related to traumatic etiology, which may mimic MMP clinically with the presentation of blood-filled blisters usually located on the soft palate but unlike MMP is minimally painful and most often solitary in nature. Microscopically, angina bullosa hemorrhagica may mimic MMP with subepithelial separation and chronically inflamed connective tissue; however, DIF testing is usually negative.[34]

Diagnosis

MMP and related lesions require careful clinical history and evaluation of the extent of disease involvement along with light microscopy and a tissue evaluation with DIF. DIF of MMP shows antibody deposition along the BMZ of any of the following: C3, IgG, and IgA (Fig. 6C, D).[32] LIGA shows linear antibody deposition of IgA along the BMZ, with accompanying IgM in some cases (Fig. 7).[31] EBA shows linear deposition of IgG and sometimes C3 at the BMZ.[30] LPP displays IgA, IgG, and C3 deposition at the BMZ.[28] Salt split testing may be required to differentiate EBA from variants of pemphigoid with the antibodies binding to the connective tissue (floor) of the bulla in EBA but the basal epithelial cells (roof) of the blister in the skin predominant variant of pemphigoid, bullous pemphigoid, which may rarely affect the oral cavity.[35]

Prognosis

MMP is treated according to severity with cases that affect only the oral mucosa considered mild and those affecting other or multiple mucosal locations more severe. Mild cases affecting only the oral cavity are generally treated first with topical steroids, with unsuccessful cases then followed by systemic treatment with dapsone and prednisone. For severe cases, systemic therapy may consist of dapsone and prednisone, azathioprine and mycophenolate mofetil, cyclophosphamide, or rituximab.[29] Ocular lesions in MMP may lead to blindness; therefore, regular examinations with an ophthalmologist are necessary. A subtype of

MMP with antibodies against laminin 332 has been demonstrated to be associated with an increased risk of cancer.[29] LIGA and EBA are treated similarly to severe or widespread MMP.[30,31] Although LIGA disease has occasionally shown an association with IBD,[36,37] the spectrum of immunopathology related to lesions of pyostomatitis vegetans (PyV) (discussed later) has not been well documented.[38,39]

> ### Pathologic Key Features
> #### VESICULOBULLOUS SUBEPITHELIAL SEPARATION PATTERN OF ORAL MUCOSA
>
> - Clinical history of relapsing and recurring blistering and ulcerative lesions involving the oral mucosa with or without skin or other mucosal sites of involvement
>
> - Microscopic findings of subepithelial separation and varying degrees of inflammation of connective tissue
>
> - DIF confirmation required for biopsy to determine variant of subepithelial separation disease

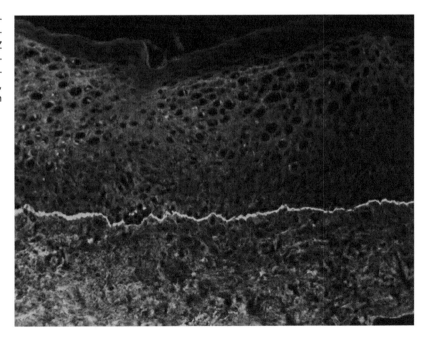

Fig. 7. DIF pattern characteristic of LIGA demonstrates IgA along BMZ (×200). (*Courtesy of* University of Florida Oral Pathology Image Archive, Gaineville, FL; with permission.)

Differential Diagnosis
VESICULOBULLOUS SUBEPITHELIAL SEPARATION PATTERN OF ORAL MUCOSA

Differential Diagnosis of Mucous Membrane Pemphigoid	
Distinguishing Features	
LIGA	• Predominantly skin disorder, oral lesions rare whereas MMP always involves mucosal surfaces with oral lesions common and rarely involves skin
	• Clinical and histologic features similar to MMP
	• DIF findings show IgA with or without IgM at BMZ whereas MMP shows C3, IgG, or IgA at BMZ
EBA	• Skin generally involved, whereas MMP less commonly involves skin
	• Clinical and histologic features similar to MMP
	• DIF findings similar to MMP with IgG and C3 at BMZ, but salt split testing can be useful to differentiate
LPP	• Generally younger than MMP patients
	• Areas of both lichenoid-appearing lesions along with bulla noted on clinical and microscopic examination whereas MMP does not show lichenoid areas
	• DIF findings similar to MMP with C3, IgG, and/or IgA at BMZ

Pitfalls
VESICULOBULLOUS SUBEPITHELIAL SEPARATION PATTERN OF ORAL MUCOSA

! Clinically may overlap with oral lichen planus (OLP) when presenting as desquamative gingivitis

! Biopsy is technically difficult due to separation of epithelium and may lead to inconclusive results on DIF testing due to loss of epithelium

! Histologic overlap of several types of subepithelial separation disorder is present necessitating DIF testing to determine diagnosis

---

SPONGIOTIC AND PSORIASIFORM REACTION PATTERNS

PYOSTOMATITIS VEGETANS

PyV is a painless oral mucosal condition often arising in association with underlying inflammatory bowel disease (IBD), most commonly ulcerative colitis. Although ulcerative colitis is considered within the autoimmune disease spectrum, the oral mucosal alterations of PyV are not presently considered an autoimmune disease. Extraintestinal manifestations (EIMs) of IBD affecting orocutaneous surfaces can be grouped by their associated etiopathology: specific EIMs exhibit similar or identical histopathology to the associated gastrointestinal disease (GID); reactive EIMs, such as PyV, lack histologic overlap with the GID and may arise when immune processes target similar antigens; and associated EIMs arise via mechanisms similar to the underlying GID, such as HLA commonalities. When PyV develops in the absence of a known diagnosis of IBD, the strength of the association between the oral/orocutaneous presentation and IBD is so compelling that formal evaluation for IBD is recommended.[38] In rare cases, PyV may develop years prior to definite confirmation of IBD.[40] PyV affects adults within the age range of 20 to 50 years, with a slight male predilection.[41] Lesions may be limited to the oral mucosa or in combination with *pyodermatitis vegetans*, the cutaneous counterpart characterized by exudative and vegetating plaques affecting intertriginous surfaces, the scalp, trunk, and extremities.[40,42] The combined presentation of skin and oral findings is termed, *pyodermatitis-PyV (PPV)*.

Gross/Clinical Features

Numerous pinpoint, painless, superficial yellow pustules appear on an edematous and erythematous oral mucosal surface.[43] Pustules are distributed along the gingiva, labial or buccal mucosa and palate, with sparing of the tongue and floor of mouth.[43,44] In some patients, the erythematous, edematous mucosa develops a thickened granular morphology leading to a folded, hyperplastic fissured appearance. Ulcerated confluent pustules can appear as superficial erosions or snail track ulcerations.[45] Involvement of both upper and lower lip vermillion imparts a striking clinical appearance.[39] Pyodermatitis vegetans presents as crusted, erythematous papulopustular eruptions that coalesce to form large vegetating asymmetric plaques. Ocular involvement or pyoblepharitis vegetans is uncommon and may present as vegetating plaques of the eyelids, blepharitis, and/or conjunctivitis.[39,46]

Microscopic Features

Microscopic examination of an oral mucosal biopsy exhibits thickening of the stratified squamous epithelium, including acanthosis, or hyperplasia.[39] In some patients, the epithelial surface changes may impart a subtle papillated silhouette at low magnification. ES, exocytosis of eosinophils and neutrophils, and/or intraepithelial abscess formation are identified.[43] Spongiotic changes contribute to the appearance of epithelial

dissociation or even focal acantholysis and mild suprabasilar clefting.[40] A moderately dense, mixed inflammatory infiltrate develops in the underlying connective tissue with eosinophils, neutrophils, plasma cells, and lymphocytes present (Fig. 8). Perivascular inflammation has been reported. In addition to intraepithelial abscess formation, subepithelial abscesses may form within the connective tissue papillae.[40,42]

Differential Diagnosis

Epithelial hyperplasia, spongiosis, and neutrophilic pustules may lead to diagnostic consideration of geographic tongue (GT) or, in extraglossal sites, ectopic GT. The conspicuous eosinophilic spongiosis and/or eosinophilic microabscess formation of PyV are atypical in GT and ectopic GT, most commonly a neutrophil-rich response (Fig. 9). Contact-, drug-, or medication-related spongiotic mucositis may occur, with or without eosinophils, and a search for flask-shaped Langerhans cell microabscess formation within the epithelium is a helpful finding and weighs against PyV (see Fig. 9A, B).[47] Separation of PyV from some forms of pemphigus, in particular, PV, pemphigus vegetans, and IgAP, may be problematic. By

Fig. 8. Histologic appearance of PyV. (*A*) Mild papillated surface silhouette (*arrows*) at low magnification (H&E, ×50). (*B*) ES, exocytosis of eosinophils (*arrows*) and neutrophils, and intraepithelial abscess formation are identified (H&E, ×200).

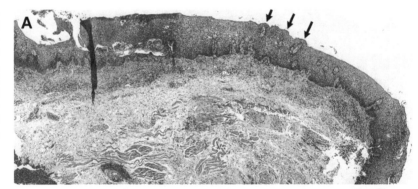
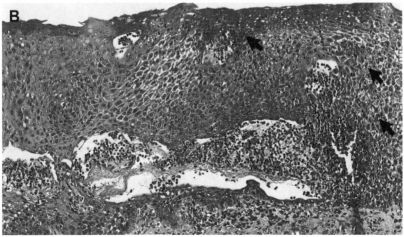

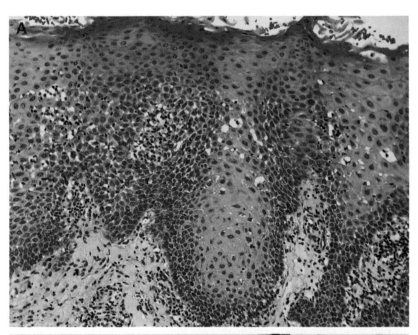

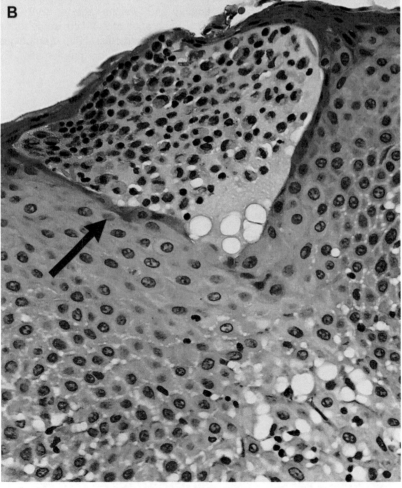

Fig. 9. Histologic appearance of contact/drug-related spongiotic mucositis. (*A*) Epithelial hyperplasia and spongiosis with intraepithelial and subepithelial inflammation (H&E, ×200). (*B*) Flask-shaped Langerhans cell microabscess formation within the epithelium (*arrow*) weighs against PyV (H&E, ×400).

light microscopic examination, PyV and early pemphigus share the feature of eosinophilic spongiosis, although identification of multiple or large intraepithelial eosinophilic abscesses supports PyV, particularly in an oral mucosal biopsy where eosinophil-rich variants of pemphigus, such as pemphigus vegetans, are decidedly uncommon. IgAP is a variant of pemphigus characterized by recurrent cutaneous lesions of the trunk, extremities, scalp, and intertriginous areas, sites similarly affected by PyV, although IgAP spares the mucous membranes.[48] Similar to PyV, IgAP exhibits epithelial acantholysis and extensive neutrophilic infiltration. IgAP demonstrates both intercellular epithelial tissue–bound IgA antibodies and circulating IgA antibodies.[40]

Diagnosis

Because some cases of mucocutaneous lesions of PyV exhibit overlap with vesiculobullous disease, immunofluorescence testing may be an appropriate recommendation. Negative immunofluorescence studies have long been regarded as the key to distinguishing PyV from pemphigus, but the strength of this assertion is tempered by a paucity of immunostudies in PyV.[38,39] In some cases, a positive IgG or IgA reaction has been identified in PyV similar to what is expected in PV and IgAP.[39,40,42] The DIF response in PyV is weak in comparison to the strong positive reaction of pemphigus, and the weak response in PyV is regarded as an aberrant finding related to epithelial damage and subsequent exposure of antigens.[40] Nonetheless, the presence of an intraepithelial and/or subepithelial reaction to IgG or IgA seems sufficient to suggest additional serologic testing be performed to exclude diagnostic considerations, such as PV, IgAP, or, in rare cases, LIGA.[42] In the setting of weak positive DIF results, low titers of circulating antibodies in an IIF study and/or discordant ELISA testing weigh against forms of pemphigus and favor PyV in the correct clinical setting.[40] One particularly instructive case involves the misdiagnosis of PPV as IgAP for 8 years due to an absence of correlative IBD history combined with positive IgA DIF studies, with IIF demonstrating very low circulating titers. Revision of the IgAP diagnosis to PPV was prompted after a diagnosis of ulcerative colitis later established on a repeat gastrointestinal examination.[40]

The association between PyV or PPV with an underlying GID is strong, and follow-up testing and gastrointestinal examination are recommended.[38–40] Abnormalities in serum laboratory values, such as peripheral eosinophilia, are not uncommon

in PyV.[38] Less frequently, laboratory values suggesting liver dysfunction have been reported in PyV, which may be related to abnormal liver biochemistry in underlying IBD.[38,49] When the appearance of PyV or lesions of PPV follows an established diagnosis of IBD or occurs in association with a flare of known IBD, the clinical diagnosis is most often supported by the histologic findings.[38,39] Tissue biopsy sampling for DIF, and/or serologic studies may still be appropriate in individual cases.

Prognosis

Once a diagnosis of PyV is established, the approach to treatment of the oral lesions may depend on control or alterations in management of the underlying IBD. Treatment of the bowel disease is often effective in curtailing most oral and skin lesions.[38] In the absence of IBD, topical therapy with topical CS can be successful in some cases, yet repeat mucosal, skin, and bowel evaluations may be a prudent approach to exclude an underlying or evolving GID. The mucosal lesions of PyV have no reported association with clinically significant hard or soft tissue destruction and are devoid of malignant potential.

GEOGRAPHIC TONGUE

GT is an immunologically mediated benign, chronic inflammatory oral condition involving tongue surface,[50] alternately designated as benign migratory glossitis given variation in distribution of disease at different time points. GT is a common condition and most often affects younger age groups, although any age can be affected.[51] Several different causes have been associated with GT, including autoimmune, hereditary, stress and/or anxiety, and allergic or atopic conditions. Psoriasis, a chronic inflammatory disease with an immunologic basis, is the most common systemic condition associated with GT. Although GT is more frequent with psoriasis,[50,52] a *specific* lesion of oral psoriasis is a matter of debate.[53] More recently, an increased prevalence of iron-deficiency anemia and celiac disease has been identified in patients with GT.[54] Most cases of GT are asymptomatic, with dysgeusia or mild burning reported in some cases.[51,55]

Gross/Clinical Features

GT is clinically characterized by the presence of variably sized demarcated annular, polycyclic, or irregular erythematous areas surrounded by a narrow, pale, yellow-white border along the tongue tip and dorsal and lateral margins of the oral tongue. Many times GT can be recognized by direct clinical examination alone, but a biopsy sample may be submitted under several circumstances: histologic confirmation, even with the clinical suspicion of GT; extraglossal lesions with clinical features of GT; deviation from the well-developed serpiginous yellow border (ie, erythematous lesions); and lesions that fail to resolve or demonstrate associated pain.

Microscopic Features

Microscopically, GT is characterized by an 'irregularly-irregular' or uneven epithelial hyperplasia of psoriasiform mucositis. Stratified squamous epithelium exhibits hyperparakeratosis, variable spongiosis, acanthosis with downward elongation and expansion of rete ridges, and basal layer hyperplasia. Thinning of the epithelium overlying the connective tissue (suprapapillary plates) is often present (Fig. 10A, B). Collections of neutrophils in the parakeratotic layer are termed, *Munro microabscesses*, and in some patients, spongiform pustules within the stratum spinosum can occur, similar to the spongiform pustules of Kogoj (Fig. 10C, D).[50] Spores and/or hyphal forms of Candida species are rarely present in the

superficial keratin layers. In samples obtained from the dorsal tongue, most filiform papillae are absent. Despite the repeated cycles of developing, healing and migratory lesions, GT is a non-scarring process and, in most cases, the underlying stroma shows only mild inflammation.

Differential Diagnosis

Oral mucosal lesions of secondary syphilis (SS) involving the oral tongue may demonstrate clinical and histologic overlap with GT. Similar to GT, SS may exhibit psoriasiform epithelial hyperplasia, spongiosis, and exocytosis of neutrophils (Fig. 11A).[56,57] The subjacent lamina propria is comparably more inflamed in SS, exhibiting a dense lichenoid patterned infiltrate composed of lymphocytes and plasma cells seen obscuring the epithelial-connective tissue junction. The stromal inflammation extends deeply into the connective tissue with conspicuous perivascular inflammation highlighting plump endothelial cells. In some patients, a perineural infiltrate may be present (Fig. 11B).[56,57] Although plasma cells are characteristic of SS,

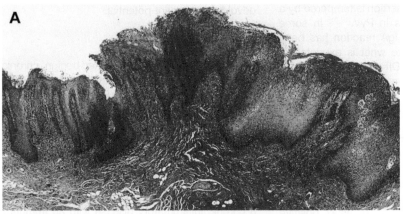

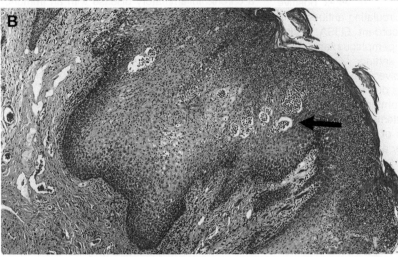

Fig. 10. Histologic appearance of GT. (*A*) Uneven epithelial hyperplasia of psoriasiform mucositis with mild stromal inflammation (H&E, ×20). (*B*) Stratified squamous epithelium exhibits hyperparakeratosis, variable spongiosis, acanthosis with downward elongation and expansion of rete ridges, and basal layer hyperplasia. Spongiform pustules within the stratum spinosum (*arrow*), similar to spongiform pustules of Kogoj (H&E, ×100).

Fig. 10. *(continued).* *(C)* Higher magnification of spongiform pustules *(arrows)* (H&E, ×200). *(D)* Collections of neutrophils in the parakeratotic layer are termed, Munro microabscesses *(arrow)* (H&E, ×300).

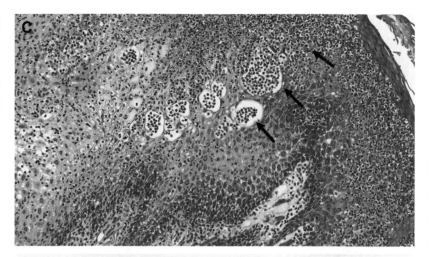

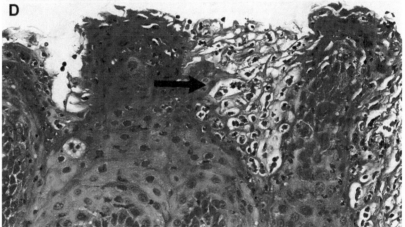

they are often nonspecific and should be correlated with other morphologic features.[56,58] Oral hyperplastic candidiasis may enter diagnostic consideration in the presence of neutrophils in the keratin layer and/or spongiform pustules. Although visible with light microscopy, Gomori methenamine silver (GMS) or periodic acid–Schiff (PAS) special staining facilitates a search for spores and hyphal forms colonizing the superficial keratin layer (**Fig. 12**). Identification of candida may represent an incidental finding, can correlate with an isolated lesion of hyperplastic candidiasis, or, when present in the midline dorsal tongue location, can represent median rhomboid glossitis (MRG). MRG is a solitary, clinically erythematous lesion often rhomboid in shape, centered along the midline of the tongue, and devoid of a yellow serpiginous border. The lesion is not migratory and generally resolves with antifungal treatment. Psoriasiform hyperplasia with Munro-type microabscess formation is occasionally reported in allergic contact-type reactions and may be indistinguishable from GT, necessitating clinical correlation.[59]

Diagnosis

Biopsy sampling can confirm the presence of psoriasiform mucositis, supportive of GT in the correct clinical context. Even in cases lacking clinical evidence of the yellow circinate border, most or all microscopic findings are present histologically, and, at minimum, the biopsy material is sufficient to exclude a clinical query of squamous dysplasia. Ancillary testing, such as GMS, PAS, or IHC staining for the presence of spirochetes, such as *Treponema pallidum*, can be useful in the diagnostic work-up for some cases. *Treponema pallidum* is most likely found

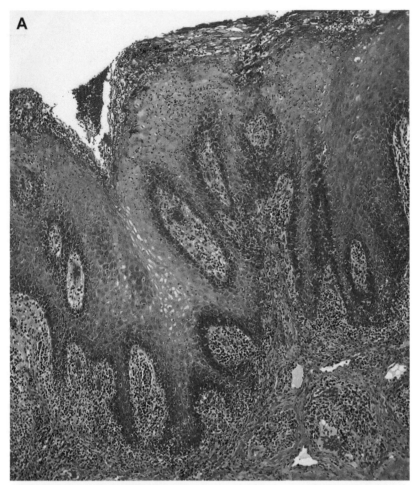

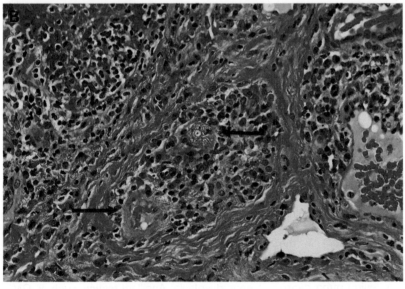

Fig. 11. Histologic appearance of SS along lateral oral tongue. (*A*) Psoriasiform epithelial hyperplasia, spongiosis, and exocytosis of neutrophils and inflamed subjacent lamina propria (H&E, ×70). (*B*) Stromal inflammation extends deeply into the connective tissue with perineural (*top arrow*) and perivascular inflammation (*bottom arrow*) (H&E, ×400).

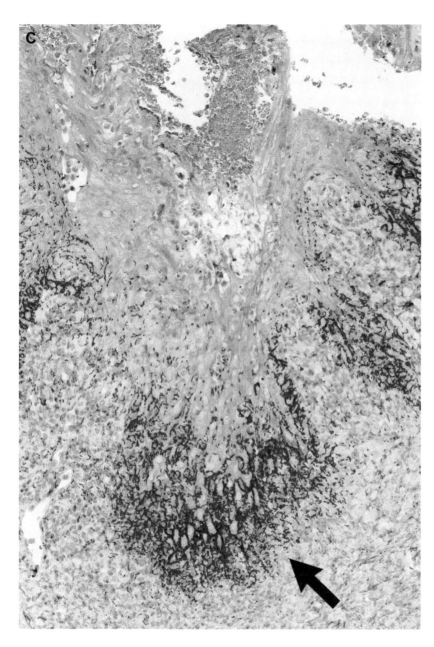

Fig. 11. (continued). (C) IHC stain (*red chromogen*) highlighting spirochetes within the epithelium and subjacent connective tissue (*arrow*) (×250).

within the epithelial areas exhibiting exocytosis (Fig. 11C), but organisms may be present within connective tissue.[57] A positive IHC reaction with a spirochete stain should be followed by serologic confirmation of syphilis. The spirochetal immunostain is not specific for *Treponema pallidum*, and the oral cavity environment may host numerous spirochetal organisms.

Prognosis

GT is a benign chronic condition and lesions can be expected to wax and wane, with periods of relative activity. GT is associated with a good prognosis and, once the lesions have clinically resolved in the affected site, there is no scar formation or lasting local sequelae, because this represents a superficially located process. GT is a common condition and at present, there are no defined clinical criteria or thresholds to guide clinicians regarding testing for associated conditions, such as allergies, anemia, psoriasis, celiac disease, and or nutritional disorder.[54]

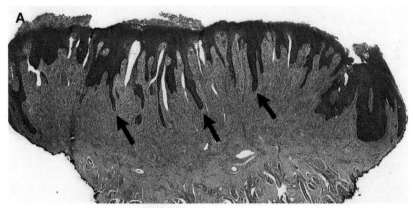

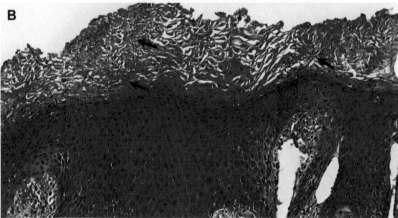

Fig. 12. Histologic appearance of MRG. (*A*) Pseudoepitheliomatous hyperplasia (*arrows*) of surface epithelium with brisk stromal inflammatory response (H&E, ×20). (*B*) Hyphae of Candida species within the superficial keratin layers (*arrows*) (H&E, ×200).

Pathologic Key Features
SPONGIOTIC AND PSORIASIFORM REACTION PATTERNS IN ORAL MUCOSA

Pyostomatitis vegetans
- Acanthosis, spongiosis, epithelial hyperplasia
- Eosinophilic exocytosis or spongiosis
- Connective tissue inflamed, neutrophils and eosinophils dominate

Geographic tongue
- Psoriasiform epithelial hyperplasia
- Thinning of suprapapillary epithelial plates
- Neutrophilic microabscesses within the keratin layer (Munro microabscess)
- Neutrophilic spongiosis within epithelium (spongiform pustules of Kogoj)
- Connective tissue relatively uninflamed

LICHENOID REACTION PATTERN

ORAL LICHEN PLANUS

OLP affects 0.5% to 2% of the adult population.[60] Adults are most commonly affected, with a female predilection. Definitive etiopathology is unknown but speculated to be related to immune dysregulation.[61] Establishing a diagnosis of OLP can be challenging because the histopathologic features are not specific,[61] and, although clinicopathologic correlation is regarded as essential to the diagnosis of OLP, the criteria can be difficult to definitively apply (**Box 1**).[61,62] Lichenoid lesions that fail to fulfill criteria of OLP are often associated with other clinically classifiable entities, but some remain without a more specific diagnosis. Cases associated with use of systemic medication are termed, *oral lichenoid drug reactions*, whereas local contact hypersensitivity reactions, such as amalgam restorations, *are oral lichenoid contact hypersensivity*

Differential Diagnosis
SPONGIOTIC AND PSORIASIFORM REACTION PATTERNS IN ORAL MUCOSA

Differential Diagnosis of Pyostomatitis Vegetans

	Distinguishing Features
GT	• Clinically favors dorsal tongue unlike PyV
	• Psoriasiform and spongiotic, neutrophils dominant, rare eosinophils
	• Connective tissue uninflamed
Drug or medication	• Any oral mucosa surface possible
	• Scattered eosinophils in stroma, unlikely microabscess formation
	• Connective tissue inflamed, perivasculitis possible
PV	• Acantholysis, basal layer tombstoning, villous silhouette
	• DIF with intracellular reaction to IgG and/or C3
	• IIF and/or ELISA-positive for IgG or C3
IgAP	• Oral mucosal lesions uncommon
	• Acantholysis, with neutrophilic infiltration
	• DIF with intracellular reaction to IgA
	• IIF and/or ELISA-positive for IgA
SS	• Psoriasiform hyperplasia
	• Neutrophils in keratin layer with microabscess possible
	• Connective tissue inflamed, blurring epitheilial/connective tissue interface
	• Perivascular and perineural inflammation
MRG	• Pseudoepitheliomatous hyperplasia with tapered rete ridge formation
	• Connective tissue inflamed
	• Yeast spores or hyphal forms in keratin layer
	• Neutrophils in keratin layer

Pitfalls
SPONGIOTIC AND PSORIASIFORM REACTION PATTERNS IN ORAL MUCOSA

! Spongiotic and psoriasiform reaction patterns are more nonspecific than vesiculobullous reaction patterns, necessitating additional clinical correlation.

! Spongiotic and psoriasiform reaction patterns exhibit histologic overlap with each other and occur in association with inflammatory, infectious, and autoimmune mediated diseases.

! DIF and IIF or immunoassays are supportive for autoimmune disease and distinguishing from microscopic mimics.

reactions.[61] Collectively, this group is referred to as *oral lichenoid lesions (OLLs)* for purposes of this discussion. Graft-versus-host disease (GVHD) represents another clinical and histologic mimic of OLP occurring in patients with a history of transplantation.[63] Lupus erythematosus (LE) and erythema multiforme (EM) may result in oral lesions with remarkable similarity to OLP. Chronic ulcerative stomatitis (CUS) is an autoimmune mucosal disease that may be clinically and histologically indistinguishable from OLP but through the use of DIF testing results, a specific diagnosis can be established.[64]

Gross Features

OLP appears clinically as striated white lesions (reticular variant) with or without erythematous

---

Box 1
Modified World Health Organization (2003) criteria for the diagnosis of oral lichen planus/oral lichenoid lesions

Clinical criteria[a]

Presence of bilateral, mostly symmetric lesions

Presence of lacelike network of slightly raised gray-white lines (reticular pattern)

Erosive, atrophic, bullous, and plaque-type lesions (accepted as a subtype only in presence of reticular lesions elsewhere in the oral mucosa)

Histopathologic criteria[b]

Presence of well-defined bandlike zone of cellular infiltration confined to the superficial part of the connective tissue, consisting mainly of lymphocytes

Signs of liquefaction degeneration in the basal cell layer

Absence of epithelial dysplasia

Final diagnosis of OLP or OLL

To arrive at a final diagnosis, the clinical and histopathologic criteria should be included.

A diagnosis of OLP requires the fulfillment of both clinical and histopathologic criteria.

The term OLL is used under the following conditions:

1. Clinically typical of OLP but histopathologically only compatible with OLP

2. Histopathologically typical of OLP but clinically only compatible with OLP

3. Clinically compatible with OLP and histopathologically compatible with OLP.

[a] In all other lesions that resemble OLP but that do not complete the clinical criteria, the phrase, *clinically compatible with*, should be used.
[b] When the histopathologic features are less obvious, the phrase, *histopathologically compatible with*, should be used.

Data from van der Meij EH, van der Waal I. Lack of clinicopathologic correlation in the diagnosis of oral lichen planus based on the presently available diagnostic criteria and suggestions for modifications. J Oral Pathol Med 2003;32(9):507–12.

---

atrophy or painful ulceration (erosive/ulcerative variant).[62] Other variants less commonly seen are plaque-like, papular, and rarely bullous.[60] Patients may be affected with oral cavity lesions only (estimated at 25% of cases), skin lesions only (35%), or both skin and oral lesions (40%).[65] In 20% to 25% of female patients with OLP, vaginal tissues may also be affected.[65] Changes to the nails may also be seen in affected patients.[65] OLP is most often present in a bilateral and symmetric distribution, favoring areas of the oral mucosa, which are susceptible to trauma, such as the buccal mucosa and lateral tongue along the occlusal plane.[61] Involvement of the gingiva is not uncommon and may present as desquamative gingivitis, a nonspecific clinical term describing atrophic erythematous gingival tissues with clinically observed or reported sloughing of the involved area. CUS is similar if not clinically identical to OLP; however, CUS is unresponsive to topical steroid therapy, unlike

OLP.[61] Oral GVHD can develop in patients with a history of hematopoietic stem cell transplant, and these lesions may be clinically indistinguishable from OLP.[66] LE involves cutaneous sites and may be combined with systemic organ involvement, with only occasional oral involvement, but the latter is similar in appearance to OLP.[67] OLLs are more often unilateral and localized in presentation and arise without any accompanying skin lesions.[62] EM may be a sudden-onset response to a medication, viral, or unknown agent and may commonly affect the oral cavity, often affecting a younger age group than classic OLP.[68]

Microscopic Features

On light microscopy, the lichenoid patterned reaction includes liquefactive degeneration of cells in the basal layer of epithelium; the formation of eosinophilic globular bodies in the epithelium, termed *cytoid bodies*, *colloid bodies*, or *Civatte bodies*; sawtooth rete ridge formation; a bandlike infiltration of lymphocytes in the superficial lamina propria immediately adjacent to the BMZ; and hyperkeratosis (**Fig. 13**A).[60–62] Ulceration may or may not be present, and the architectural and cytomorphologic criteria of squamous epithelial dysplasia should be absent.[69]

Differential Diagnosis

In general, there are no reliable histologic features to differentiate OLP from other entities such as OLLs, GVHD, LE, CUS, EM, and PNP, known to exhibit a lichenoid reaction pattern based on light microscopy alone.[68] OLL cases have also been reported to show a more diffuse and mixed chronic inflammatory infiltrate, with plasma cells mixed with eosinophils and lymphocytes and an increase in the number of cytoid/colloid/Civatte bodies, but these features are not definitive diagnostic findings.[61,68] Differentiation of OLP from OLL may not be possible on a histologic basis, but a temporal association with medication use, proximal location close to a restoration, or the incomplete presence of clinical or histologic criteria of OLP favors OLL.[62] Some cases of GVHD, OLLs, and LE exhibit a perivascular inflammatory infiltrate, although this is a nonspecific finding (**Fig. 14**).[65] To distinguish OLP from CUS, the most reliable mechanism is the pattern of DIF results (discussed later). In some instances, squamous epithelial dysplasia may exhibit a lichenoid patterned

Fig. 13. Histologic appearance of OLP. (*A*) Interface vacuolar change (*arrow*); eosinophilic globular bodies in the epithelium, termed cytoid/colloid/Civatte bodies; and bandlike infiltration of lymphocytes in the superficial lamina propria immediately adjacent to the BMZ (×200, H&E stain). (*B*) DIF demonstrates deposition of fibrinogen at the BMZ of OLP lesion (×200). (*Courtesy of* [*B*] University of Florida Oral Pathology Image Archive, Gaineville, FL; with permission.)

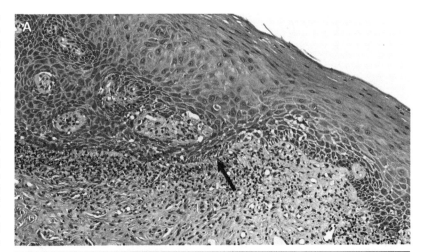
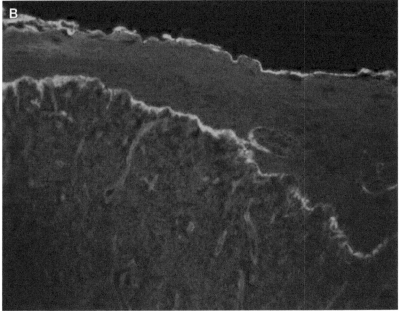

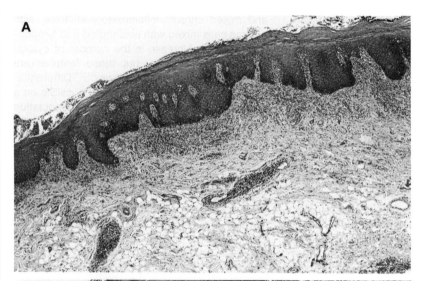

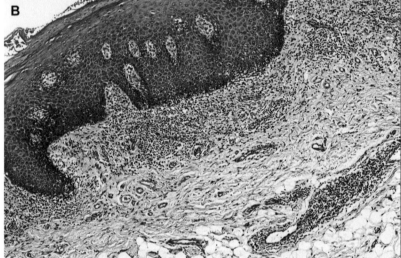

Fig. 14. Histologic appearance of an oral mucosal lichenoid lesion. (*A, B*) Squamous epithelium exhibiting surface keratosis, vacuolar interface change, and a perivascular inflammatory infiltrate (H&E, ×100 and H&E, ×200, respectively).

inflammatory response and may enter diagnostic consideration. Although originally termed *lichenoid dysplasia*, the use of this terminology is discouraged to avoid confusion.[70] The presence of architectural and/or cytologic atypia argues against OLP, even in the presence of a strikingly similar subepithelial bandlike chronic inflammatory infiltrate.[71] DIF is not helpful in differentiating true OLP from squamous dysplasia with a lichenoid patterned inflammatory infiltrate, because dysplastic lesions can exhibit fibrinogen positivity on DIF.[72] In rare cases of PNP, the lichenoid reaction pattern may be the dominant finding, without any evidence of acantholysis. Although the presence of dyskeratosis may represent a subtle clue, this finding may be interpreted as

cytoid body formation; therefore, correlation with immunopathologic, serologic results and clinical history (discussed previously) is essential.[15,19]

Diagnosis

DIF testing to secure the specific diagnosis of OLP is not regarded as essential, and the benefit of DIF is in excluding other histologically similar entities within the differential diagnosis.[60,61] The expected DIF pattern for classic OLP includes the deposition of fibrinogen at the BMZ and occasional deposition of IgM in the cytoid/Civatte/colloid bodies (**Fig. 13**B).[60] The sensitivity of DIF testing for the diagnosis of OLP ranges between 48% and 66%.[73-75] Unfortunately, OLLs and GVHD lesions may show similar results to OLP on DIF testing. Testing of DIF on CUS lesions, however, generally shows speckled intranuclear IgG positivity in the basilar and para basilar areas (**Fig. 15A**).[61,64] Deposits of IgG, IgM, or C3 along the BMZ often in a shaggy pattern are characteristic of LE (**Fig. 15B**).[35] EM is generally nonspecific on DIF testing but may show IgM, C3, or fibrinogen deposition at the BMZ or in a perivascular pattern.[68] The final diagnosis of OLP and/or related lichenoid patterned diseases uses analysis of medical history, clinical history of lesions, clinical appearance, light microscopy histology, and, in many cases, immunofluorescence testing. Diagnostic criteria for OLP was established by the World Health Organization in 1978 and modified in 2003.[62,76]

Prognosis

Unlike cutaneous LP, OLP lesions tend to be longstanding in duration, often persisting over 20 years.[65] Many patients present with asymptomatic lesions, which do not require treatment

Fig. 15. DIF patterns in the differential diagnosis of OLP. (*A*) CUS demonstrates speckled intranuclear IgG positivity in the basal and parabasal layers (×200). (*B*) Deposits of IgM along the BMZ often in a shaggy pattern is characteristic of LE (×200). (*Courtesy of* University of Florida Oral Pathology Image Archive, Gaineville, FL; with permission.)

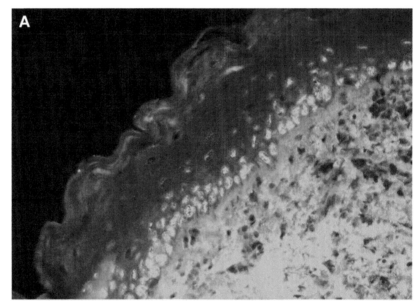

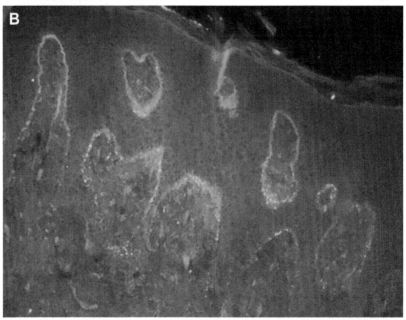

but do merit regular follow-up to monitor appearance and progression of lesions. For patients who have symptomatic erosive or ulcerated forms of OLP, topical steroids are the first-choice therapy, ranging from moderate (such as triamcinolone) to potent strengths (such as clobetasol), either in ointment form for localized lesions or suspension for diffuse involvement.[60] Topical steroid therapy generally shows minimal systemic absorption but may lead to side effects, such as secondary oral candida infection and mucosal atrophy.[60] Other treatment options

---

Pathologic Key Features
LICHENOID REACTION PATTERN

- Chronic disease with clinical presentation showing unilateral or bilateral white striated lesions with or without mucosal atrophy, erythema, and ulceration. Bilateral and symmetric lesions may be more supportive of a diagnosis of OLP, whereas isolated or unilateral lesions may be more suggestive of OLLs. A temporal relationship with medication use or close proximity to dental restoration may be indicative of OLLs.

- Histologic features include subepithelial bandlike chronic inflammatory infiltrate in the superficial lamina propria, degeneration of the basal layer of epithelium, presence of Civatte/colloid/cytoid bodies, and sawtooth rete ridges. Epithelial dysplasia should not be present.

- If DIF testing is performed, fibrinogen deposition along the basement membrane zone supports a diagnosis of OLP/OLL.

ΔΔ

Differential Diagnosis
LICHENOID REACTION PATTERN

	Distinguishing Features
OLL	• Often asymmetric clinical presentation
	• May be associated with local dental material (contact) or systemic medication
	• May be histologically indistinguishable
CUS	• Clinically and histologically indistinguishable
	• CUS may not respond to topical steroids whereas OLP generally is responsive.
	• DIF findings in CUS show perinuclear IgG in basal/suprabasilar layers whereas OLP shows fibrinogen positivity at BMZ.
GVHD	• Clinically and histologically indistinguishable, although perivascular infiltrate may be present on GVHD H&E biopsies.
	• History of allogenic stem cell transplant
LE	• LE patients younger than OLP patients
	• Skin lesions present in most cases, oral lesions rare
	• Systemic involvement may be present.
	• Perivascular inflammation may be present on H&E biopsy.
	• DIF findings in LE show IgG, IgM, or C3 deposition at the BMZ whereas OLP shows fibrinogen positivity at BMZ.
EM	• Abrupt onset of symptoms
	• Skin lesions present in most cases
	• DIF findings in EM are nonspecific but may show IgM, C3, or fibrinogen at the BMZ or in a perivascular pattern whereas OLP shows fibrinogen positivity at BMZ.

include systemic corticosteroids in cases of widespread involvement or lesions failing to resolve with topical therapy or calcineurin inhibitors, such as cyclosporine, tacrolimus, or pimecrolimus.[77] The potential for transformation of OLP to oral squamous cell carcinoma (OSCC) has been a long-standing controversy and the risk is estimated to range between 0% and 3.5%.[61,78] Difficulties in classification between OLP and OLL and exclusion of epithelial dysplasia with lichenoid patterned inflammation have made calculation of the exact risk unclear. Patients with oral GVHD lesions may be at an increased risk of the development of OSCC, likely in relation to immunosuppression.[65] With these considerations, OLP patients are recommended to be re-evaluated every 2 to 12 months depending on stability of disease to monitor for clinical alterations.[60]

(!) Pitfalls
LICHENOID REACTION PATTERN

! Oral dysplastic lesions may mimic lichenoid disease clinically and histologically; therefore, architectural and cytomorphologic alterations of dysplasia must be excluded to suggest OLP/OLL.

! Lesions confined to the gingiva may lack characteristic features and present similarly to vesiculobullous disease, such as MMP; therefore, DIF testing may be required for diagnosis.

! Careful clinical and medical history and presence of skin involvement should be evaluated to exclude GVHD, LE, and EM.

! CUS may present clinically and histologically identical to OLP and must be differentiated by DIF testing.

REFERENCES

1. Ghanadan A, Saghazadeh A, Daneshpazhooh M, et al. Direct immunofluorescence for immunobullous and other skin diseases. Expert Rev Clin Immunol 2015;11(5):589–96.
2. Elston DM, Stratman EJ, Miller SJ. Skin biopsy: biopsy issues in specific diseases. J Am Acad Dermatol 2016;74(1):1–16, [quiz: 17–8].
3. Pohla-Gubo G, Hintner H. Direct and indirect immunofluorescence for the diagnosis of bullous autoimmune diseases. Dermatol Clin 2011;29(3):365–72, vii.
4. McMillan R, Taylor J, Shephard M, et al. World Workshop on Oral Medicine VI: a systematic review of the treatment of mucocutaneous pemphigus vulgaris. Oral Surg Oral Med Oral Pathol Oral Radiol 2015;120(2):132–42.e1.
5. Svecova D. Pemphigus vulgaris: a clinical study of 44 cases over a 20-year period. Int J Dermatol 2015;54(10):1138–44.
6. Beutner EH, Jordon RE. Demonstration of skin antibodies in sera of pemphigus vulgaris patients by indirect immunofluorescent staining. Proc Soc Exp Biol Med 1964;117:505–10.
7. Ruocco V, Ruocco E, Lo Schiavo A, et al. Pemphigus: etiology, pathogenesis, and inducing or triggering factors: facts and controversies. Clin Dermatol 2013;31(4):374–81.
8. Yong AA, Tey HL. Paraneoplastic pemphigus. Australas J Dermatol 2013;54(4):241–50.
9. Anhalt GJ, Kim SC, Stanley JR, et al. Paraneoplastic pemphigus. An autoimmune mucocutaneous disease associated with neoplasia. N Engl J Med 1990;323(25):1729–35.
10. Ohzono A, Sogame R, Li X, et al. Clinical and immunological findings in 104 cases of paraneoplastic pemphigus. Br J Dermatol 2015;173(6):1447–52.
11. Frew JW, Murrell DF. Paraneoplastic pemphigus (paraneoplastic autoimmune multiorgan syndrome): clinical presentations and pathogenesis. Dermatol Clin 2011;29(3):419–25, viii.
12. Hertl M, Jedlickova H, Karpati S, et al. Pemphigus. S2 guideline for diagnosis and treatment–guided by the European Dermatology Forum (EDF) in cooperation with the European Academy of Dermatology and Venereology (EADV). J Eur Acad Dermatol Venereol 2015;29(3):405–14.
13. Leger S, Picard D, Ingen-Housz-Oro S, et al. Prognostic factors of paraneoplastic pemphigus. Arch Dermatol 2012;148(10):1165–72.
14. Poot AM, Diercks GF, Kramer D, et al. Laboratory diagnosis of paraneoplastic pemphigus. Br J Dermatol 2013;169(5):1016–24.
15. Zimmermann J, Bahmer F, Rose C, et al. Clinical and immunopathological spectrum of paraneoplastic pemphigus. J Dtsch Dermatol Ges 2010;8(8):598–606.
16. Poot AM, Siland J, Jonkman MF, et al. Direct and indirect immunofluorescence staining patterns in the diagnosis of paraneoplastic pemphigus. Br J Dermatol 2016;174(4):912–5.
17. Joly P, Richard C, Gilbert D, et al. Sensitivity and specificity of clinical, histologic, and immunologic features in the diagnosis of paraneoplastic pemphigus. J Am Acad Dermatol 2000;43(4):619–26.
18. Santoro FA, Stoopler ET, Werth VP. Pemphigus. Dent Clin North Am 2013;57(4):597–610.

19. Nguyen VT, Ndoye A, Bassler KD, et al. Classification, clinical manifestations, and immunopathological mechanisms of the epithelial variant of paraneoplastic autoimmune multiorgan syndrome: a reappraisal of paraneoplastic pemphigus. Arch Dermatol 2001;137(2):193–206.

20. Gallo E, Garcia-Martin P, Fraga J, et al. Paraneoplastic pemphigus with eosinophilic spongiosis and autoantibodies against desmocollins 2 and 3. Clin Exp Dermatol 2014;39(3):323–6.

21. Bunn B, Hunter K, Khurram SA, et al. Adenoid dysplasia of the oral mucosa. Oral Surg Oral Med Oral Pathol Oral Radiol 2014;118(5):586–92.

22. Weir JC, Weathers DR. A fixation artifact simulating acantholytic disease. Oral Surg Oral Med Oral Pathol 1976;41(1):105–8.

23. Joly P, Litrowski N. Pemphigus group (vulgaris, vegetans, foliaceus, herpetiformis, brasiliensis). Clin Dermatol 2011;29(4):432–6.

24. Abe T, Maruyama S, Babkair H, et al. Simultaneous immunolocalization of desmoglein 3 and IgG4 in oral pemphigus vulgaris: IgG4 predominant autoantibodies in its pathogenesis. J Oral Pathol Med 2015;44(10):850–6.

25. Powell JG, Grover RK, Plunkett RW, et al. Evaluation of a newly available ELISA for envoplakin autoantibodies for the diagnosis of paraneoplastic pemphigus. J Drugs Dermatol 2015;14(10):1103–6.

26. Ellebrecht CT, Bhoj VG, Nace A, et al. Reengineering chimeric antigen receptor T cells for targeted therapy of autoimmune disease. Science 2016;353(6295):179–84.

27. Zhang J, Qiao QL, Chen XX, et al. Improved outcomes after complete resection of underlying tumors for patients with paraneoplastic pemphigus: a single-center experience of 22 cases. J Cancer Res Clin Oncol 2011;137(2):229–34.

28. Sultan A, Stojanov IJ, Lerman MA, et al. Oral lichen planus pemphigoides: a series of four cases. Oral Surg Oral Med Oral Pathol Oral Radiol 2015;120(1):58–68.

29. Chan LS. Ocular and oral mucous membrane pemphigoid (cicatricial pemphigoid). Clin Dermatol 2012;30(1):34–7.

30. Iranzo P, Herrero-Gonzalez JE, Mascaro-Galy JM, et al. Epidermolysis bullosa acquisita: a retrospective analysis of 12 patients evaluated in four tertiary hospitals in Spain. Br J Dermatol 2014;171(5):1022–30.

31. Eguia del Valle A, Aguirre Urizar JM, Martinez Sahuquillo A. Oral manifestations caused by the linear IgA disease. Med Oral 2004;9(1):39–44.

32. Chan LS, Ahmed AR, Anhalt GJ, et al. The first international consensus on mucous membrane pemphigoid: definition, diagnostic criteria, pathogenic factors, medical treatment, and prognostic indicators. Arch Dermatol 2002;138(3):370–9.

33. Bindhu P, Krishnapillai R, Thomas P, et al. Facts in artifacts. J Oral Maxillofac Pathol 2013;17(3):397–401.

34. Beguerie JR, Gonzalez S. Angina bullosa hemorrhagica: report of 11 cases. Dermatol Reports 2014;6(1):5282.

35. Rastogi V, Sharma R, Misra SR, et al. Diagnostic procedures for autoimmune vesiculobullous diseases: a review. J Oral Maxillofac Pathol 2014;18(3):390–7.

36. Shipman AR, Reddy H, Wojnarowska F. Association between the subepidermal autoimmune blistering diseases linear IgA disease and the pemphigoid group and inflammatory bowel disease: two case reports and literature review. Clin Exp Dermatol 2012;37(5):461–8.

37. Watchorn RE, Ma S, Gulmann C, et al. Linear IgA disease associated with ulcerative colitis: the role of surgery. Clin Exp Dermatol 2014;39(3):327–9.

38. Hegarty AM, Barrett AW, Scully C. Pyostomatitis vegetans. Clin Exp Dermatol 2004;29(1):1–7.

39. Wang H, Qiao S, Zhang X, et al. A case of pyodermatitis-pyostomatitis vegetans. Am J Med Sci 2013;345(2):168–71.

40. Abellaneda C, Mascaro JM Jr, Vazquez MG, et al. All that glitters is not pemphigus: pyodermatitis-pyostomatitis vegetans misdiagnosed as IgA pemphigus for 8 years. Am J Dermatopathol 2011;33(1):e1–6.

41. Hansen LS, Silverman S Jr, Daniels TE. The differential diagnosis of pyostomatitis vegetans and its relation to bowel disease. Oral Surg Oral Med Oral Pathol 1983;55(4):363–73.

42. Wolz MM, Camilleri MJ, McEvoy MT, et al. Pemphigus vegetans variant of IgA pemphigus, a variant of IgA pemphigus and other autoimmune blistering disorders. Am J Dermatopathol 2013;35(3):e53–6.

43. Neville BW, Smith SE, Maize JC, et al. Pyostomatitis vegetans. Am J Dermatopathol 1985;7(1):69–77.

44. Nico MM, Hussein TP, Aoki V, et al. Pyostomatitis vegetans and its relation to inflammatory bowel disease, pyoderma gangrenosum, pyodermatitis vegetans, and pemphigus. J Oral Pathol Med 2012;41(8):584–8.

45. Femiano F, Lanza A, Buonaiuto C, et al. Pyostomatitis vegetans: a review of the literature. Med Oral Patol Oral Cir Bucal 2009;14(3):E114–7.

46. Dupuis EC, Haber RM, Robertson LH. Pyoblepharitis vegetans in association with pyodermatitis-pyostomatitis vegetans: expanding the spectrum of a rare, multisystem disorder. J Cutan Med Surg 2016;20(2):163–5.

47. Rosa G, Fernandez AP, Vij A, et al. Langerhans cell collections, but not eosinophils, are clues to a diagnosis of allergic contact dermatitis in appropriate skin biopsies. J Cutan Pathol 2016; 43(6):498–504.

48. Porro AM, Caetano Lde V, Maehara Lde S, et al. Non-classical forms of pemphigus: pemphigus herpetiformis, IgA pemphigus, paraneoplastic pemphigus and IgG/IgA pemphigus. An Bras Dermatol 2014;89(1): 96–106.

49. Valentino PL, Feldman BM, Walters TD, et al. Abnormal liver biochemistry is common in pediatric inflammatory bowel disease: prevalence and associations. Inflamm Bowel Dis 2015;21(12): 2848–56.

50. Picciani BL, Domingos TA, Teixeira-Souza T, et al. Geographic tongue and psoriasis: clinical, histopathological, immunohistochemical and genetic correlation - a literature review. An Bras Dermatol 2016;91(4):410–21.

51. Miloglu O, Goregen M, Akgul HM, et al. The prevalence and risk factors associated with benign migratory glossitis lesions in 7619 Turkish dental outpatients. Oral Surg Oral Med Oral Pathol Oral Radiol Endod 2009;107(2):e29–33.

52. Yesudian PD, Chalmers RJ, Warren RB, et al. In search of oral psoriasis. Arch Dermatol Res 2012; 304(1):1–5.

53. Fatahzadeh M, Schwartz RA. Oral psoriasis: an overlooked enigma. Dermatology 2016;232(3): 319–25.

54. Cigic L, Galic T, Kero D, et al. The prevalence of celiac disease in patients with geographic tongue. J Oral Pathol Med 2016;45(10):791–6.

55. Gavrilovic IT, Balagula Y, Rosen AC, et al. Characteristics of oral mucosal events related to bevacizumab treatment. Oncologist 2012;17(2): 274–8.

56. Ficarra G, Carlos R. Syphilis: the renaissance of an old disease with oral implications. Head Neck Pathol 2009;3(3):195–206.

57. Siqueira CS, Saturno JL, de Sousa SC, et al. Diagnostic approaches in unsuspected oral lesions of syphilis. Int J Oral Maxillofac Surg 2014;43(12): 1436–40.

58. Barrett AW, Villarroel Dorrego M, Hodgson TA, et al. The histopathology of syphilis of the oral mucosa. J Oral Pathol Med 2004;33(5): 286–91.

59. Allen CM, Blozis GG. Oral mucosal reactions to cinnamon-flavored chewing gum. J Am Dent Assoc 1988;116(6):664–7.

60. Alrashdan MS, Cirillo N, McCullough M. Oral lichen planus: a literature review and update. Arch Dermatol Res 2016;308(8):539–51.

61. Cheng YS, Gould A, Kurago Z, et al. Diagnosis of oral lichen planus: a position paper of the American Academy of Oral and Maxillofacial Pathology. Oral Surg Oral Med Oral Pathol Oral Radiol 2016; 122(3):332–54.

62. van der Meij EH, van der Waal I. Lack of clinicopathologic correlation in the diagnosis of oral lichen planus based on the presently available diagnostic criteria and suggestions for modifications. J Oral Pathol Med 2003;32(9): 507–12.

63. Hull K, Kerridge I, Avery S, et al. Oral chronic graft-versus-host disease in Australia: clinical features and challenges in management. Intern Med J 2015;45(7):702–10.

64. Qari H, Villasante C, Richert J, et al. The diagnostic challenges of separating chronic ulcerative stomatitis from oral lichen planus. Oral Surg Oral Med Oral Pathol Oral Radiol 2015;120(5): 622–7.

65. Dudhia BB, Dudhia SB, Patel PS, et al. Oral lichen planus to oral lichenoid lesions: Evolution or revolution. J Oral Maxillofac Pathol 2015; 19(3):364–70.

66. Mays JW, Fassil H, Edwards DA, et al. Oral chronic graft-versus-host disease: current pathogenesis, therapy, and research. Oral Dis 2013; 19(4):327–46.

67. Mays JW, Sarmadi M, Moutsopoulos NM. Oral manifestations of systemic autoimmune and inflammatory diseases: diagnosis and clinical management. J Evid Based Dental Pract 2012;12(3 Suppl): 265–82.

68. Scully C, Bagan J. Oral mucosal diseases: erythema multiforme. Br J Oral Maxillofac Surg 2008;46(2): 90–5.

69. van der Meij EH, Schepman KP, van der Waal I. The possible premalignant character of oral lichen planus and oral lichenoid lesions: a prospective study. Oral Surg Oral Med Oral Pathol Oral Radiol Endod 2003;96(2):164–71.

70. Krutchkoff DJ, Eisenberg E. Lichenoid dysplasia: a distinct histopathologic entity. Oral Surg Oral Med Oral Pathol 1985;60(3):308–15.

71. Fitzpatrick SG, Honda KS, Sattar A, et al. Histologic lichenoid features in oral dysplasia and squamous cell carcinoma. Oral Surg Oral Med Oral Pathol Oral Radiol 2014;117(4):511–20.

72. Montague LJ, Bhattacharyya I, Islam MN, et al. Direct immunofluorescence testing results in cases of premalignant and malignant oral lesions. Oral Surg Oral Med Oral Pathol Oral Radiol 2015; 119(6):675–83.

73. Helander SD, Rogers RS 3rd. The sensitivity and specificity of direct immunofluorescence testing in disorders of mucous membranes. J Am Acad Dermatol 1994;30(1):65–75.

74. Sano SM, Quarracino MC, Aguas SC, et al. Sensitivity of direct immunofluorescence in oral diseases.

Study of 125 cases. Med Oral Patol Oral Cir Bucal 2008;13(5):E287–91.

75. Rogers RS 3rd, Van Hale HM. Immunopathologic diagnosis of oral mucosal inflammatory diseases. Australas J Dermatol 1986;27(2):51–7.

76. Rad M, Hashemipoor MA, Mojtahedi A, et al. Correlation between clinical and histopathologic diagnoses of oral lichen planus based on modified WHO diagnostic criteria. Oral Surg Oral Med Oral Pathol Oral Radiol Endod 2009;107(6): 796–800.

77. Suresh SS, Chokshi K, Desai S, et al. Medical management of oral lichen planus: a systematic review. J Clin Diagn Res 2016;10(2):ZE10–5.

78. Fitzpatrick SG, Hirsch SA, Gordon SC. The malignant transformation of oral lichen planus and oral lichenoid lesions: a systematic review. J Am Dent Assoc 2014;145(1):45–56.

Glandular Neoplasia of the Sinonasal Tract

Edward B. Stelow, MD*

KEYWORDS

- Adenocarcinoma • Nasal • Papillary • Intestinal • Respiratory epithelial adenomatoid hamartoma
- Seromucinous hamartoma • Sinonasal • Sinus

Key Features

- A few well-described glandular lesions have been described that occur within the sinonasal tract. These include so-called hamartomas as well as adenocarcinomas.

- The pathologist must be able to distinguish these lesions from one another and from other sinonasal lesions owing to the vastly different prognoses and treatments for these lesions.

ABSTRACT

Glandular lesions that cannot be diagnosed readily as salivary gland tumors occur uncommonly in the upper aerodigestive tract. They occur only with some frequency within the sinonasal tract. Well-characterized lesions at this site include the respiratory epithelial adenomatoid hamartoma, seromucinous hamartoma, and intestinal and non–intestinal-type adenocarcinomas. This article reviews the clinicopathologic features of these fascinating lesions.

OVERVIEW

As with the mouth, the sinonasal tract forms during embryogenesis from the ectoderm, although true skin appendageal structures extend only into the distal nares.[1] The majority of the remaining tract is covered with a ciliated columnar or respiratory-type epithelium with occasional goblet cells and underlying seromucinous glands. Squamous and mucinous metaplasia can be present in varying quantities and degrees throughout the tract, usually as a response to injury. Focally, usually at the very apex of the tract, the mucosa is lined by olfactory mucosa. This layer is a specialized mucosa composed of tall, eosinophilic supporting cells, elongated, ciliated olfactory neurons, and small, basally located cells.

As with other sites of the upper aerodigestive tract, squamous cell carcinoma is the most common malignancy and even neoplasm of the sinonasal tract. At this site, however, squamous cell carcinoma accounts for a lesser percentage of overall neoplasia and malignancy than it does throughout other components of the upper aerodigestive tract. Not surprising, salivary gland–type neoplasia account for the second most frequent neoplasia seen here and the majority of the array of named salivary gland tumors have been identified at this site.

After excluding squamous cell carcinoma and salivary gland–type neoplasia, things get quite interesting, however. Within the sinonasal tract, a variety of distinct and less distinct glandular neoplasms occur, lesions that are almost unheard of within the remainder of the tract. This article explores the fascinating array of benign and malignant glandular tumors that have described primary to the sinonasal tract.

BENIGN TUMORS

Benign glandular tumors unique to the sinonasal tract have, for better or worse, been generally termed "hamartomas." These include the respiratory epithelial adenomatoid hamartoma (REAH) and the seromucinous hamartoma (SMH).

Department of Pathology, University of Virginia, Charlottesville, VA, USA
* Surgical Pathology, UVA Health Services, Box 800214, Jefferson Park Avenue, Charlottesville, VA 22908.
E-mail address: es7yj@virginia.edu

Surgical Pathology 10 (2017) 89–102
http://dx.doi.org/10.1016/j.path.2016.10.004

RESPIRATORY EPITHELIAL ADENOMATOID HAMARTOMA

The term "hamartoma" has been used to describe a number of disparate lesions of the nasopharynx and sinonasal tract throughout the years. The first major synthesis and potential identification of a unique entity was made by Wenig and Heffner.[2] They identified 31 lesions with consistent histologic features that they named REAH.

Nearly 90% of patients with REAHs are men and the reported patient ages have ranged from 27 to 81 years (median, 58).[2–6] Symptoms include obstruction, stuffiness, epistaxis, post-nasal drainage, and chronic rhinosinusitis. Sites of occurrence include the nasal septum, lateral nasal wall, ethmoid sinus, maxillary sinus, frontal sinus, and nasopharynx. Approximately 70% of REAHs occur in the nasal cavity, usually along the posterior nasal septum–olfactory cleft.[7,8]

REAHs are circumscribed and polypoid, and have been reported to measure up to 5 cm in size. A stalk has sometimes been noted. On cut surface, lesions are firm, tan-white, and solid with occasional cystic foci. The surfaces are covered by ciliated respiratory epithelium, which is in direct continuity with well-developed, branching glands lined chiefly with ciliated respiratory epithelial cells (Fig. 1).[2,6] Sometimes, the epithelium is cuboidal or flat and mucous gland metaplasia may also be present (see Fig. 1). Numerous glands with mucinous luminal contents may be observed, and these are sometimes dilated. A seromucinous gland hyperplasia is sometimes seen and there may be stromal hyalinization. Other nonspecific changes include stromal edema, increased vascularity, and a mixed acute and chronic inflammatory infiltrate. Noted conditions found coincidentally have included inverted papilloma and solitary fibrous tumor. Lymphangiomatous proliferation and osseous metaplasia have been seen rarely within the REAH. Foci of squamous metaplasia may be present. The fibrovascular stroma sometimes has foci of metaplastic bone or lymphoid follicles.[5] When bone is present, some have referred to such lesions as chondroosseous respiratory epithelial hamartomas.[5]

As mentioned, there is some controversy as to whether these lesions are hyperplastic or neoplastic. The distribution of disease and association with chronic rhinosinusitis suggest a reactive process, but an early study by Ozolek and Hunt[9] showed REAHs to have increased fractional allelic loss (31%) when compared with polypoid sinusitis. The most loss occurred on 9p and 18q near the p16 and SMAD4 genes, respectively.

The typical REAH should be distinguished from an inflammatory polyp and Schneiderian papilloma. Unlike inflammatory polyps, REAHs occur as single lesions and are usually present on the posterior nasal septum. Other features that favor a diagnosis of REAH over inflammatory polyp include a greater quantity of glandular proliferation, basement membrane material enveloping the glands, and atrophic epithelial changes. Schneiderian papillomas have a thickened, proliferating epithelium with intraepithelial mucous cysts and acute inflammation. Another very important consideration in the differential diagnosis is chondromesenchymal hamartoma.[10] These lesions frequently have a REAH-like glandular proliferation associated with nests of differentiated chondroid material and loose stromal elements (Fig. 2). These lesions typically occur in children and may be a manifestation of a germline

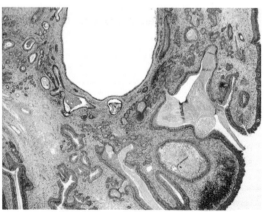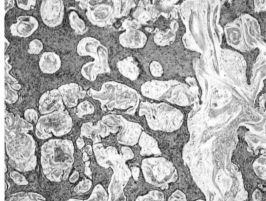

Fig. 1. Respiratory epithelial adenomatoid hamartoma (REAH). (*Left*) Typical low-power image of REAH with numerous dilated glands lined by a respiratory-type epithelium (H&E, ×40). (*Right*) Mucinous change may be prominent (H&E, ×100).

Fig.2. Chondromesenchymal hamartoma. The lesions characteristically have small islands of chondroid material within the stroma. They must be distinguished from respiratory epithelial adenomatoid hamartoma owing to their association with germline DICER1 mutations (H&E, ×100).

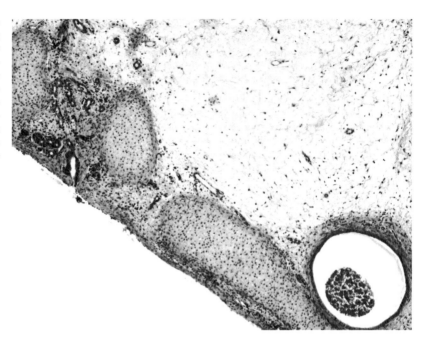

DICER1 mutation and associated with pleuropulmonary blastoma. One approach to the diagnosis of REAH would suggest that it should only be made when the features alone explain the entity observed and that when a different lesion is truly present, the REAH features should simply be considered nonspecific and/or secondary.

Complete excision cures REAH. No recurrences have been noted to date.[2,8]

SEROMUCINOUS HAMARTOMAS

In 1974, Baillie and Batsakis[11] described a glandular proliferation of the nasopharynx that they termed glandular (SMH). Weinreb and colleagues[12] have since described 7 cases of SMH involving the sinonasal tract. Patients were 4 men and 3 women and ages ranged from 14 to 85 years with a mean age of 56 years. As with REAHs, the majority of lesions occurred on the posterior nasal septum and one occurred on the lateral nasal wall. Nasal obstruction and epistaxis were the most common presenting symptoms.

Unlike with REAHs, with SMHs the underlying glandular component consists predominately of seromucinous glands. Larger glands lined by a respiratory-type epithelium, however, are invariably present.[12] Smaller tubules, ducts, and glands are present in lobular and more haphazard arrangements, lined by bland cuboidal cells that rarely contain dark, eosinophilic granular material (**Fig. 3**). The smaller glands may have little

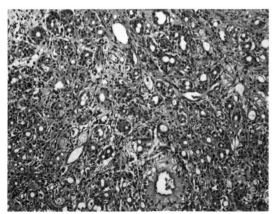
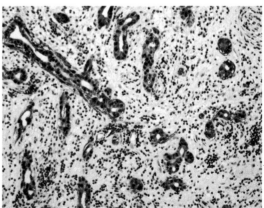

Fig. 3. Seromucinous hamartoma. A somewhat haphazard proliferation of seromucinous glands predominated is SMHs (H&E, ×100) (*left*). These glands are typically immunoreactive with antibodies to S100 protein (H&E, ×200) (*right*).

intervening stroma and can seem to be back to back. The glands may be surrounded by stromal hyalinization. A chronic lymphoplasmacellular infiltrate is typically present.

The immunohistochemical findings overlap with REAH, and additionally highlight the seromucinous glands. Both respiratory and seromucinous glands are CK7 and CK19 positive, and CK20 negative CK20.[12,13] The p63 and high-molecular-weight cytokeratins highlight the basal and myoepithelial cells surrounding the large glands and some of the seromucinous glands, whereas muscle markers are negative in basal cells. Of note, the seromucinous glandular proliferation typical of SMH shows little or no basal cell staining.[12] In contrast with REAH, the seromucinous glands are variably S100 protein positive (see **Fig. 3**), and uniformly SOX-10 and DOG1 positive.[12–14]

Good criteria do not exist for the definitive distinction between REAHs with florid seromucinous glandular proliferation, SMHs, and lobular patterned low-grade nonintestinal adenocarcinomas. In our series of 29 low-grade nonintestinal adenocarcinomas, 6 were associated with polypoid lesions with features typical of REAH.[15] That said, the SMHs described by Weinreb et al[12] have similar histologic and immunohistochemical features, including a lack of myoepithelial cells surrounding the seromucinous glandular proliferations. Recurrence for either lesion is uncommon (only 20% of the lesions reported by Weinreb et al recurred) and metastases are only very rarely seen with sinonasal low-grade nonintestinal adenocarcinomas. Some authors have likened the glandular proliferation of SMH to microglandular adenosis of the breast.[16] Indeed, it may be that "adenosis" or "adenoma" is truly the best appellations for these benign glandular proliferations.

MALIGNANCIES

Adenocarcinomas of the sinonasal tract that are not best classified as salivary-gland type malignancies include intestinal-type sinonasal adenocarcinoma (ITAC) and nonintestinal type sinonasal adenocarcinomas (SNAC).

INTESTINAL-TYPE SINONASAL ADENOCARCINOMA

ITACs represent the largest and most histologically consistent group of nonsalivary gland–type sinonasal adenocarcinomas. They consist of glandular or mucin-producing neoplasms composed of intestinal-type epithelial cells. Included in this group is a spectrum of neoplasia ranging from tumors resembling conventional colonic adenocarcinomas and mucinous adenocarcinomas to deceptively bland-appearing neoplasms resembling normal intestinal mucosa.

In a comprehensive series and literature review, Barnes[17] notes the existence of this entity for more than 100 years. In the late 1960s and early 1970s, Hadfield and colleagues[18–23] demonstrated a strong association with exposure to hardwood dust in the English furniture making industry, subsequently confirmed in England and other countries.[24–28] Exposures to softwood dusts in the logging and milling industries, as well as leather dust in the shoemaking industry, and possibly flour dust, have also been implicated as risk factors for the development of these neoplasms.[17,25,27] In older studies, before the institution of dust control measures, the incidence of this tumor in longtime wood-workers was noted to approach 500 to 1000 times that of the general population.[18] About 20% of these tumors have historically arisen in individuals with industrial wood dust exposure.[19] Recently, formaldehyde has been suggested as a risk factor for the disease.[29]

Approximately 80% of reported ITACs have occurred in men.[17] Reported sites of origin have included the ethmoid sinuses (40%), the nasal cavity (28%), and the maxillary antrum (23%). Typical presenting symptoms include unilateral nasal obstruction, epistaxis, rhinorrhea, mass in the cheek or change in facial contour, exophthalmos, or, less commonly, vision impairment or symptoms relating to facial nerve involvement.[17,30] Symptoms are typically present for less than 1 year, but may have been up to 5 years in duration. Often the initial clinical diagnosis is nasal polyps or chronic sinusitis, rather than malignancy.

Barnes' study[17] suggested some clinical differences between sporadic tumors and those arising in individuals occupationally exposed to dust. Not surprisingly, tumors related to occupational exposure affect men in 85% to 95% of cases. In this setting, the tumors show a strong tendency to arise in the ethmoid sinuses.[20,21,28] Sporadic tumors frequently arise in women and involve the maxillary antrum in 20% to 50% of cases.[17]

The gross appearance of these tumors is not dissimilar from that of colonic adenocarcinomas, and occasionally may mimic the appearance of ulcerated or hemorrhagic inflammatory polyps.[17] A fungating, grossly polypoid, or papillary mass with a hemorrhagic to pink–white color is seen commonly. Areas of mucosal ulceration are typical and may have associated hemorrhage. Some tumors will have a grossly mucoid or gelatinous appearance.

These tumors can recapitulate the entire spectrum of appearances assumed by normal, adenomatous and overtly malignant small and large intestinal mucosa. At one extreme are neoplasms composed of multiple cell types native to the normal small intestine, including Paneth cells, goblet cells, resorptive cells, argentaffin cells, villi formation, and even apparent underlying muscularis mucosae.[22,31] More typical papillary tumors consist of elongated fronds lined by stratified, mitotically active, dysplastic columnar cells and goblet cells, creating an appearance similar to that of an intestinal tubular or villous adenoma (Fig. 4). The papillary neoplasms may be confined to the surface mucosa or obviously invasive.[17,32]

The most common variant of ITAC resembles typical gland-forming colonic adenocarcinoma (see Fig. 4). Pleomorphic columnar cells line irregular, back-to-back glands. Mitotic figures, including atypical forms, are identified easily in the glandular cells. Areas of "dirty necrosis" are common, with necrotic cellular debris partially filling glandular lumens. Intracellular and intraluminal mucin is present focally, but goblet cells are not a prominent component of the tumor. With more poorly differentiated

tumors, gland formation becomes less obvious and the tumors acquire more prominent solid and cribriform components. Less frequently, ITACs will have abundant mucus production, which may accumulate in large extracellular pools in a pattern identical to that of colonic colloid carcinoma, or may be present predominantly intracellularly, forming prominent signet ring cells (see Fig. 4).[17,32]

The grading of ITACs has been the subject of several studies.[17,32–34] Batsakis and colleagues[32] divided these tumors into papillary, sessile, and alveolar–mucoid neoplasms. Papillary tumors were similar in appearance to colonic adenomas, often lacking clear-cut features of malignancy using criteria applied to analogous colonic lesions. Sessile carcinomas resembled conventional colonic adenocarcinomas, and alveolar–mucoid tumors were analogous to colloid or mucinous-type colonic neoplasms. Barnes,[17] in an extensive review of the topic, recognized 5 variants of ITACs: papillary, colonic, solid, mucinous, and mixed. Papillary and colonic tumors were equivalent essentially to the papillary and sessile designations of Batsakis

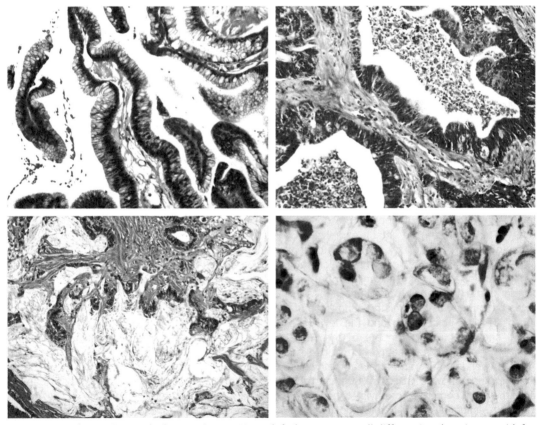

Fig. 4. Intestinal-type sinonasal adenocarcinoma. Upper left shows a very well-differentiated carcinoma with features similar to a villous adenoma of the colon (H&E, ×200); Tumors generally seems to be identical to typical colonic adenocarcinomas (*upper right* [H&E, ×200]), sometimes with abundant extracellular mucus (*lower left* [H&E, ×100]). Uncommonly, tumors can be composed of signet ring cells (*lower right* [H&E, ×400]).

and colleagues. Solid tumors were more poorly differentiated neoplasms with less obvious gland formation, and mucinous tumors included both extracellular mucinous (colloid) and intracellular mucinous (signet ring) types. In a review of 79 ITACs arising in woodworkers, Kleinsasser and Schroeder[34] recognized 4 primary tumor types, and total of 6 tumor types and grades. These included papillary–tubular cylinder cell, grades I, II, and III; alveolar goblet cell; solid signet ring cell; and transitional type neoplasms. The grade I tumors closely resemble the papillary designation of Batsakis and colleagues, grade II tumors are similar to the sessile designation of Batsakis and colleagues, and the grade III tumors resemble the solid tumors or Barnes.

ITACs express specific antigens of colonic differentiation.[35–39] ITACs have been shown to express CDX-2 (80%–88%) and CK20 (67%–100%). A single study showed tumor cell immunoreactivity with antibodies to villin.[39] MUC2 immunoreactivity has been noted in 88% of cases.[36] Also, of note, CK7 immunoreactivity has been noted in 43% to 100% of cases and has been described as "variable."[35–39]

The molecular pathogenesis of ITACs remains poorly understood. A number of studies have investigated the status of antigens typical of colonic adenocarcinomas. Studies have varied significantly in the identification of beta-catenin nuclear localization.[40,41] Other studies have demonstrated KRAS mutations in up to 43% of cases, although results have varied widely.[42–45] HRAS mutations were identified in 1 study, but not in another.[43,46] BRAF mutations seem to be very uncommon.[47–49] Although overexpression of epidermal growth factor receptor has been demonstrated to be "high" in up to 30% of cases by immunohistochemistry and gene copy gains have been identified, mutations of the gene are rare.[49] The tumors have intact expression of mismatch repair proteins by immunohistochemistry and the vast majority do not have microsatellite instability.[40,45,50] Overexpression of p53 protein and HER-2 has been noted in some cases by immunohistochemistry, although mutation of TP53 is uncommon and the few cases tested showed normal numbers of the *HER-2* gene.[35,46,51,52] Promoter methylation of p14 and p16 has been identified and a recent methylation profiling study showed CDH13, ESR1, and APC to be the most commonly methylated genes.[46,53] A study investigating loss of heterozygosity at multiple sites found deletions at 3p25, 3p14, 4q25, 5q14, 8p23, 10q25, 11p13, 17p13, and 18q21.[54] Comparative genomic hybridization has shown gains at 1q, 5p, 7q, 8q, 12p, 12q, 18q, 19q, 20q, 22, and X with losses at 4, 5q, 6q, 8p, 9p, 17p, and 18q.[55–57]

When confronted with a histologically malignant-appearing intestinal-type adenocarcinoma in the sinonasal region, pathologists will undoubtedly consider the possibility of metastatic disease, particularly if they have not previously encountered primary sinonasal tumors of this type. Gastrointestinal adenocarcinomas have been documented to metastasize to this region and this concern is therefore reasonable.[58] Although there is considerable immunohistochemical overlap, strong staining for carcinoembryonic antigen is more common in colonic adenocarcinomas and would lend some support to the possibility of metastatic disease and, conversely, strong staining for chromogranin would be more often encountered in primary sinonasal tumors.[59] This distinction is not a problem with the well-differentiated ITACs resembling colonic adenomas or even normal colonic mucosa.

Because of the presence of mucin-secreting cells, ITACs occasionally may be confused with mucoepidermoid carcinomas. However, the former tumors lack the multiple, distinct cell types, including squamous cells, clear cells, and intermediate cells, as well as mucinous cells that typify mucoepidermoid carcinoma.

There can obviously be some confusion with nonintestinal SNACs, both at the low and high grades of the spectrum. Low-grade nonintestinal SNACs can be exophytic and papillary and are lined by columnar epithelial cells occasionally with more mucinous or goblet-type cells. These tumors, however, have round and bland, basally located nuclei instead of the hyperchromatic, elongated, atypical, and stratified nuclei seen with ITACs. Immunohistochemistry can also be helpful because nonintestinal SNACs react with antibodies to CK7 but not with antibodies to CK20, MUC2, CDX-2, or villin.[36,38,39] A subset of nonintestinal SNAC are also S100, SOX-10, and/or DOG1 positive.[14] High-grade nonintestinal SNACs sometimes have a cribriform growth pattern with an intestinal appearance. These tumors typically produce much less mucin (both intracellular and extracellular) than ITACs and will not react with antibodies to CK20, MUC2, CDX-2, or villin.

ITACs are characterized by 1 or more local recurrences in more than one-half of patients.[17,60] Regional lymph node and distant metastases are less common, being seen in less than 8% and 13% of patients, respectively. The optimal treatment for ITAC is complete surgical resection (open or endoscopic), with adjuvant radiation therapy to the region of the tumor.[61] Given the low rate of regional lymph node metastases, routine radical neck dissections are not recommended.[62] Individual enlarged or suspicious lymph nodes may be evaluated initially by fine needle aspiration, followed by resection if necessary. Barnes[17] reviewed the clinical features of 213 cases, at least 19% of which occurred in woodworkers. Overall, 60% of patients were known to have died of disease, and 80% of these did so within 3 years of diagnosis. Survival of up to 9 years before death from disease was noted.

Some studies have shown a slight survival difference for dust-related versus sporadic tumors. Dust-related intestinal-type adenocarcinomas have a 5-year survival of approximately 50%.[28] Sporadic tumors seem to have a poorer prognosis with a 20% to 40% survival at 5 years.[17] A more recent multicenter study also suggests that patients with dust exposure fare better than those without.[60] Regardless of pathogenesis, the clinical course for these tumors can be quite protracted and 5-year disease-free survival cannot be equated with cure. A recent study limited to ethmoid sinus adenocarcinomas showed an overall 5-year survival of 64% and a 10-year survival of 49%.[60] Most of the tumors occurred in patients with dust exposure, although the histologic features were characterized somewhat poorly. Patients with very large tumors that extended into the cranial cavity fared worse.

Several studies have shown that grading and subtyping of these tumors correlates with patients' overall survival rate and duration of survival.[17,28,32–34] Despite the complexity of the grading systems and their relationships with prognosis, studies may be summarized in this way: Some ITACs are very papillary and well-differentiated, and seem to behave better than most, whereas those tumors with solid growth or signet ring cell morphology do worse than most. Regardless of the degree of differentiation, all forms of ITAC should be considered as locally aggressive proliferations. Even tumors deceptively resembling normal intestinal epithelial are known to be locally destructive, ultimately fatal neoplasms.[22,31]

LOW-GRADE NONINTESTINAL SINONASAL ADENOCARCINOMA

Low-grade nonintestinal SNACs are microscopically somewhat heterogeneous. They are well-differentiated, often papillary, adenocarcinomas arising in the sinonasal tract that lack intestinal-like features. They are distinguished from high-grade nonintestinal SNACs by their lack of necrosis and lack of significant mitotic activity and cytologic atypia, although definitive criteria are lacking.[63] No risk factors have not been identified for these low-grade neoplasms.[15] There is no apparent association with tobacco use or alcohol consumption and no genetic, occupational, or environmental factors have been identified.[64]

In Heffner and colleagues's[65] review of 23 low-grade lesions from the sinonasal region, the patients had a broad age distribution from 9 to 75 years, with most being in their fifth through seventh decades of life. There was no sex or racial predilection. Patients typically presented with nasal obstruction or epistaxis. Fewer than 10% of patients complained of pain. Symptom duration averaged 5.5 months, but was up to 5 years in 1 case. Tumor location included the ethmoid sinus (30%), the nasal cavity (22%), the nasal septum (17.5%), multiple sinuses (17.5%), and the maxillary antrum (13%). Although early reports indicate a male predilection,[66,67] subsequent series show a more even sex predilection.[14,15,68]

Gross descriptions of these tumors are often lacking. Some sinonasal cases have been described as "raspberry-like."[66] The consistency ranges from soft to firm, and some cases may be gritty. Tumors have ranged in size from 0.3 to 4.0 cm.[64]

In Heffner and colleagues's[65] early report of low-grade nonintestinal SNACs, some tumors resembling salivary gland carcinomas were included. Even once named salivary gland–type tumors are excluded, there is some variation is histologic features from case to case. In general, the features are those of a very well-differentiated glandular neoplasm with papilla and small glands lined by a single layer of bland columnar to cuboidal cells (**Fig. 5**).[15,65–68] Most tumors have prominent exophytic growth; however, other tumors may be predominately infiltrative and tubular. Glands are frequently "back to back" and generally have lightly eosinophilic, mucinous cytoplasm; however, squamous, morular, or oncocytic cells are sometimes present. The lumen may be dilated and filled with mucous. Mitotic figures are rare and nuclear atypia and prominent nucleoli are not seen generally. Psammoma bodies have been identified in some cases.

Low-grade nonintestinal SNACs are universally immunoreactive with antibodies to CK7 and are not immunoreactive with antibodies to typically intestinal epithelial antigens, such as CK20, CDX2 and MUC2.[36–38,68] Although many have been immunoreactive with antibodies to S100 protein, they have not been immunoreactive with antibodies to smooth muscle actin, calponin, CD10, or p63 (except in areas of squamous metaplasia).[68] SOX-10 and DOG-1 immunoreactivity have been noted in a subset suggesting seromucinous differentiation.[14] Endocrine immunoreactivity has not

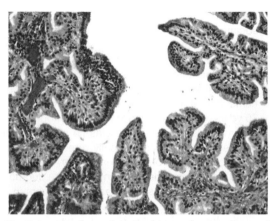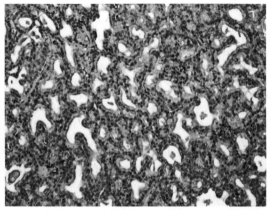

Fig. 5. Low-grade nonintestinal-type adenocarcinoma. These are low-grade glandular lesions usually with papillary (*left*) and/or tubular (*right*) formations (H&E, ×100).

been demonstrated in the few cases stained with antibodies to chromogranin or CD57.[68] Morules that are CDX2 and beta catenin positive in a nuclear fashion are rarely noted, the former of which may be a pitfall if taken out of morphologic context.[14]

Low-grade nonintestinal SNACs have been subjected rarely to genetic testing. By immunohistochemistry in 1 study, 40% showed abundant nuclear staining with antibodies to p53 protein whereas none stained with antibodies to HER2/neu.[68] KRAS, APC, beta-catenin, hMLH1, and hMSH2 mutations have not been identified in the few cases tested.[45]

Low-grade nonintestinal SNACs should be distinguished from ITACs because of their considerably less aggressive clinical course and better survival. This process is usually a straightforward determination. Low-grade SNACs, by definition, lack an "intestinal" microscopic appearance. Except for the rare ITACs mimicking adenomas or even normal intestinal mucosa, the majority of the intestinal-type adenocarcinomas are considerably more pleomorphic than low-grade nonintestinal SNACs. Immunohistochemistry can be used when needed because ITACs will be immunoreactive with antibodies to CK20, CDX-2, and MUC2.[36–39,68,69]

Although some tumors have a seromucinous appearance, they should also be distinguished from named salivary-type neoplasms. Immunohistochemistry can be used to demonstrate myoepithelial differentiation with pleomorphic adenomas, epithelial myoepithelial carcinomas, and adenoid cystic carcinomas. Polymorphous low-grade adenocarcinomas should, in general, show more heterogeneity in their growth patterns. Acinic cell carcinomas should be composed of small acinar structures and definite serous differentiation should be seen.

Finally, low-grade nonintestinal SNACs should also be distinguished from REAHs and SMHs.[2,6] These lesions grossly resemble inflammatory polyps, but microscopically contain often complex glandlike epithelial proliferations. Most often, the epithelial component resembles normal respiratory mucosa with a pseudostratified appearance composed of ciliated and scattered mucinous cells (REAH). The epithelial nests are often surrounded by prominent cuffs of stromal hyalinization. The overall appearance is distinguished easily from the uniform, nonstratified epithelium of low-grade adenocarcinoma. Uncommonly, hamartomas may contain a predominance of seromucinous glands (SMH). Such lesions may lack a prominent basal/myoepithelial cell layer and even a lobular growth pattern.[6,15] As mentioned, definitive criteria for distinguishing such tumors for low-grade nonintestinal SNACs are lacking.

Treatment for these tumors has been complete surgical resection via an appropriate approach. Lesions may require a lateral rhinotomy, Caldwell-Luc procedure, and removal of the affected sinus or intranasal tumor.[65] A few patients have received adjuvant radiation therapy, but given the overall good prognosis and limited number of cases, there is no evidence that this has affected survival.

Of the 66 cases of low-grade nonintestinal SNAC in the literature, recurrences were noted in 16 cases, metastases in 2 cases, and 3 patients died of their disease.[15,36,65–68,70] Most of the recurrences were noted in Heffner and colleagues's[65] early report, in which some tumors that would now be diagnosed as salivary gland–type tumors were included. At least one of the patients noted to have had a metastasis and to have died of disease was noted in retrospect to have had a high-grade component to their original tumor.[66]

HIGH-GRADE NONINTESTINAL SINONASAL ADENOCARCINOMA

High-grade nonintestinal SNACs are relatively poorly described. By definition they (1) cannot be better diagnosed as salivary gland neoplasia (2), do not have an intestinal phenotype, and (3) are high grade with moderate to marked cytologic pleomorphism, high mitotic activity, and necrosis.[63]

No definitive risk factors have not been identified for high-grade nonintestinal SNACs. Cases have been described, however, that were associated with Schneiderian papillomas.[71–75] Since our published series of high-grade nonintestinal SNACs, we have seen a few cases of tumors related to high-risk human papillomavirus. Bishop and colleagues[76] described human papilloma virus–associated sinonasal carcinomas that resemble adenoid cystic carcinomas should also be noted here as the described histomorphology of human papilloma virus–associated carcinoma continues to expand.

Heffner and colleagues[65] reviewed adenocarcinomas from the sinonasal region, and 14 of the 27 cases were considered high grade and not noted to seem to be intestinal. Of these, 10 neoplasms occurred in men and 4 in women; the age range was 15 to 80 years. The most common symptoms included nasal obstruction and/or facial "swelling" or deformity. The most common sites of involvement included the nasal cavity and maxillary antrum, although tumors also occurred in the maxillary, frontal, ethmoid, and sphenoid sinuses. Of 28 cases seen at the University of Virginia and Memorial Sloan-Kettering Cancer Center, 23 were from men and the age range was 19 to 83 years.[75] Thirteen cases involved the nasal cavity and sinuses, whereas 11 involved the nasal cavity only and 4 involved the sinuses only.

The histology for high-grade nonintestinal SNACs is variable (Fig. 6).[75] Many cases have solid and trabecular growth with occasional small cystic spaces, and are composed of neoplastic cells that have a small amount of amphiphilic cytoplasm. These tumors resemble the blastomatous components sometimes seen in teratocarcinosarcomas.[77] Occasional cases are more nested and composed of larger cells, with more abundant

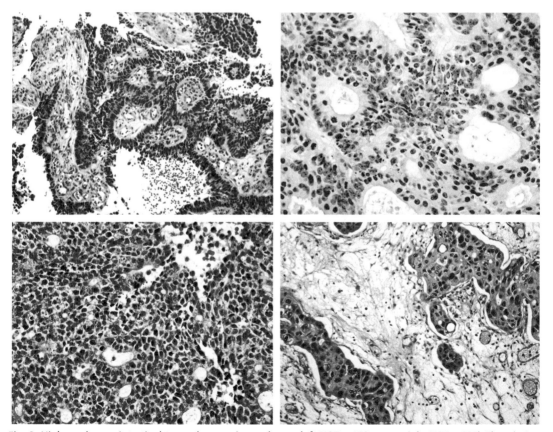

Fig. 6. High-grade non–intestinal-type adenocarcinoma (*upper left*, H&E, ×100; *upper right*, H&E, ×200). These lesions show diverse morphology with some showing abundant solid growth akin to sinonasal undifferentiated carcinomas (*lower left* [H&E, ×200]) and occasional cases showing a somewhat apocrine phenotype (*lower right* [H&E, ×200]).

eosinophilic cytoplasm (somewhat akin to salivary duct carcinoma). Many cases will have focal areas of solid growth with areas that are akin to those of sinonasal undifferentiated carcinoma. Uncommonly, some cases may be composed of clear cells and resemble renal cell carcinoma (RCC), and some investigators have attempted to designate these are their own tumor type given the relative reproducibility of the histologic and immunohistochemical features (**Fig. 7**).[78,79] Finally, we and others have noted that some cases may seem to be akin to high-grade mucoepidermoid carcinomas and to be associated with oncocytic Schneiderian papillomas.[71,72,74] Most cases, by definition, have marked cytologic and nuclear pleomorphic, abundant mitotic activity, and necrosis; however, these features were not uniform.

Tumors generally lack CDX2 and CK20 immunoreactivity (aside from rare CK20 immunoreactive cells).[75] Diffuse, strong CK7 immunoreactivity has been seen in 43% of cases. S100, p63, and neuroendocrine antigen reactivity was only seen is rare cell in occasional cases. Rare cases also express seromucinous markers such as SOX-10 and DOG1.[14] Cases that resemble RCC have been noted to stain with antibodies to CA-IX, although antibodies to RCC and CD10 are less reliable.[80,81] The few cases we have seen secondary to high-risk human papilloma virus infection as well as those cases described by Bishop and colleagues[76] that resemble adenoid cystic carcinoma, are diffusely immunoreactive with antibodies to p16.

High-grade nonintestinal SNACs should be distinguished from low-grade nonintestinal SNACs because of their marked difference in prognosis. Low-grade lesions should be predominately papillary or tubular, unlike high-grade lesions which are frequently solid or trabecular. Although focal cytologic atypia is sometimes seen with low-grade lesions, abundant mitotic figures or tumor necrosis is seen with high-grade lesions.

High-grade nonintestinal SNACs should also be distinguished from ITACs. Most ITACs are gland forming and the tumors frequently produce extracellular mucus. Immunohistochemistry may be helpful, especially with small biopsies. ITACs frequently are immunoreactive with antibodies to CK20, CDX-2, and MUC2, whereas high-grade, nonintestinal SNACs rarely are immunoreactive with these antibodies (rare focal CK20 immunoreactivity has been noted).

Sinonasal undifferentiated carcinoma is sometimes considered in the differential diagnosis. For a diagnosis of SNUC, no or very, very limited glandular differentiation should be seen by routine histology. Finally, the distinction of these tumors from high-grade salivary duct carcinoma can be very difficult and, indeed, may be semantic. Some tumors seem to be akin to salivary duct carcinomas with infiltrating islands of pleomorphic glandular cells, sometimes with abundant eosinophilic cytoplasm. Furthermore, within the current World Health Organization classification system of salivary gland tumors is the diagnosis "adenocarcinoma, not otherwise specified," a waste basket

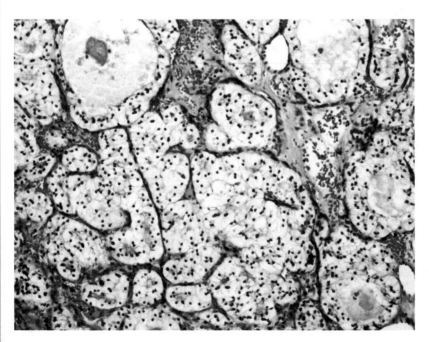

Fig. 7. Renal cell like sinonasal adenocarcinoma. These tumors seem to be identical to clear cell carcinomas of the kidney (H&E, ×200).

diagnosis that could easily be made to include these tumors.

Most patients with high-grade nonintestinal SNACs have undergone resection and radiation therapy.[65,70] Occasional patients have also received chemotherapy. Twelve of the 14 patients reported by Heffner et al[65] died of their disease at 0.5 to 5 years after their diagnosis. One patient was alive with disease at 3 years and one with no evidence of disease at 11 years. In a report of sinonasal adenocarcinomas authored by Orvidas and colleagues,[70] 3 of 9 patients with high-grade nonintestinal SNACs recurred and 4 of 9 died of disease at 0.6 to 4 years. Patients with adenocarcinomas that seem to be similar to renal cell carcinoma have fared much better, again suggesting that such tumors may be best classified as their own entity.[81]

SUMMARY

Glandular lesions that cannot best be classified as salivary gland–type neoplasia are most common in the sinonasal tract when compared with the remaining upper aerodigestive tract. It is important to recognize the benign and low-grade nonintestinal SNACs and to distinguish them from high-grade nonintestinal SNACs and ITACs because of the severe difference in prognosis and treatments. Although a strong link has been made between ITAC and industrial exposure, the etiologies to the other tumors remain mostly unknown.

REFERENCES

1. Stelow EB, Mills SE. Normal anatomy and histology. Biopsy interpretation of the upper aerodigestive tract and ear. 2nd edition. Philadelphia: Wolters Kluwer/Lippincott Williams and Wilkins; 2013. p. 1–5.
2. Wenig BM, Heffner DK. Respiratory epithelial adenomatoid hamartomas of the sinonasal tract and nasopharynx: a clinicopathologic study of 31 cases. Ann Otol Rhinol Laryngol 1995;104(8):639–45.
3. Liang J, O'Malley BW Jr, Feldman M, et al. A case of respiratory epithelial adenomatoid hamartoma. Am J Otolaryngol 2007;28(4):277–9.
4. Mortuaire G, Pasquesoone X, Leroy X, et al. Respiratory epithelial adenomatoid hamartomas of the sinonasal tract. Eur Arch Otorhinolaryngol 2007;264(4):451–3.
5. Roffman E, Baredes S, Mirani N. Respiratory epithelial adenomatoid hamartomas and chondroosseous respiratory epithelial hamartomas of the sinonasal tract: a case series and literature review. Am J Rhinol 2006;20(6):586–90.
6. Sangoi AR, Berry G. Respiratory epithelial adenomatoid hamartoma: diagnostic pitfalls with emphasis on differential diagnosis. Adv Anat Pathol 2007;14(1):11–6.
7. Gauchotte G, Marie B, Gallet P, et al. Respiratory epithelial adenomatoid hamartoma: a poorly recognized entity with mast cell recruitment and frequently associated with nasal polyposis. Am J Surg Pathol 2013;37(11):1678–85.
8. Lee JT, Garg R, Brunworth J, et al. Sinonasal respiratory epithelial adenomatoid hamartomas: series of 51 cases and literature review. Am J Rhinol Allergy 2013;27(4):322–8.
9. Ozolek JA, Hunt JL. Tumor suppressor gene alterations in respiratory epithelial adenomatoid hamartoma (REAH): comparison to sinonasal adenocarcinoma and inflamed sinonasal mucosa. Am J Surg Pathol 2006;30(12):1576–80.
10. Stewart DR, Messinger Y, Williams GM, et al. Nasal chondromesenchymal hamartomas arise secondary to germline and somatic mutations of DICER1 in the pleuropulmonary blastoma tumor predisposition disorder. Hum Genet 2014;133(11):1443–50.
11. Baillie EE, Batsakis JG. Glandular (seromucinous) hamartoma of the nasopharynx. Oral Surg Oral Med Oral Pathol 1974;38(5):760–2.
12. Weinreb I, Gnepp DR, Laver NM, et al. Seromucinous hamartomas: a clinicopathological study of a sinonasal glandular lesion lacking myoepithelial cells. Histopathology 2009;54(2):205–13.
13. Ozolek JA, Barnes EL, Hunt JL. Basal/myoepithelial cells in chronic sinusitis, respiratory epithelial adenomatoid hamartoma, inverted papilloma, and intestinal-type and nonintestinal-type sinonasal adenocarcinoma: an immunohistochemical study. Arch Pathol Lab Med 2007;131(4):530–7.
14. Purgina B, Bastaki JM, Duvvuri U, et al. A subset of sinonasal non-intestinal type adenocarcinomas are truly seromucinous adenocarcinomas: a morphologic and immunophenotypic assessment and description of a novel pitfall. Head Neck Pathol 2015;9(4):436–46.
15. Jo VY, Mills SE, Cathro HP, et al. Low-grade sinonasal adenocarcinomas: the association with and distinction from respiratory epithelial adenomatoid hamartomas and other glandular lesions. Am J Surg Pathol 2009;33(3):401–8.
16. Ambrosini-Spaltro A, Morandi L, Spagnolo DV, et al. Nasal seromucinous hamartoma (microglandular adenosis of the nose): a morphological and molecular study of five cases. Virchows Arch 2010;457(6):727–34.
17. Barnes L. Intestinal-type adenocarcinoma of the nasal cavity and paranasal sinuses. Am J Surg Pathol 1986;10(3):192–202.
18. Acheson ED, Cowdell RH, Hadfield E, et al. Nasal cancer in woodworkers in the furniture industry. Br Med J 1968;2(5605):587–96.

19. Acheson ED, Cowdell RH, Jolles B. Nasal cancer in the Northamptonshire boot and shoe industry. Br Med J 1970;1(5693):385–93.

20. Hadfield EH. A study of adenocarcinoma of the paranasal sinuses in woodworkers in the furniture industry. Ann R Coll Surg Engl 1970;46(6):301–19.

21. Hadfield EH, Macbeth RG. Adenocarcinoma of ethmoids in furniture workers. Ann Otol Rhinol Laryngol 1971;80(5):699–703.

22. Jarvi O. Heterotopic tumors with an intestinal mucous membrane structure in the nasal cavity. Acta Otolaryngol 1945;33:471–5.

23. McDonald JR, Havens FZ. A study of malignant tumors of glandular nature found in the nose, throat, and mouth. Surg Clin North Am 1948;28:1087–106.

24. Andersen HC, Andersen I, Solgaard J. Nasal cancers, symptoms and upper airway function in woodworkers. Br J Ind Med 1977;34(3):201–7.

25. Cecchi F, Buiatti E, Kriebel D, et al. Adenocarcinoma of the nose and paranasal sinuses in shoemakers and woodworkers in the province of Florence, Italy (1963-77). Br J Ind Med 1980;37(3):222–5.

26. Imbus HR, Dyson WL. A review of nasal cancer in furniture manufacturing and woodworking in North Carolina, the United States, and other countries. J Occup Med 1987;29(9):734–40.

27. Ironside P, Matthews J. Adenocarcinoma of the nose and paranasal sinuses in woodworkers in the state of Victoria, Australia. Cancer 1975;36(3):1115–24.

28. Klintenberg C, Olofsson J, Hellquist H, et al. Adenocarcinoma of the ethmoid sinuses. A review of 28 cases with special reference to wood dust exposure. Cancer 1984;54(3):482–8.

29. Luce D, Leclerc A, Begin D, et al. Sinonasal cancer and occupational exposures: a pooled analysis of 12 case-control studies. Cancer Causes Control 2002;13(2):147–57.

30. Sanchez-Casis G, Devine KD, Weiland LH. Nasal adenocarcinomas that closely simulate colonic carcinomas. Cancer 1971;28(3):714–20.

31. Mills SE, Fechner RE, Cantrell RW. Aggressive sinonasal lesion resembling normal intestinal mucosa. Am J Surg Pathol 1982;6(8):803–9.

32. Batsakis JG, Holtz F, Sueper RH. Adenocarcinoma of nasal and paranasal cavities. Arch Otolaryngol 1963;77:625–33.

33. Franquemont DW, Fechner RE, Mills SE. Histologic classification of sinonasal intestinal-type adenocarcinoma. Am J Surg Pathol 1991;15(4):368–75.

34. Kleinsasser O, Schroeder HG. Adenocarcinomas of the inner nose after exposure to wood dust. Morphological findings and relationships between histopathology and clinical behavior in 79 cases. Arch Otorhinolaryngol 1988;245(1):1–15.

35. Bashir AA, Robinson RA, Benda JA, et al. Sinonasal adenocarcinoma: immunohistochemical marking and expression of oncoproteins. Head Neck 2003;25(9):763–71.

36. Cathro HP, Mills SE. Immunophenotypic differences between intestinal-type and low-grade papillary sinonasal adenocarcinomas: an immunohistochemical study of 22 cases utilizing CDX2 and MUC2. Am J Surg Pathol 2004;28(8):1026–32.

37. Choi HR, Sturgis EM, Rashid A, et al. Sinonasal adenocarcinoma: evidence for histogenetic divergence of the enteric and nonenteric phenotypes. Hum Pathol 2003;34(11):1101–7.

38. Franchi A, Massi D, Palomba A, et al. CDX-2, cytokeratin 7 and cytokeratin 20 immunohistochemical expression in the differential diagnosis of primary adenocarcinomas of the sinonasal tract. Virchows Arch 2004;445(1):63–7.

39. Kennedy MT, Jordan RC, Berean KW, et al. Expression pattern of CK7, CK20, CDX-2, and villin in intestinal-type sinonasal adenocarcinoma. J Clin Pathol 2004;57(9):932–7.

40. Perez-Ordonez B, Huynh NN, Berean KW, et al. Expression of mismatch repair proteins, beta catenin, and E cadherin in intestinal-type sinonasal adenocarcinoma. J Clin Pathol 2004;57(10):1080–3.

41. Diaz-Molina JP, Llorente JL, Vivanco B, et al. Wnt-pathway activation in intestinal-type sinonasal adenocarcinoma. Rhinology 2011;49(5):593–9.

42. Bornholdt J, Hansen J, Steiniche T, et al. K-ras mutations in sinonasal cancers in relation to wood dust exposure. BMC Cancer 2008;8:53.

43. Perez P, Dominguez O, Gonzalez S, et al. Ras gene mutations in ethmoid sinus adenocarcinoma: prognostic implications. Cancer 1999;86(2):255–64.

44. Saber AT, Nielsen LR, Dictor M, et al. K-ras mutations in sinonasal adenocarcinomas in patients occupationally exposed to wood or leather dust. Cancer Lett 1998;126(1):59–65.

45. Yom SS, Rashid A, Rosenthal DI, et al. Genetic analysis of sinonasal adenocarcinoma phenotypes: distinct alterations of histogenetic significance. Mod Pathol 2005;18(3):315–9.

46. Perrone F, Oggionni M, Birindelli S, et al. TP53, p14ARF, p16INK4a and H-ras gene molecular analysis in intestinal-type adenocarcinoma of the nasal cavity and paranasal sinuses. Int J Cancer 2003;105(2):196–203.

47. Franchi A, Innocenti DR, Palomba A, et al. Low prevalence of K-RAS, EGF-R and BRAF mutations in sinonasal adenocarcinomas. Implications for anti-EGFR treatments. Pathol Oncol Res 2014;20(3):571–9.

48. Lopez F, Garcia Inclan C, Perez-Escuredo J, et al. KRAS and BRAF mutations in sinonasal cancer. Oral Oncol 2012;48(8):692–7.

49. Szablewski V, Solassol J, Poizat F, et al. EGFR expression and KRAS and BRAF mutational status

in intestinal-type sinonasal adenocarcinoma. Int J Mol Sci 2013;14(3):5170–81.

50. Martinez JG, Perez-Escuredo J, Lopez F, et al. Microsatellite instability analysis of sinonasal carcinomas. Otolaryngol Head Neck Surg 2009;140(1): 55–60.

51. Holmila R, Cyr D, Luce D, et al. COX-2 and p53 in human sinonasal cancer: COX-2 expression is associated with adenocarcinoma histology and wood-dust exposure. Int J Cancer 2008;122(9):2154–9.

52. Nazar G, Gonzalez MV, Garcia JM, et al. Amplification of CCND1, EMS1, PIK3CA, and ERBB oncogenes in ethmoid sinus adenocarcinomas. Otolaryngol Head Neck Surg 2006;135(1):135–9.

53. Costales M, Lopez-Hernandez A, Garcia-Inclan C, et al. Gene methylation profiling in sinonasal adenocarcinoma and squamous cell carcinoma. Otolaryngol Head Neck Surg 2016;155:808–15.

54. Gotte K, Riedel F, Schafer C, et al. Cylindrical cell carcinomas of the paranasal sinuses do not show p53 alterations but loss of heterozygosity at 3p and 17p. Int J Cancer 2000;85(5):740–2.

55. Ariza M, Llorente JL, Alvarez-Marcas C, et al. Comparative genomic hybridization in primary sinonasal adenocarcinomas. Cancer 2004;100(2): 335–41.

56. Hermsen MA, Llorente JL, Perez-Escuredo J, et al. Genome-wide analysis of genetic changes in intestinal-type sinonasal adenocarcinoma. Head Neck 2009;31(3):290–7.

57. Korinth D, Pacyna-Gengelbach M, Deutschmann N, et al. Chromosomal imbalances in wood dust-related adenocarcinomas of the inner nose and their associations with pathological parameters. J Pathol 2005;207(2):207–15.

58. Bernstein JM, Montgomery WW, Balogh K Jr. Metastatic tumors to the maxilla, nose, and paranasal sinuses. Laryngoscope 1966;76(4):621–50.

59. McKinney CD, Mills SE, Franquemont DW. Sinonasal intestinal-type adenocarcinoma: immunohistochemical profile and comparison with colonic adenocarcinoma. Mod Pathol 1995;8(4):421–6.

60. Choussy O, Ferron C, Vedrine PO, et al. Adenocarcinoma of Ethmoid: a GETTEC retrospective multicenter study of 418 cases. Laryngoscope 2008; 118(3):437–43.

61. Nicolai P, Schreiber A, Bolzoni Villaret A, et al. Intestinal type adenocarcinoma of the ethmoid: outcomes of a treatment regimen based on endoscopic surgery with or without radiotherapy. Head Neck 2016;38(Suppl 1):E996–1003.

62. Donhuijsen K, Kollecker I, Petersen P, et al. Metastatic behaviour of sinonasal adenocarcinomas of the intestinal type (ITAC). Eur Arch Otorhinolaryngol 2016;273(3):649–54.

63. Franchi A, Santucci M, Wenig BM. Adenocarcinoma. In: Barnes L, Eveson JW, Reichart P, et al, editors.

Pathology and genetics of head and neck tumours. Lyon (France): IARC Press; 2005. p. 20–3.

64. Wenig BM, Hyams VJ, Heffner DK. Nasopharyngeal papillary adenocarcinoma. A clinicopathologic study of a low-grade carcinoma. Am J Surg Pathol 1988;12(12):946–53.

65. Heffner DK, Hyams VJ, Hauck KW, et al. Low-grade adenocarcinoma of the nasal cavity and paranasal sinuses. Cancer 1982;50(2):312–22.

66. Kleinsasser O. Terminal tubulus adenocarcinoma of the nasal seromucous glands. A specific entity. Arch Otorhinolaryngol 1985;241(2):183–93.

67. Neto AG, Pineda-Daboin K, Luna MA. Sinonasal tract seromucous adenocarcinomas: a report of 12 cases. Ann Diagn Pathol 2003;7(3):154–9.

68. Skalova A, Cardesa A, Leivo I, et al. Sinonasal tubulopapillary low-grade adenocarcinoma: histopathological, immunohistochemical and ultrastructural features of poorly recognised entity. Virchows Arch 2003;443(2):152–8.

69. Zeizafoun N, Elmberger G, Wenig BM. Thyroid transcription factor (TTF-1) immunoreactivity in low-grade nasopharyngeal papillary adenocarcinomas (LGNPPA): a report of three cases. Mod Pathol 2007;20(Suppl 2):231–232A.

70. Orvidas LJ, Lewis JE, Weaver AL, et al. Adenocarcinoma of the nose and paranasal sinuses: a retrospective study of diagnosis, histologic characteristics, and outcomes in 24 patients. Head Neck 2005;27(5):370–5.

71. Barnes L, Bedetti C. Oncocytic Schneiderian papilloma: a reappraisal of cylindrical cell papilloma of the sinonasal tract. Hum Pathol 1984; 15(4):344–51.

72. Kapadia SB, Barnes L, Pelzman K, et al. Carcinoma ex oncocytic Schneiderian (cylindrical cell) papilloma. Am J Otolaryngol 1993;14(5): 332–8.

73. Kaufman MR, Brandwein MS, Lawson W. Sinonasal papillomas: clinicopathologic review of 40 patients with inverted and oncocytic Schneiderian papillomas. Laryngoscope 2002;112(8 Pt 1):1372–7.

74. Maitra A, Baskin LB, Lee EL. Malignancies arising in oncocytic Schneiderian papillomas: a report of 2 cases and review of the literature. Arch Pathol Lab Med 2001;125(10):1365–7.

75. Stelow EB, Jo VY, Mills SE, et al. A histologic and immunohistochemical study of high-grade non-intestinal sinonasal adenocarcinomas. Mod Pathol 2009;22(Suppl1):252A.

76. Bishop JA, Ogawa T, Stelow EB, et al. Human papillomavirus-related carcinoma with adenoid cystic-like features: a peculiar variant of head and neck cancer restricted to the sinonasal tract. Am J Surg Pathol 2013;37(6):836–44.

77. Heffner DK, Hyams VJ. Teratocarcinosarcoma (malignant teratoma?) of the nasal cavity and

paranasal sinuses a clinicopathologic study of 20 cases. Cancer 1984;53(10):2140–54.

78. Zur KB, Brandwein M, Wang B, et al. Primary description of a new entity, renal cell-like carcinoma of the nasal cavity: van Meegeren in the house of Vermeer. Arch Otolaryngol Head Neck Surg 2002;128(4):441–7.

79. Ash JE, Beck MR, Wilkes JD. Tumors originating in epithelial tissues. Tumors of the upper respiratory tract and ear, vol. 12 and 13. Washington, DC: Armed Forces Institute of Pathology; 1964. p. 34.

80. Shen T, Shi Q, Velosa C, et al. Sinonasal renal cell-like adenocarcinomas: robust carbonic anhydrase expression. Hum Pathol 2015;46(11):1598–606.

81. Storck K, Hadi UM, Simpson R, et al. Sinonasal renal cell-like adenocarcinoma: a report on four patients. Head Neck Pathol 2008;2(2):75–80.

Sinonasal Small Round Blue Cell Tumors

An Immunohistochemical Approach

Lisa M. Rooper, MD[a], Justin A. Bishop, MD[b,c],*

KEYWORDS

- Sinonasal tumors • Small round blue cell tumors • Immunohistochemistry • Cytokeratin
- Squamous differentiation • Neuroendocrine differentiation

Key points

- The sinonasal small round blue cell tumor (SRBCT) differential diagnosis is extensive and fraught with pitfalls, necessitating a thoughtful immunohistochemical approach.
- A reasonable initial immunohistochemical panel for undifferentiated sinonasal SRBCT might include pancytokeratin, p63 (or p40), synaptophysin, chromogranin, S100, desmin, CD45, and CD99.
- Patchy pancytokeratin expression is frequently seen in nonepithelial SRBCTs and should not be interpreted as definitive evidence of epithelial differentiation.
- p63 or p40 positivity, although helpful, does not equate to squamous cell carcinoma; other SRBCTs may have similar staining but vastly different treatment and prognosis.
- Focal neuroendocrine marker reactivity is common in sinonasal SRBCTs and should not be mistaken for definitive evidence of a neuroendocrine neoplasm.

ABSTRACT

Although clinical history and morphologic appearance should be the initial considerations when evaluating small round blue cell tumors of the sinonasal tract, the final diagnosis often hinges on immunohistochemical findings. Unfortunately, interpretation of stains in these tumors is fraught with numerous pitfalls and limitations. This article presents an approach to sinonasal small round blue cell tumors based on four common immunohistochemical patterns: cytokeratin positivity, squamous marker positivity, neuroendocrine marker positivity, and cytokeratin negativity.

OVERVIEW

The so-called "small round blue cell tumors" (SRBCT) of the sinonasal tract encompass a wide range of epithelial, mesenchymal, neuroectodermal, and hematolymphoid neoplasms. Recently, the differential diagnosis of these challenging tumors has become even broader with description of several new entities.[1–6] In evaluating SRBCT, such clinical characteristics as age, location, and radiographic appearance can provide important diagnostic clues. Furthermore, the hematoxylin and eosin (H&E) appearance of architectural, cytoplasmic, chromatin, and stromal characteristics can significantly narrow the differential diagnosis.

Disclosures: The authors have no disclosures.
a Department of Pathology, The Johns Hopkins Medical Institutions, 401 North Broadway, Weinberg 2242, Baltimore, MD 21231-2410, USA; b Department of Pathology, The Johns Hopkins Medical Institutions, 401 North Broadway, Weinberg 2249, Baltimore, MD 21231-2410, USA; c Department of Otolaryngology-Head and Neck Surgery, The Johns Hopkins Medical Institutions, 401 North Broadway, Weinberg 2249, Baltimore, MD 21231-2410, USA
* Corresponding author. The Johns Hopkins Medical Institutions, 401 North Broadway, Weinberg 2249, Baltimore, MD 21231-2410.
E-mail address: jbishop@jhmi.edu

Surgical Pathology 10 (2017) 103–123
http://dx.doi.org/10.1016/j.path.2016.10.005

Despite this guidance, diagnosis of SRBCT almost always necessitates performance of immunohisto-chemistry (IHC). In the many cases with limited tissue, extensive crush artifact, nonspecific clinical presentation, or minimal differentiation, a broad panel of stains is often necessary. A reasonable initial work-up for such cases might include pancy-tokeratin, p63 (or p40), synaptophysin, chromogranin, S100, desmin, CD45, and CD99. Although several excellent thematic overviews of SRBTC have recently been published,[7–10] this article approaches this group of tumors as most practicing pathologists will: through the lens of IHC. Here, we discuss subclassification of cytokeratin-positive, squamous marker–positive, neuroendo-crine marker–positive, and cytokeratin-negative sinonasal SRBCT, with particular focus on navigating pitfalls and limitations of each category.

CYTOKERATIN-POSITIVE SMALL ROUND BLUE CELL TUMORS

One of the most important distinctions in sinonasal SRBCTs is between tumors that demonstrate or lack epithelial differentiation. A strict definition of cytokeratin positivity is necessary to accurately separate these groups. Epithelial differentiation is best proven by diffuse, strong positivity for

Differential Diagnosis
CYTOKERATIN-POSITIVE
TUMORS

Consistent pancytokeratin positivity
- Adenoid cystic carcinoma (ACC)

- Adamantinoma-like EFT

- Human papilloma virus (HPV)-related ACC-like carcinoma

- Nonkeratinizing squamous cell carcinoma (SCC)

- Nasopharyngeal carcinomas (NPC)/lymphoe-pithelial-like carcinomas (LELC)

- NUT midline carcinoma

- SMARCB1-deficient carcinoma

- Sinonasal undifferentiated carcinoma (SNUC)

Focal nonspecific pancytokeratin staining

- EFT

- MMM

- ONB

- RMS

pancytokeratins, such as AE1/AE3; expression of low-molecular-weight cytokeratins (LMWCK), such as CAM 5.2, or high-molecular-weight cyto-keratins (HMWCK), such as CK903 or CK5/6, is variable.[8] Although epithelial membrane antigen (EMA) reactivity may support individual diagnoses, EMA expression by itself is not specific for epithelial differentiation. Furthermore, it must be recognized that focal cytokeratin positivity is not sufficient evidence of definitive epithelial origin, because nonepithelial lesions, such as rhabdomyosarcoma (RMS), olfactory neuroblastoma (ONB), Ewing family tumors (EFT), and mucosal malignant mela-nomas (MMM), frequently display patchy reac-tivity.[11,12] This section presents the subset of cytokeratin-positive SRBCT that lack reliable squa-mous or neuroendocrine differentiation.

Pitfalls
CYTOKERATIN-POSITIVE
TUMORS

! Focal reactivity for cytokeratin does not prove epithelial differentiation and can be seen in EFT, MMM, ONB, and RMS

! Although EMA can help confirm certain diag-noses, true cytokeratin positivity is required to prove epithelial differentiation in the sino-nasal tract

! SNUC is a diagnosis of exclusion and should not be made if there is more than focal squa-mous or neuroendocrine reactivity

SINONASAL UNDIFFERENTIATED CARCINOMA

SNUC is an aggressive sinonasal tumor that charac-teristically develops over weeks[13] and causes death within a year of diagnosis.[14,15] SNUC is morpholog-ically and immunohistochemically a diagnosis of exclusion and has become less common with devel-opment of better immunohistochemical markers and description of more specific tumor types. SNUC demonstrates sheets of nondescript malig-nant cells with prominent nucleoli, abundant mitoses, and extensive necrosis (**Fig. 1**). No overt squamous, glandular, or neuroendocrine differentia-tion should be present.[14] SNUC expresses pancyto-keratin and LMWCK but usually not HMWCK.[13,14,16] Although focal reactivity for p40, p63, chromogra-nin, and synaptophysin should not be taken as evi-dence of squamous or neuroendocrine lineage in SNUC, diffuse positivity for any such markers essen-tially negates this diagnosis.[17,18] Nonspecific stain-ing for CD99 has been reported,[19] but SNUC lacks S100 or Epstein-Barr virus (EBV) positivity.[8,14,19]

| | **Key Features** | | |
| | Sɪɴᴏɴᴀsᴀʟ **SRBCT** | | |

Diagnosis	Clinical Clues	H&E Hints	Diagnostic IHC
ACC	Nonspecific	Biphasic cells with cribriforming Basement membrane–like material	Pancytokeratin+ S100+, p63+ in basal cells C-kit+, CK7+ in ductal cells
Adamantinoma-like EFT	More common in children and young adults	Peripheral palisading Basement membrane–like material	Pancytokeratin+, p63+, p40+ Membranous CD99+, NKX2.2+, Fli1+
EFT	More common in children and young adults	Clear cytoplasm	Membranous CD99+ NKX2.2+, Fli1+
HPV-related ACC-like carcinoma	Nonspecific	Biphasic cells with cribriforming Surface squamous dysplasia	Pancytokeratin+ S100+, p63+ in basal cells C-kit+, CK7+ in ductal cells p16, HR HPV in situ hybridization+
Mesenchymal chondrosarcoma	More common in young adults	Central hyaline cartilage Hemangiopericytoma-like vessels	S100+ in cartilage
MMM	Brown/black pigmentation	Melanin pigment Prominent nucleoli	S100+, SOX10+, HMB45+, MelanA+
Natural killer (NK)/ T-cell lymphoma	More common in Asia, Central and South America	Angiocentric and angioinvasive growth	CD56+, CD57+, TIA+ EBV-encoded early RNA+
NUT midline carcinoma	More common in young adults	Foci of abrupt keratinization	Pancytokeratin+, p63+, p40+ NUT1+
Nonkeratinizing SCC	Nonspecific	Focal keratinization	Pancytokeratin+, p63+, p40+ HR HPV variable
NPC/LELC	More common in Southeast Asia and Northeast Africa	Syncytial cells Interspersed lymphocytes	Pancytokeratin+, p63+, p40+ EBV-encoded early RNA+
ONB	Dumbbell-shaped mass at cribriform plate	Lobulated with vascular stroma True rosettes or pseudorosettes	Chromogranin+, synaptophysin+ Sustentacular S100+
Pituitary adenoma	Can produce active hormones	No mitoses	Pancytokeratin+, chromogranin+, synaptophyin+ Prolactin, HGH, ACTH variable
Plasmacytoma	Nonspecific	True plasma cells	CD138+, MUM1+ Kappa or lambda restricted
RMS	More common in children	Rhabdomyoblastic differentiation	Desmin+, myogenin+
Small cell carcinoma	Nonspecific	Nuclear molding High mitotic rate	Dotlike pancytokeratin+ Chromogranin+, synaptophysin+
SMARCB1-deficient CA	Nonspecific	Rhabdoid or plasmacytoid cells	Pancytokeratin+ Loss of INI1
SNUC	Grows over weeks	Nonspecific	Pancytokeratin+

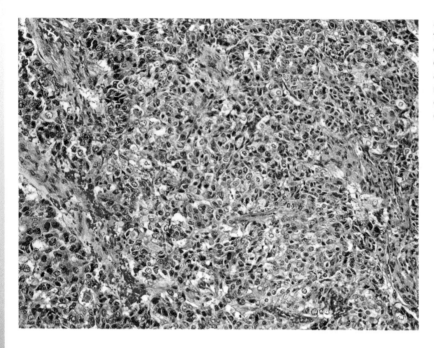

Fig. 1. Sinonasal undifferentiated carcinoma demonstrates sheets of cells with vesicular nuclei and numerous mitoses; no squamous, glandular, or neuroendocrine differentiation is identifiable.

SOLID VARIANT OF ADENOID CYSTIC CARCINOMA

ACC is the most common salivary gland tumor of the sinonasal tract[20,21]; the 10% of tumors that demonstrate predominantly solid architecture are associated with the worst outcomes.[20,22] On H&E, focal areas of cribriform differentiation and distinct ductal (luminal) and basal (myoepithelial) cell populations can suggest ACC (**Fig. 2**). Even in solid ACC, where two cell populations are not evident morphologically, the presence of tumor cells with biphasic immunophenotypes strongly support this diagnosis. Solid ACC typically result from an overgrowth of the ductal cells, which express CK7, c-kit, and EMA. The abluminal basal cells, however, are usually sparse and demonstrate S100, p63, p40, SMA, and calponin.[21,23]

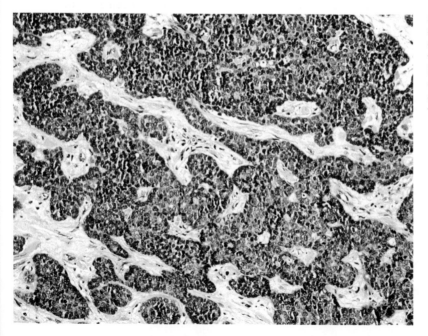

Fig. 2. The solid variant of adenoid cystic carcinoma displays only focal cribriform growth, but a subtle biphasic population of ductal and myoepithelial cells are typically evident throughout.

p63 or Δnp63(p40) positivity in these basal cells should not be considered evidence of squamous differentiation (discussed later).

HUMAN PAPILLOMA VIRUS–RELATED CARCINOMA WITH ADENOID CYSTIC-LIKE FEATURES

One recently described sinonasal carcinoma demonstrates morphology similar to ACC but is strongly HPV-positive.[4] As in conventional ACC, HPV-related carcinoma with ACC-like features demonstrates a dual population of ductal and basal cells with solid and cribriform growth (Fig. 3). This tumor shows squamous dysplasia in the overlying surface epithelium without infiltrating squamous carcinoma.[4] Immunohisto-chemically, HPV-related carcinoma with ACC-like features demonstrates biphasic staining identical to ACC, including CK7 and c-kit positivity in ductal cells and S100, p63, and calponin expression in basal cells.[4] However, these tumors

also are strongly p16 positive by IHC and HPV positive by in situ hybridization (ISH) or polymer-ase chain reaction–based detection methods.[4]

SMARCB1-DEFICIENT CARCINOMA

SMARCB1-deficient carcinoma is another recently described sinonasal tumor that is defined by inactivation of the SMARCB1 (INI1) tumor-suppressor gene.[1,3] Like tumors that share this alteration at other anatomic sites, SMARCB1-deficient sinonasal carcinomas frequently demon-strate rhabdoid or plasmacytoid morphology (Fig. 4). On IHC, SMARCB1-deficient carcinomas are defined by loss of INI1, the protein product of the SMARCB1 gene that is expressed in all normal cells.[1,3,24] These tumors also demonstrate strong and diffuse pancytokeratin positivity. However, SMARCB1-deficient carcinomas display some immunohistochemical heterogeneity, with variable positivity for squamous markers, such as p40 and p63, and neuroendocrine markers, such as chro-mogranin and synaptophysin.[1,3,24]

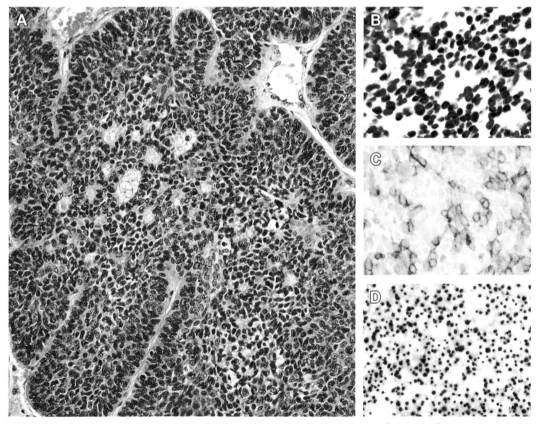

Fig. 3. HPV-related sinonasal carcinoma with adenoid cystic-like features shows a focal cribriform pattern (A). P63 is positive in the myoepithelial-like cells (B), c-kit stains ductal cells (C), and HPV RNA in situ hybridization is diffusely positive (D).

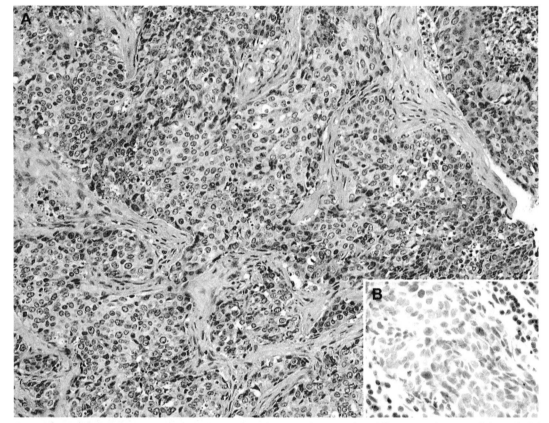

Fig. 4. SMARCB1-deficient sinonasal carcinoma has sheets and nests of undifferentiated eosinophilic cells (*A*) with loss of INI1 expression by immunohistochemistry (*B*).

TUMORS WITH SQUAMOUS MARKER-POSITIVITY

The next main category of sinonasal SRBCT is those that display positivity for squamous markers. Although these tumors are virtually always cytokeratin-positive, HMWCK expression alone is not sufficient to prove squamous differentiation.[25] But even the most specific squamous markers, such as p63 and p40, show cross reactivity with some nonsquamous tumors, requiring alternate lineages to be ruled out. p63 demonstrates varying degrees of expression in SNUC, RMS, ONB, small cell neuroendocrine carcinoma (SCNEC), and extranodal NK/T-cell lymphoma.[17,25,26] The newer antibody p40 demonstrates identical sensitivity and superior sensitivity to p63 but still occasionally stains nonsquamous neoplasms.[18,27] Importantly, p63 and p40 are also markers of basal/myoepithelial differentiation; biphasic staining is seen in salivary tumors, such as ACC, and should not suggest true squamous positivity. Although it is tempting to classify all tumors positive for squamous markers as SCC, this category includes other entities with vastly different treatments and prognoses, and more precise subclassification is essential.

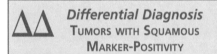

Differential Diagnosis
TUMORS WITH SQUAMOUS MARKER-POSITIVITY

Consistent p63/p40 positivity
- Adamantinoma-like EFT
- Nonkeratinizing SCC
- NPC/LELC
- NUT midline carcinoma

Variable p63/p40 positivity
- ACC (basal cells)
- HPV-related ACC-like (basal cells)
- SMARCB1-deficient carcinoma

Focal nonspecific p63/p40 staining
- NK/T-cell lymphoma
- ONB
- RMS
- SCNEC
- SNUC

Pitfalls
TUMORS WITH SQUAMOUS MARKER POSITIVITY

! P63 demonstrates varying degrees of positivity in NK/T cell lymphoma, ONB, RMS, SCNEC, and SNUC; p40 is more specific for squamous differentiation but not entirely so

! Basal/myoepithelial cells in salivary lesions, such as ACC or HPV-related ACC-like carcinoma, also demonstrate p63/p40 positivity, but ductal cells are negative

! All tumors with true squamous positivity are not SCC; adamantinoma-like EWS, NUT midline carcinoma, and NPC/LELC are essential to distinguish because of vastly different treatment and prognosis

NONKERATINIZING SQUAMOUS CELL CARCINOMA

SCC comprises 40% to 50% of all malignant neoplasms in the sinonasal tract; its behavior is heavily dependent on location and stage at presentation.[28] The nonkeratinizing variant of SCC often falls into the SRBCT category. On H&E, nonkeratinizing SCC is characterized by broad nests and ribbons of atypical cells with a pushing border (**Fig. 5**); despite the name, focal keratinization can support the diagnosis.[28] Nonkeratinizing SCC almost always exhibits diffuse, strong positivity for pancytokeratin, HMWCK, p63, and p40.[16,27] Although HPV has been detected in approximately 20% of nonkeratinizing sinonasal SCC, its implications for treatment and prognosis are unclear at this time.[29] Importantly, p16 is suboptimally specific for HPV outside the oropharynx,

and is not a good surrogate for the presence of high-risk HPV. If HPV testing is performed, a more specific testing method, such as ISH or polymerase chain reaction–based detection, is required.

NASOPHARYNGEAL CARCINOMA/ LYMPHOEPITHELIAL-LIKE CARCINOMA

Although NPC are, by definition, centered on the nasopharynx, they may extend into the sinonasal tract secondarily and are often included in the sinonasal SRBCT differential diagnosis. LELC that appear similar to NPC also rarely can arise as primary sinonasal neoplasms.[30] These tumors are most common in Southeast Asian and Northeast African patients; their exquisite radiosensitivity facilitates 80% to 90% survival even in advanced disease.[31,32] The nonkeratinizing

Fig. 5. Nonkeratinizing squamous cell carcinoma demonstrates broad ribbons of malignant cells without identifiable keratinization.

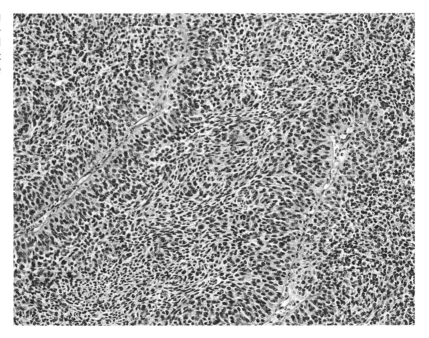

subtype of NPC/LELC is the most likely to fall into the SRBCT spectrum. On H&E, these tumors show a lymphoepithelial pattern, including syncytial cells with vesicular nuclei, prominent nucleoli, and numerous interspersed lymphocytes (**Fig. 6**). NPC/LELC typically demonstrate diffuse strong positivity for pancytokeratin, HMWCK, p63, and p40; LMWCK may only be focally positive.[16,27,30] NPC/LELC are almost always EBV-driven, and EBV-encoded early RNA (EBER) ISH is a helpful means for confirming the diagnosis.[30] Distinguishing NPC extending into the sinonasal tract from a primary LELC requires clinical and radiographic correlation.

NUT MIDLINE CARCINOMA

NUT midline carcinoma is an aggressive tumor that primarily affects young adults and occurs in a wide range of midline sites including the sinonasal tract.[5,6] It is defined by abnormalities in the nuclear protein in testis (NUT) gene, most commonly a t(15;19); BRD4-NUT gene

fusion.[16,33] Although NUT midline carcinoma has a uniformly fatal prognosis, the availability of clinical trials for promising targeted therapies makes specific diagnosis essential.[34] On H&E, NUT midline carcinoma is characterized by primitive small round blue cells that may demonstrate foci of abrupt keratinization (**Fig. 7**). NUT midline carcinoma shows positivity for pancytokeratin, EMA, p63, and p40 in most cases.[5,6,27] Monoclonal NUT1 protein expression by IHC has excellent sensitivity and specificity for NUT midline carcinoma, obviating molecular analysis in most cases.[35]

ADAMANTINOMA-LIKE EWING FAMILY TUMORS

Although EFT is discussed in detail later, divergent complex epithelial differentiation in the adamantinoma-like variant merits separate consideration here. Adamantinoma-like EFT is a sarcoma characterized by the same EWSR1 alterations seen in conventional EFT.[36] However,

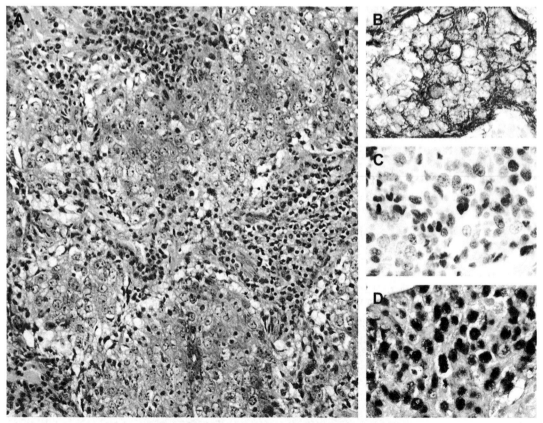

Fig. 6. Nasopharyngeal carcinoma/lymphoepithelial-like carcinoma displays interspersed lymphocytes and syncytial cells with vesicular nuclei (*A*) that are positive for AE1/AE3 (*B*), p40 (*C*), and EBV-encoded early RNA (*D*).

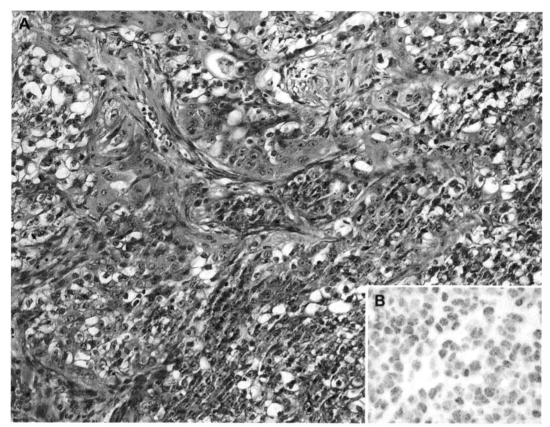

Fig. 7. NUT midline carcinoma grows as sheets of undifferentiated, primitive cells (*A*); NUT1 is diffusely positive in a nuclear distribution (*B*).

it demonstrates well-developed epithelial morphology, including nested architecture with peripheral nuclear palisading, interspersed basement-membrane material, and occasional overt keratinization (**Fig. 8**). Concordantly, adamantinoma-like EFT is diffusely positive for cytokeratin, p63, and p40.[2] Like other EFT, however, these tumors demonstrate strong membranous staining for CD99, occasional synaptophysin and chromogranin positivity, and rare reactivity for S100.[2] Its considerable overlap with carcinomas argues for the inclusion of CD99 in any SRBCT immunohistochemical panel, because it only rarely demonstrates membranous labeling in primary sinonasal carcinomas.[2]

TUMORS WITH NEUROENDOCRINE MARKER POSITIVITY

The category of neuroendocrine-positive sinonasal SRBCT includes cytokeratin-positive and -negative neoplasms and tumors of true neuroendocrine and neuroectodermal lineages.[12,37] Importantly, the only benign tumor in the SRBCT differential, pituitary adenoma (PA), is neuroendocrine marker positive. Appropriate selection and interpretation of IHC is essential to reaching an accurate identification of these tumors. Although historically popular, CD56 and neuron-specific enolase (NSE) are nonspecific markers that should not be used in isolation as evidence of neuroendocrine differentiation.[38] Although synaptophysin and chromogranin are more specific, they still show some cross reactivity with nonneuroendocrine neoplasms. For example, focal chromogranin and synaptophysin staining is commonly seen in SNUC, RMS, and MMM and should not be interpreted as definitive evidence neuroendocrine positivity.[9,38] Furthermore, SMARCB1-deficient carcinomas and EFTs can display variable degrees of synaptophysin and chromogranin expression.

△△ Differential Diagnosis
TUMORS WITH
NEUROENDOCRINE MARKER POSITIVITY

Consistent chromogranin/synaptophysin positivity
- ONB

- PA

- SCNEC

Variable chromogranin/synaptophysin positivity

- EFT

- SMARCB1-deficient carcinoma

Focal nonspecific chromogranin/synaptophysin staining

- MMM

- RMS

- SNUC

! Pitfalls
TUMORS WITH
NEUROENDOCRINE
MARKER POSITIVITY

! CD56 and NSE are expressed in a wide range of SRBCT; determination of true neuroendocrine differentiation should require chromogranin and/or synaptophysin staining

! Focal reactivity for neuroendocrine markers is common in SNUC, RMS, and melanoma and should not be interpreted as neuroendocrine positivity

! All SRBCT with neuroendocrine positivity are not malignant; remember to consider PA in low-grade lesions

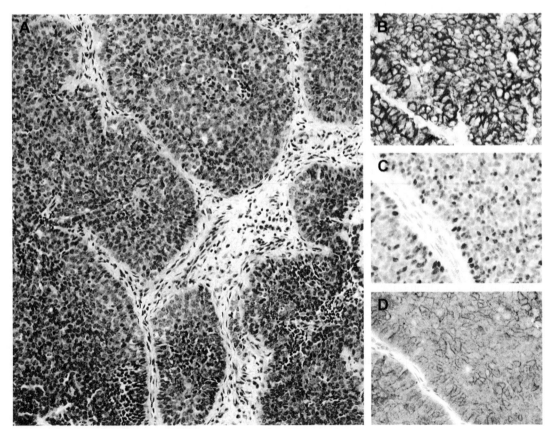

Fig. 8. Adamantinoma-like Ewing family tumor displays nests of cells with peripheral palisading (*A*). Although AE1/AE3 (*B*) and p40 (*C*) are strongly positive, diffuse membranous CD99 staining is evident (*D*).

OLFACTORY NEUROBLASTOMA

ONB originates from the olfactory neuroepithe-lium and creates a characteristic dumbbell-shaped mass across the cribriform plate on imaging.[12] The clinical Kadish stage has tradition-ally dictated ONB outcomes, although histopath-ologic Hyams grading also has some prognostic value.[12,15] Low-grade ONB displays lobules of uniform tumor cells with speckled chromatin, prominent neuropil, and occasional Homer Wright pseudorosettes separated by richly vascular stroma (Fig. 9). In contrast, high-grade tumors demonstrate diffuse growth with true Flexner-Wintersteiner rosettes, minimal neuropil, nuclear pleomorphism, prominent mitoses, and necrosis. ONB classically express synaptophysin and chromogranin with characteristic S100 staining in sustentacular cells lining lobules; this staining pattern is best developed in lower-grade exam-ples. Although occasional ONB show patchy cytokeratin reactivity, they are consistently EMA

negative.[12] Most but not all ONBs are also nega-tive for p63 and p40.[17]

PITUITARY ADENOMA

Although PA is usually an intracranial tumor, up to 2% involve the sinonasal tract by direct exten-sion,[39] and rare cases arise from ectopic pituitary tissue in the sphenoid sinus.[40,41] In contrast to other SRBCTs, PA is fundamentally a benign neoplasm, and a high index of suspicion is neces-sary to avoid misdiagnosis and overtreatment. On H&E, PA is identified by variably nested, trabecular, or glandular arrangements of bland cells with eosinophilic granular cytoplasm, speckled chromatin, and usually no mitotic figures (Fig. 10). PA displays diffuse, or dotlike strong positivity for pancytokeratin and chromogranin and synaptophysin. PA is most likely to be confused with ONB. Because low-grade ONB and PA show considerable histologic overlap, when confronted with this differential diagnosis,

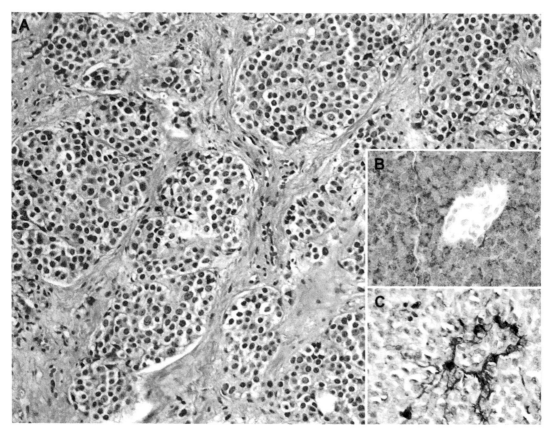

Fig. 9. Olfactory neuroblastoma demonstrates lobules of uniform cells with specked chromatin (*A*). Tumor cells are synaptophysin-positive (*B*), and S100 stains sustentacular cells (*C*).

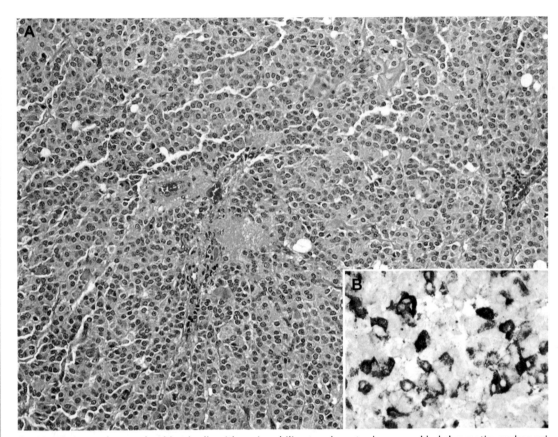

Fig. 10. Pituitary adenoma has bland cells with eosinophilic granular cytoplasm, speckled chromatin, and no mitoses (*A*) that express prolactin (*B*).

location is perhaps the single most important distinguishing feature. ONB usually involve the ethmoid sinus, whereas PA are almost invariably centered in the sphenoid sinus. Immunohistochemically, ONB are far less frequently cytokeratin positive, and demonstrate a well-formed sustentacular layer around nests. Although S100-positive folliculostellate cells (modified glial cells) may be noted in PA, they are uncommon, and when present are more focal and randomly distributed than seen in ONB. Expression of pituitary hormones is inconsistent but when present can confirm the diagnosis, with prolactin staining in 60% of cases.[41]

SMALL CELL CARCINOMA

Although primary neuroendocrine carcinomas are rare in the sinonasal tract, most can be classified as small cell carcinoma. They behave aggressively, with a particular predisposition for intercranial metastases.[42] On H&E, sinonasal small cell carcinoma is indistinguishable from its pulmonary counterpart, with sheets of small to intermediate-sized cells with minimal cytoplasm, hyperchromatic chromatin, nuclear molding, and abundant mitoses (**Fig. 11**). Small cell carcinoma express pancytokeratin and LMWCK with a frequent paranuclear dotlike pattern but are negative for HMWCK.[8] Although neuroendocrine positivity is variable, small cell carcinomas generally demonstrate clear positivity for either synaptophysin or chromogranin.[37] Aberrant weak and/or patchy positivity for p63 is also frequently seen,[25] whereas TTF1 expression seems to be rare in the sinonasal tract small cell carcinomas.[9]

CYTOKERATIN-NEGATIVE TUMORS

The category of cytokeratin-negative SRBCT encompasses melanomas, sarcomas, and hematolymphoid malignancies. EFT, MMM, ONB, and RMS frequently display focal cytokeratin reactivity that should not be interpreted as epithelial differentiation.[11,12] Furthermore, other key markers used to subclassify this group also show cross reactivity. Diffuse S100 positivity is seen not only in MMM, but also in cartilage of mesenchymal chondrosarcoma (MC), basal cells of ACC, and sustentacular cells of ONB.[8,10] Although desmin expression suggests RMS, MMM and MC candemonstrate heterogeneous staining.[43] Even CD99, the pathognomonic marker for EFT, is identified in MC, RMS, and SNUC, although usually not in a diffuse, membranous pattern.[43] Conversely, NK/T-cell lymphoma and plasmacytoma, which show variable CD45 positivity, and the cellular component of MC, which is S100-negative, may be entirely negative on an IHC screening panel.[44,45] Additional specific stains are almost always necessary to prove a diagnosis in this category.

Differential Diagnosis
CYTOKERATIN-NEGATIVE TUMORS

Consistent S100 positivity

• MMM

Variable S100 positivity

• ACC (basal cells)

• HPV-related ACC-like (basal cells)

• MC (cartilage)

• ONB (sustentacular cells)

Consistent desmin positivity

• RMS

Focal nonspecific desmin staining

• MC

• MMM

Consistent CD99 positivity

• Adamantinoma-like EFT

• EFT

Focal nonspecific CD99 staining

• MC

• RMS

• SNUC

Pitfalls
CYTOKERATIN-NEGATIVE TUMORS

! Focal reactivity for cytokeratin does not prove epithelial differentiation and is frequently seen in EFT, MMM, ONB, and RMS

! S100, desmin, and CD99 positivity are not entirely specific for subclassifying cytokeratin-negative sinonasal SRBCT and should be confirmed with additional markers

! MC, NK/T-cell lymphoma, and plasmacytoma can be entirely negative on an initial screening IHC panel

---

MUCOSAL MALIGNANT MELANOMA

The sinonasal tract is one of the most common sites for MMM, a rare and aggressive melanoma subtype with a 5-year survival of just 20%.[46,47] Sinonasal melanoma shares the protean appearance of other melanomas, with variably epithelioid, spindle cell, or small cell histology.[12] Nevertheless, an in situ component can support the diagnosis in up to 80% of cases.[46] Tumor cells frequently demonstrate prominent, cherry-red nucleoli (**Fig. 12**). S100 and SOX10 are the most sensitive markers of MMM, whereas HMB45 and Melan A offer improved specificity.[47,48] In our experience, S100 positivity is variable, and in the setting of an SRBCT where suspicion for MMM is high (eg, prominent nucleoli or pagetoid intraepithelial growth), multiple melanoma markers should be attempted even if S100 is weak or patchy (Bishop JA, unpublished observations). In addition to the aberrant cytokeratin staining previously described, MMM can rarely show heterogeneous staining with desmin, chromogranin, synaptophysin, and calponin.[49,50]

RHABDOMYOSARCOMA

The two most common subtypes of RMS to affect the sinonasal tract are embryonal, which has a relatively good prognosis, and alveolar, which demonstrates aggressive behavior.[51,52] Although RMS more frequently affects children, usually in embryonal form,[51] the alveolar subtype is the most common sinonasal sarcoma in adults and is the most likely to enter into the SRBCT differential diagnosis.[53] The presence of rhabdomyoblastic differentiation with cytoplasmic cross-striations is strongly suggestive of RMS (**Fig. 13**), although this finding is not entirely specific.[54] On IHC, RMS consistently demonstrates positivity for desmin,

116

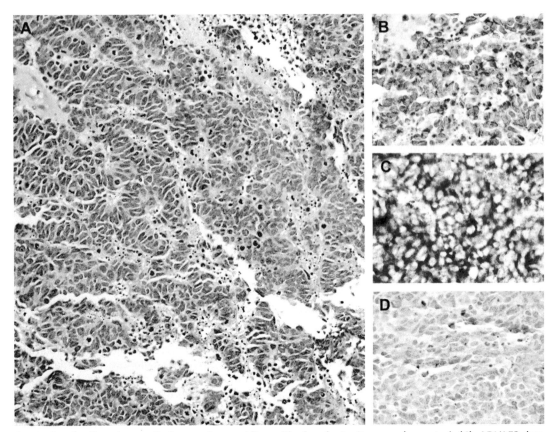

Fig. 11. Small cell carcinoma displays nuclear molding with abundant mitoses and apoptosis (*A*). AE1/AE3 demonstrates dotlike positivity (*B*) with synaptophysin (*C*) and chromogranin staining (*D*).

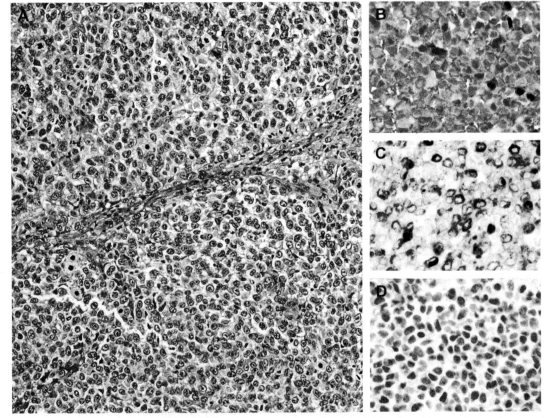

Fig. 12. Sinonasal malignant melanoma demonstrates sheets of epithelioid cells with prominent cherry-red nucleoli (*A*); S100 (*B*), Melan A (*C*), and SOX10 (*D*) are strongly positive.

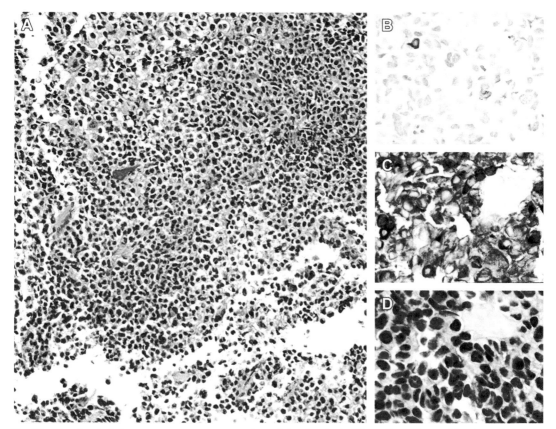

Fig. 13. Alveolar rhabdomyosarcoma grows as nests and sheets of primitive cells, with or without overt rhabdomytoblasts on routine staining (*A*). Rhabdomyosarcoma may exhibit focal AE1/AE3 positivity (*B*), but desmin (*C*) and myogenin (*D*) are strongly and diffusely positive.

myogenin, and MyoD1.[11] RMS is particularly notorious for aberrant immunohistochemical reactivity, with focal pancytokeratin, synaptophysin, and chromogranin straining in 30% to 40%; CD99 staining can also be seen.[43,55,56] A diagnosis of alveolar RMS should be confirmed by molecular testing for *PAX3-FOX01* or *PAX7-FOX01* gene fusions.[11]

EWING FAMILY TUMORS

EFT, previously known as Ewing sarcoma and primitive neuroectodermal tumor, is defined by recurrent fusions involving the *EWSR1* gene, most commonly t(11;22) EWS-FLI1.[12] Sinonasal EFT predominantly occurs in children and young adults and seems to demonstrate better outcomes than other anatomic sites.[57] On H&E, EFT displays lobules and sheets of uniform clear cells with vesicular nuclei (**Fig. 14**). Strong, membranous positivity for CD99 is pathognomonic for EFT[12,58,59]; nuclear expression of newer markers Fli-1 and NKX 2.2 also supports the diagnosis.[60,61]

A significant subset of EFT demonstrates synaptophysin, chromogranin, or LMWCK positivity.[12,57,62] The adamantinoma-like variant is strongly positive for HMWCK and p63. Weak, nonspecific S100 reactivity has also been reported in EFT.[57]

MESENCHYMAL CHONDROSARCOMA

MC is an aggressive subtype of chondrosarcoma that tends to affect young adults and rarely arises in the sinonasal tract.[63] Although overt cartilaginous differentiation is not always present, the entire tumor should be evaluated for diagnostic islands of hyaline cartilage if MC is suspected.[45] MC also displays small round to spindled cells with hemangiopericytoma-like vessels (**Fig. 15**). Unfortunately, the MC immunophenotype does not facilitate easy diagnosis in cases without overt cartilage production. Although the cartilaginous component is generally S100 positive, expression is rarely seen in the cellular component.[64] Moreover, MC frequently shows aberrant desmin,

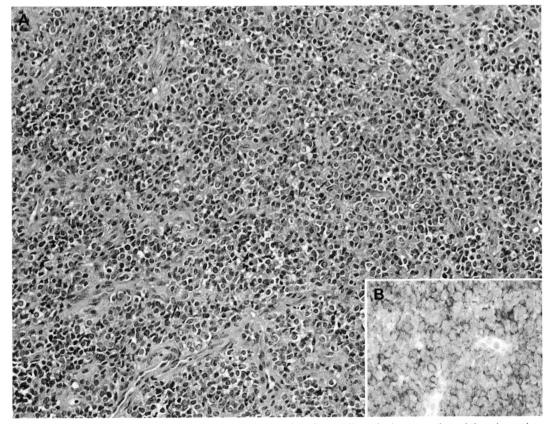

Fig. 14. Ewing family tumors demonstrate vague lobules of uniform cells with clear cytoplasm (*A*) and membranous CD99 positivity (*B*).

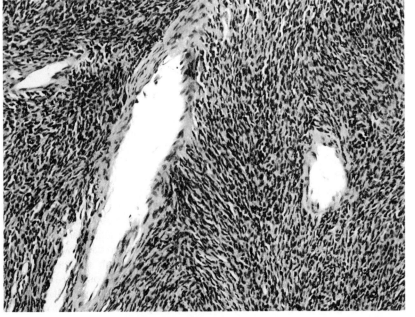

Fig. 15. Mesenchymal chondrosarcoma is a spindled to round cell malignancy with prominent hemangiopericytoma-like blood vessels. The diagnostic finding (not depicted) is foci of well-differentiated cartilage.

EMA, SMA, and CD99 staining.[64,65] SOX9 has been reported as a sensitive and specific marker for MC.[66,67] Recently a recurrent HEY1-NCOA2 gene fusion has been described in MC and may show promise as a diagnosis-defining marker[68]

EXTRANODAL NK/T-CELL LYMPHOMA, NASAL TYPE

Extranodal NK/T-cell lymphoma, nasal type, is an aggressive subtype of lymphoma that is most commonly encountered in Asia and Central and South America.[44] The key morphologic feature of this neoplasm is angiocentric and angioinvasive growth with associated fibrinoid necrosis (Fig. 16); variable cellularity and associated mixed inflammation can cause overlap with inflammatory processes and SRBCT. NK/T cell lymphomas are well-established to be EBV-driven and should be EBER-positive.[44] Most arise from activated NK cells and therefore express CD56, CD57, cytoplasmic CD3, TIA1, granzyme, and perforin[69]; CD45 is positive in most but not all cases.[44] They are generally negative for T-cell markers, such as surface CD3, CD4, CD5, and CD8.[69]

PLASMACYTOMA

The sinonasal tract is the most common site of solitary extramedullary plasmacytomas, comprising approximately 75% of such lesions.[70] These tumors are much less likely to progress to systemic myeloma than plasmacytomas of bone and respond well to radiation therapy.[71] In many cases, plasmacytic morphology is apparent on H&E (Fig. 17), and the chief diagnostic consideration is a florid inflammatory process. However, poorly differentiated or badly preserved tumors fall into the SRBCT spectrum. Plasmacytomas should demonstrate positivity with CD138 and MUM1, and kappa or lambda light-chain restriction; CD45 staining is variable.[71] Although plasmacytomas are cytokeratin-negative, positivity for EMA is a well-recognized pitfall that should not be interpreted as evidence of epithelial differentiation.[44]

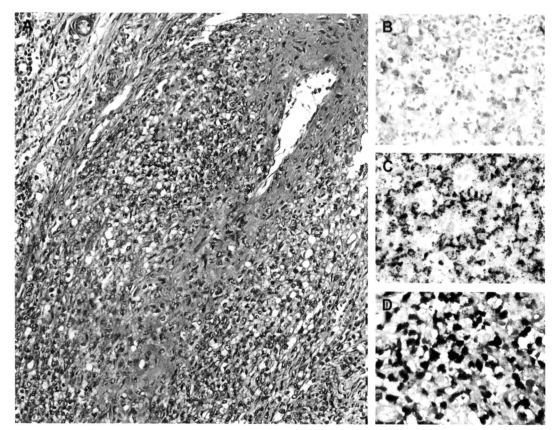

Fig. 16. NK-T cell lymphoma displays angioinvasive growth with fibrinoid necrosis (A). Tumor cells are positive for CD56 (B), TIA (C), and EBER (D).

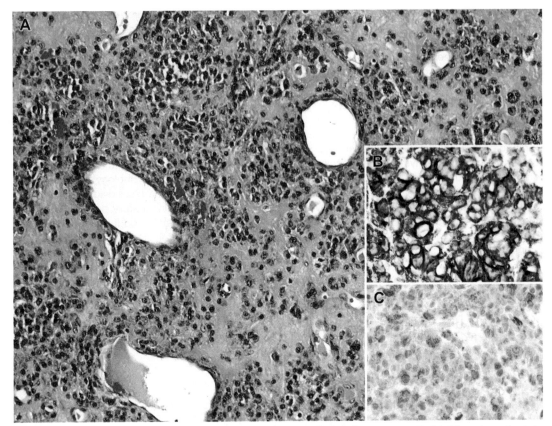

Fig. 17. Plasmacytoma demonstrates discohesive plasmacytic cells (*A*) that express CD138 (*B*) and are lambda-restricted (*C*).

REFERENCES

1. Agaimy A, Koch M, Lell M, et al. SMARCB1(INI1)-deficient sinonasal basaloid carcinoma: a novel member of the expanding family of SMARCB1-deficient neoplasms. Am J Surg Pathol 2014;38(9):1274–81.

2. Bishop JA, Alaggio R, Zhang L, et al. Adamantinoma-like Ewing family tumors of the head and neck: a pitfall in the differential diagnosis of basaloid and myoepithelial carcinomas. Am J Surg Pathol 2015;39(9):1267–74.

3. Bishop JA, Antonescu CR, Westra WH. SMARCB1 (INI-1)-deficient carcinomas of the sinonasal tract. Am J Surg Pathol 2014;38(9):1282–9.

4. Bishop JA, Ogawa T, Stelow EB, et al. Human papillomavirus-related carcinoma with adenoid cystic-like features: a peculiar variant of head and neck cancer restricted to the sinonasal tract. Am J Surg Pathol 2013;37(6):836–44.

5. Syed R, Bishop JA, Ali SZ. Sacral and presacral lesions: cytopathologic analysis and clinical correlates. Diagn Cytopathol 2012;40(1):7–13.

6. Stelow EB, Bellizzi AM, Taneja K, et al. NUT rearrangement in undifferentiated carcinomas of the upper aerodigestive tract. Am J Surg Pathol 2008;32(6):828–34.

7. Bridge JA, Bowen JM, Smith RB. The small round blue cell tumors of the sinonasal area. Head Neck Pathol 2010;4(1):84–93.

8. Franchi A, Palomba A, Cardesa A. Current diagnostic strategies for undifferentiated tumours of the nasal cavities and paranasal sinuses. Histopathology 2011;59(6):1034–45.

9. Montone KT. The differential diagnosis of sinonasal/nasopharyngeal neuroendocrine/neuroectodermally derived tumors. Arch Pathol Lab Med 2015;139(12):1498–507.

10. Simons SA, Bridge JA, Leon ME. Sinonasal small round blue cell tumors: an approach to diagnosis. Semin Diagn Pathol 2016;33(2):91–103.

11. Thompson LDR, Fanburg-Smith JC. Malignant soft tissue tumours. In: Barnes L, Eveson JW, Reichart P, International Agency for Research on Cancer, et al, editors. Pathology and genetics of head and neck tumours. Lyon (France): IARC; 2005. p. 430.

12. Wenig BM, Dulguerov P, Kapadia SB, et al. Neuroectodermal tumours. In: Barnes L, Eveson JW, Reichart P, International Agency for Research on Cancer, et al, editors. Pathology and genetics of head and neck tumours. Lyon (France): IARC; 2005. p. 430.

13. Houston GD, Gillies E. Sinonasal undifferentiated carcinoma: a distinctive clinicopathologic entity. Adv Anat Pathol 1999;6(6):317–23.

14. Frierson HF Jr. Sinonasal undifferentiated carcinoma. In: Barnes L, Eveson JW, Reichart P, International Agency for Research on Cancer, et al, editors. Pathology and genetics of head and neck tumours. Lyon (France): IARC; 2005. p. 430.

15. Miyamoto RC, Gleich LL, Biddinger PW, et al. Esthesioneuroblastoma and sinonasal undifferentiated carcinoma: impact of histological grading and clinical staging on survival and prognosis. Laryngoscope 2000;110(8):1262–5.

16. Franchi A, Moroni M, Massi D, et al. Sinonasal undifferentiated carcinoma, nasopharyngeal-type undifferentiated carcinoma, and keratinizing and nonkeratinizing squamous cell carcinoma express different cytokeratin patterns. Am J Surg Pathol 2002;26(12):1597–604.

17. Bourne TD, Bellizzi AM, Stelow EB, et al. p63 Expression in olfactory neuroblastoma and other small cell tumors of the sinonasal tract. Am J Clin Pathol 2008;130(2):213–8.

18. Singh L, Ranjan R, Arava S, et al. Role of p40 and cytokeratin 5/6 in the differential diagnosis of sinonasal undifferentiated carcinoma. Ann Diagn Pathol 2014;18(5):261–5.

19. Cerilli LA, Holst VA, Brandwein MS, et al. Sinonasal undifferentiated carcinoma: immunohistochemical profile and lack of EBV association. Am J Surg Pathol 2001;25(2):156–63.

20. Batsakis JG, Luna MA, el-Naggar A. Histopathologic grading of salivary gland neoplasms. III. Adenoid cystic carcinomas. Ann Otol Rhinol Laryngol 1990; 99(12):1007–9.

21. Eveson JW. Salivary gland-type carcinomas. In: Barnes L, Eveson JW, Reichart P, International Agency for Research on Cancer, et al, editors. Pathology and genetics of head and neck tumours. Lyon (France): IARC; 2005. p. 430.

22. Thompson LD, Penner C, Ho NJ, et al. Sinonasal tract and nasopharyngeal adenoid cystic carcinoma: a clinicopathologic and immunophenotypic study of 86 cases. Head Neck Pathol 2014;8(1): 88–109.

23. Rooper L, Sharma R, Bishop JA. Polymorphous low grade adenocarcinoma has a consistent p63+/p40-immunophenotype that helps distinguish it from adenoid cystic carcinoma and cellular pleomorphic adenoma. Head Neck Pathol 2015;9(1):79–84.

24. Bell D, Hanna EY, Agaimy A, et al. Reappraisal of sinonasal undifferentiated carcinoma: SMARCB1 (INI1)-deficient sinonasal carcinoma: a single-institution experience. Virchows Arch 2015;467(6): 649–56.

25. Serrano MF, El-Mofty SK, Gnepp DR, et al. Utility of high molecular weight cytokeratins, but not p63, in the differential diagnosis of neuroendocrine and basaloid carcinomas of the head and neck. Hum Pathol 2008;39(4):591–8.

26. Ye Z, Cao Q, Niu G, et al. p63 and p53 expression in extranodal NK/T cell lymphoma, nasal type. J Clin Pathol 2013;66(8):676–80.

27. Tilson MP, Bishop JA. Utility of p40 in the differential diagnosis of small round blue cell tumors of the sinonasal tract. Head Neck Pathol 2014;8(2):141–5.

28. Pilch BZ, Bouquot JE, Thompson LDR. Squamous cell carcinoma. In: Barnes L, Eveson JW, Reichart P, International Agency for Research on Cancer, et al, editors. Pathology and genetics of head and neck tumours. Lyon (France): IARC; 2005. p. 430.

29. Lewis JS, Westra WH, Thompson LD, et al. The sinonasal tract: another potential "hot spot" for carcinomas with transcriptionally-active human papillomavirus. Head Neck Pathol 2014;8(3):241–9.

30. Tsang WYW, Chan JKC. Lymphoepithelial carcinoma. In: Barnes L, Eveson JW, Reichart P, International Agency for Research on Cancer, et al, editors. Pathology and genetics of head and neck tumours. Lyon (France): IARC; 2005. p. 430.

31. Lee N, Harris J, Garden AS, et al. Intensity-modulated radiation therapy with or without chemotherapy for nasopharyngeal carcinoma: radiation therapy oncology group phase II trial 0225. J Clin Oncol 2009;27(22):3684–90.

32. Tham IW, Hee SW, Yeo RM, et al. Treatment of nasopharyngeal carcinoma using intensity-modulated radiotherapy: the National Cancer Centre Singapore experience. Int J Radiat Oncol Biol Phys 2009;75(5): 1481–6.

33. Vargas SO, French CA, Faul PN, et al. Upper respiratory tract carcinoma with chromosomal translocation 15;19: evidence for a distinct disease entity of young patients with a rapidly fatal course. Cancer 2001;92(5):1195–203.

34. Stathis A, Zucca E, Bekradda M, et al. Clinical response of carcinomas harboring the BRD4-NUT oncoprotein to the targeted bromodomain inhibitor OTX015/MK-8628. Cancer Discov 2016; 6(5):492–500.

35. Haack H, Johnson LA, Fry CJ, et al. Diagnosis of NUT midline carcinoma using a NUT-specific monoclonal antibody. Am J Surg Pathol 2009;33(7): 984–91.

36. Bridge JA, Fidler ME, Neff JR, et al. Adamantinoma-like Ewing's sarcoma: genomic confirmation, phenotypic drift. Am J Surg Pathol 1999;23(2):159–65.

37. Perez-Ordonez B. Neuroendocrine tumors. In: Barnes L, Eveson JW, Reichart P, International Agency

for Research on Cancer, et al, editors. Pathology and genetics of head and neck tumours. Lyon (France): IARC; 2005. p. 430.

38. Bell D, Hanna EY, Weber RS, et al. Neuroendocrine neoplasms of the sinonasal region. Head Neck 2016;38(Suppl 1):E2259–66.

39. Cole IE, Keene M. Nasal obstruction in pituitary tumours. J Laryngol Otol 1981;95(2):183–9.

40. Luk IS, Chan JK, Chow SM, et al. Pituitary adenoma presenting as sinonasal tumor: pitfalls in diagnosis. Hum Pathol 1996;27(6):605–9.

41. Thompson LD, Seethala RR, Muller S. Ectopic sphenoid sinus pituitary adenoma (ESSPA) with normal anterior pituitary gland: a clinicopathologic and immunophenotypic study of 32 cases with a comprehensive review of the English literature. Head Neck Pathol 2012;6(1):75–100.

42. Rosenthal DI, Barker JL Jr, El-Naggar AK, et al. Sinonasal malignancies with neuroendocrine differentiation: patterns of failure according to histologic phenotype. Cancer 2004;101(11):2567–73.

43. Magro G, Longo FR, Angelico G, et al. Immunohistochemistry as potential diagnostic pitfall in the most common solid tumors of children and adolescents. Acta Histochem 2015;117(4–5):397–414.

44. Chan ACL, Chan JKC, Cheung MMC, et al. Hematolymphoid tumours. In: Barnes L, Eveson JW, Reichart P, International Agency for Research on Cancer, et al, editors. Pathology and genetics of head and neck tumours. Lyon (France): IARC; 2005. p. 430.

45. Saito K, Unni KK. Malignant tumours of bone and cartilage. In: Barnes L, Eveson JW, Reichart P, International Agency for Research on Cancer, et al, editors. Pathology and genetics of head and neck tumours. Lyon (France): IARC; 2005. p. 430.

46. Mochel MC, Duncan LM, Piris A, et al. Primary mucosal melanoma of the sinonasal tract: a clinicopathologic and immunohistochemical study of thirty-two cases. Head Neck Pathol 2015;9(2): 236–43.

47. Thompson LD, Wieneke JA, Miettinen M. Sinonasal tract and nasopharyngeal melanomas: a clinicopathologic study of 115 cases with a proposed staging system. Am J Surg Pathol 2003;27(5): 594–611.

48. Miettinen M, McCue PA, Sarlomo-Rikala M, et al. Sox10–a marker for not only schwannian and melanocytic neoplasms but also myoepithelial cell tumors of soft tissue: a systematic analysis of 5134 tumors. Am J Surg Pathol 2015;39(6):826–35.

49. Lee H, Torres FX, McLean SA, et al. Immunophenotypic heterogeneity of primary sinonasal melanoma with aberrant expression of neuroendocrine markers and calponin. Appl Immunohistochem Mol Morphol 2011;19(1):48–53.

50. Smith SM, Schmitt AC, Carrau RL, et al. Primary sinonasal mucosal melanoma with aberrant diffuse and strong desmin reactivity: a potential diagnostic pitfall! Head Neck Pathol 2015;9(1):165–71.

51. Maurer HM, Gehan EA, Beltangady M, et al. The Intergroup Rhabdomyosarcoma Study-II. Cancer 1993;71(5):1904–22.

52. Simon JH, Paulino AC, Smith RB, et al. Prognostic factors in head and neck rhabdomyosarcoma. Head Neck 2002;24(5):468–73.

53. Szablewski V, Neuville A, Terrier P, et al. Adult sinonasal soft tissue sarcoma: analysis of 48 cases from the French sarcoma group database. Laryngoscope 2015;125(3):615–23.

54. Bishop JA, Thompson LD, Cardesa A, et al. Rhabdomyoblastic differentiation in head and neck malignancies other than rhabdomyosarcoma. Head Neck Pathol 2015;9(4):507–18.

55. Bahrami A, Gown AM, Baird GS, et al. Aberrant expression of epithelial and neuroendocrine markers in alveolar rhabdomyosarcoma: a potentially serious diagnostic pitfall. Mod Pathol 2008; 21(7):795–806.

56. Yasuda T, Perry KD, Nelson M, et al. Alveolar rhabdomyosarcoma of the head and neck region in older adults: genetic characterization and a review of the literature. Hum Pathol 2009;40(3):341–8.

57. Hafezi S, Seethala RR, Stelow EB, et al. Ewing's family of tumors of the sinonasal tract and maxillary bone. Head Neck Pathol 2011;5(1):8–16.

58. Folpe AL, Goldblum JR, Rubin BP, et al. Morphologic and immunophenotypic diversity in Ewing family tumors: a study of 66 genetically confirmed cases. Am J Surg Pathol 2005;29(8):1025–33.

59. Llombart-Bosch A, Machado I, Navarro S, et al. Histological heterogeneity of Ewing's sarcoma/PNET: an immunohistochemical analysis of 415 genetically confirmed cases with clinical support. Virchows Arch 2009;455(5):397–411.

60. Hung YP, Fletcher CD, Hornick JL. Evaluation of NKX2-2 expression in round cell sarcomas and other tumors with EWSR1 rearrangement: imperfect specificity for Ewing sarcoma. Mod Pathol 2016; 29(4):370–80.

61. Lee AF, Hayes MM, Lebrun D, et al. FLI-1 distinguishes Ewing sarcoma from small cell osteosarcoma and mesenchymal chondrosarcoma. Appl Immunohistochem Mol Morphol 2011; 19(3):233–8.

62. Gu M, Antonescu CR, Guiter G, et al. Cytokeratin immunoreactivity in Ewing's sarcoma: prevalence in 50 cases confirmed by molecular diagnostic studies. Am J Surg Pathol 2000;24(3):410–6.

63. Knott PD, Gannon FH, Thompson LD. Mesenchymal chondrosarcoma of the sinonasal tract: a clinicopathological study of 13 cases with a review of the literature. Laryngoscope 2003;113(5):783–90.

64. Hoang MP, Suarez PA, Donner LR, et al. Mesenchymal chondrosarcoma: a small cell neoplasm

with polyphenotypic differentiation. Int J Surg Pathol 2000;8(4):291–301.

65. Gengler C, Letovanec I, Taminelli L, et al. Desmin and myogenin reactivity in mesenchymal chondrosarcoma: a potential diagnostic pitfall. Histopathology 2006;48(2):201–3.

66. Fanburg-Smith JC, Auerbach A, Marwaha JS, et al. Reappraisal of mesenchymal chondrosarcoma: novel morphologic observations of the hyaline cartilage and endochondral ossification and beta-catenin, Sox9, and osteocalcin immunostaining of 22 cases. Hum Pathol 2010;41(5):653–62.

67. Wehrli BM, Huang W, De Crombrugghe B, et al. Sox9, a master regulator of chondrogenesis, distinguishes mesenchymal chondrosarcoma from other small blue round cell tumors. Hum Pathol 2003; 34(3):263–9.

68. Wang L, Motoi T, Khanin R, et al. Identification of a novel, recurrent HEY1-NCOA2 fusion in mesenchymal chondrosarcoma based on a genome-wide screen of exon-level expression data. Genes Chromosomes Cancer 2012;51(2):127–39.

69. Hong M, Lee T, Young Kang S, et al. Nasal-type NK/T-cell lymphomas are more frequently T rather than NK lineage based on T-cell receptor gene, RNA, and protein studies: lineage does not predict clinical behavior. Mod Pathol 2016;29(5):430–43.

70. Wax MK, Yun KJ, Omar RA. Extramedullary plasmacytomas of the head and neck. Otolaryngol Head Neck Surg 1993;109(5):877–85.

71. Hotz MA, Schwaab G, Bosq J, et al. Extramedullary solitary plasmacytoma of the head and neck. A clinicopathological study. Ann Otol Rhinol Laryngol 1999;108(5):495–500.

Inflammatory and Infectious Lesions of the Sinonasal Tract

Kathleen T. Montone, MD*, Virginia A. LiVolsi, MD

KEYWORDS

- Sinonasal • Rhinosinusitis • Vasculitis • Midline destructive disease

---

Key points

- The sinonasal tract is affected by a variety of nonneoplastic inflammatory diseases, which may be infectious, inflammatory, or autoimmune in origin.

- The differential diagnosis of granulomatous disease of the sinonasal tract includes infection (bacterial, mycobacterial, fungal, parasitic), vasculitic disease, sarcoidosis, cocaine-induced injury, and idiopathic disease.

- Sinonasal fungal disease comprises a spectrum of diseases in which fungi are noninvasive or invasive. Allergic fungal rhinosinusitis is not a fungal infection but an inflammatory reaction to fungi in the sinonasal tract.

- The end result of many sinonasal inflammatory processes is destruction of the midline, resulting in facial deformity.

ABSTRACT

The sinonasal tract is frequently affected by nonneoplastic inflammatory diseases. Inflammatory lesions of the sinonasal tract can be divided into 3 main categories: chronic rhinosinusitis, which encompasses a heterogeneous group of entities, all of which result in mucosal inflammation with or without polyps-eosinophils; infectious diseases; and autoimmune diseases and vasculitides, which can result in midline necrosis and facial deformities. This article reviews the common inflammatory lesions of the sinonasal tract with emphasis on infectious diseases, vasculitis, iatrogenic, and diseases of unknown cause. Many of these lesions can result in midline destruction and result in facial deformity.

OVERVIEW

The sinonasal tract is frequently affected by a variety of nonneoplastic inflammatory diseases. Inflammatory lesions of the sinonasal tract can be divided into 3 main categories:

1. Chronic rhinosinusitis (CRS), which encompasses a heterogeneous group of entities, all of which result in mucosal inflammation with or without polyps-eosinophils
2. Infectious diseases
3. Autoimmune diseases and vasculitides, which can result in midline necrosis and facial deformities

This article focuses on a variety of nonneoplastic inflammatory diseases of the sinonasal tract (**Box 1**).

Disclosure Statement: The authors have nothing to disclose.
Department of Pathology and Laboratory Medicine, Hospital of the University of Pennsylvania, 3400 Spruce Street, 6 Founders, Philadelphia, PA 19104, USA
* Corresponding author.
E-mail address: Kathleen.Montone@uphs.upenn.edu

surgpath.theclinics.com

CHRONIC RHINOSINUSITIS

INTRODUCTION

Rhinosinusitis can be classified as acute (symptoms for <1 month), subacute (symptoms between 1 and 3 months), and chronic (symptoms >3 months).

Acute rhinosinusitis is usually the result of an infection or allergic process and often does not generate a pathologic specimen. Persistent acute rhinosinusitis develops into a chronic process. CRS comprises a mixture of diseases all of which lead to obstruction and mucosal inflammation.[1,2] The pathogenesis of CRS is multifactorial, with infectious, genetic, and environmental exposures all thought to be important factors.[1–3]

GROSS DESCRIPTION

The mucosa in CRS may appear thickened and edematous. Polypoid changes may be noted. There is often a lack of correlation between the clinical symptoms and the gross (as well as microscopic) pathology.

MICROSCOPIC DESCRIPTION

On histology, CRS is characterized by submucosal edema and a mixed inflammatory infiltrate consisting of lymphocytes, plasma cells, eosinophils, histiocytes, and rare neutrophils (**Fig. 1**). Recent studies have identified Rosai-Dorfman–histiocytes in some patients with CRS.[4] Fibrosis is often not seen with the exception of those undergoing repeat surgery. The surface mucosa may show squamous metaplasia and, in long-standing cases, there may be goblet cell hyperplasia, mucosal thickening, and papillary hyperplasia of the mucosa. As mentioned earlier, the histologic features do not always correlate with the severity of the clinical symptoms.

DIFFERENTIAL DIAGNOSIS

Most cases of CRS are nonspecific but histologic examination may confirm a definitive cause like specific infectious agents or autoimmune diseases. Other entities in the differential diagnosis of CRS include sinonasal inflammatory polyps (which are often found in patients with CRS) and epithelial neoplasms (particularly in the presence of mucosal hyperplasia).

DIAGNOSIS

The diagnosis of CRS is based predominantly on clinical findings. Patients present with symptoms of nasal stuffiness/blockage, headache, and rhinorrhea of more than 3 months' duration. Pathologic examination is not needed for clinical diagnosis but cases that do not respond to conservative therapy often require functional endoscopic sinus surgery (FESS). Tissue removed during these procedures should be examined in its entirety to rule out other causes of CRS symptoms, such as specific infections, vasculitides, and neoplasms. Although the cause of CRS is not completely understood, it is not surprising that infection, including bacterial and fungal, has been implicated in the pathogenesis.[1–3,5–8] A genetic basis for CRS is supported by familial tendencies as well as the association of CRS with genetic syndromes such as cystic fibrosis (CF).[1–3,9,10]

Fig. 1. CRS characterized by the presence of submucosal fibrosis, eosinophils, and lymphocytes (hematoxylin-eosin; original magnification ×100).

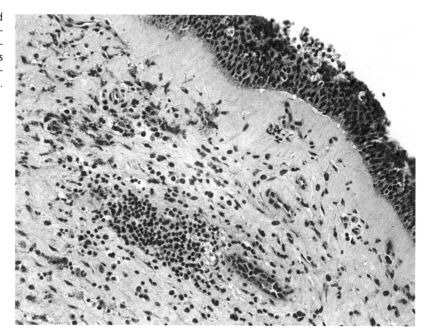

PROGNOSIS

CRS results in billions of dollars in health care costs each year. CRS represents a mixture of entities and the treatment depends on the underlying cause, which may or may not be able to be determined. Treatment options include medical therapy, such as long-term antibiotics (which may or may not be successful), and intranasal steroids. Patients who fail conservative therapy undergo FESS, which may need to be repeated multiple times before symptoms abate. The presence of Rosai-Dorfman histiocytes was associated with disease recurrence in a recent study.

SINONASAL INFLAMMATORY POLYPS

INTRODUCTION

Sinonasal inflammatory polyps (SNPs) are non-neoplastic exophytic growths in the sinonasal tract characterized by submucosal edema and inflammation. They are commonly seen in adults and are uncommon in young children, with the exception of children with CF who are at increased risk for polyps.[1,3,11] Individuals who are heterozygous for CF have increased incidence of CRS and SNPs and mutations in the CF gene (CF transmembrane regulator) have been found in patients with SNPs.[3,11] Patients with SNPs usually present with nasal obstruction and rhinorrhea. SNPs are common features of CRS, allergic rhinitis, infectious diseases, aspirin sensitivity syndrome,

allergic fungal rhinosinusitis (AFRS), and CF. A special type of SNP is the antrochoanal polyp, which is a polyp that arises in the maxillary sinus and grows posteriorly through the nasal choana to reach the nasopharynx/nasal cavity.

GROSS FEATURES

Sinonasal polyps may occur singly or multiply and may be unilateral or bilateral. They most commonly arise from the lateral nasal wall. Polyps are often myxoid, soft, and fleshy, and can grow to a size of several centimeters. Antrochoanal polyps have a similar gross appearance to SNPs with the exception of the presence of a stalk attachment to the maxillary sinus, and they are usually unilateral.

MICROSCOPIC FEATURES

On histology, SNPs are characterized by the presence of polypoid sinonasal surface mucosa with expansion of the submucosa by edema and inflammation, which usually consists of lymphocytes and plasma cells with or without eosinophils (**Fig. 2**). Submucosal glands are few to absent and the stroma may be fibrotic. The overlying mucosa is usually intact and respiratory, although squamous metaplasia (and very rarely dysplasia) may be present. Occasionally, the mucosa shows ulceration and lesions may infarct. SNPs may show glandular hyperplasia, fibrosis, infarction, and granulation tissue. The polyp stroma may

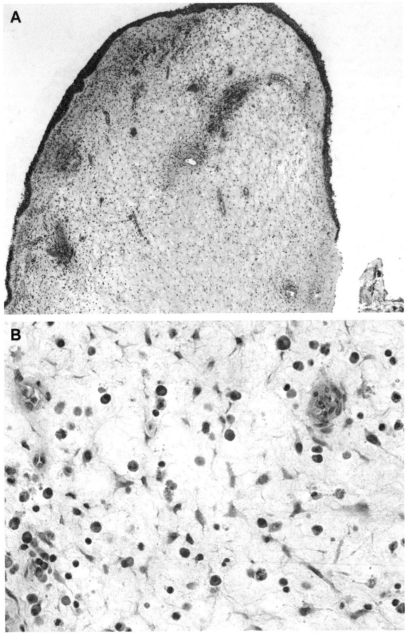

Fig. 2. Sinonasal inflammatory polyp. (*A*) Low-power view of sinonasal inflammatory polyp showing intact sinonasal mucosa and edematous, and inflamed stroma devoid of submucosal glands (hematoxylin-eosin; original magnification ×50). (*B*) Higher power shows stromal edema and mixed inflammation consisting of lymphocytes, plasma cells, and eosinophils (hematoxylin-eosin; original magnification ×200).

become hyalinized and confused with amyloid. The stroma may show enlarged atypical stromal cells (myofibroblasts), which should not be confused with malignancy.

DIFFERENTIAL DIAGNOSIS

The differential diagnosis of SNPs is broad because many disease entities, particularly infectious diseases, may produce polypoid mucosal changes. The stroma may be vascular, which can be confused with hemangiomas, and sclerotic/hyalinized, which can be confused with amyloid. Rarely, inverted papillomas may be polypoid, hence the importance of extensive histologic sampling of SNPs for microscopic examination. In SNPs with stromal cell atypia, the possibility of rhabdomyosarcoma (RMS) or other types of spindle cell malignancies can be entertained.

DIAGNOSIS

Many entities in the sinonasal tract may present in a polypoid fashion so the diagnosis of SNPs is made on histopathologic examination and exclusion, if necessary, of those lesions in the differential diagnosis described earlier. The best practice is to examine all material received because polypoid masses may harbor infectious causes, vasculitic processes, and unexpected benign and malignant neoplasms. For lesions with hyalinized stroma, Congo red to exclude amyloid may be needed. Care must be taken to evaluate the epithelium in SNPs, particularly because some inverted papillomas may present unexpectedly as polypoid masses. For lesions with stromal cell atypia, RMS may need to be excluded. However, the atypical stromal cells in SNPs have low nuclear to cytoplasmic ratios and lack atypical mitoses. Immunohistochemistry for desmin and myogenin (which are positive in RMS) may be useful in difficult cases. A genetic predisposition to nasal polyps has been reported.[1,3,11–15] DNA microarray technology has shown differential expression of several genes in CRS with and without polyps. Most of the up-regulated genes and their products seem to be related to inflammatory and immune-modulated responses.

PROGNOSIS

SNPs are treated effectively with surgery and also by treating the underlying condition, if possible, to prevent recurrence. Recurrences are common, particularly for those lesions that have been incompletely resected.

ASPIRIN SENSITIVITY SYNDROME

INTRODUCTION

About 15% of patients with SNPs have aspirin sensitivity syndrome; an under-recognized clinical entity characterized by the triad of adult-onset asthma, nasal polyps, and sensitivity to aspirin or other nonsteroidal antiinflammatory drugs (NSAIDs) (Samter triad).[1,16] The condition can present at any age but is usually seen in young adults. Following ingestion of aspirin (or other NSAIDs), affected individuals develop difficulty breathing and rhinorrhea. The pathogenesis is not thought to be allergic because patients already have CRS symptoms, but the symptoms are worsened following aspirin (or other NSAID) use.

GROSS FEATURES

Grossly patients present with nasal polyps, which are commonly bilateral, and the other findings associated with CRS.

MICROSCOPIC FEATURES

On histology, the sinonasal mucosa from patients with aspirin sensitivity shows severe chronic inflammation with numerous eosinophils and sinonasal inflammatory polyp formation (**Fig. 3**A, B). Allergic mucin (AM), without fungal elements, is a common feature[17] (**Fig. 3**C).

DIFFERENTIAL DIAGNOSIS

The diagnosis is based on the clinical history. Without clinical history, the histologic findings seen in aspirin sensitivity resemble those seen in allergic rhinitis. In addition, the presence of AM should alert the pathologist to a possible diagnosis of AFRS and requires histochemical stains for fungi.

DIAGNOSIS

The diagnosis of aspirin sensitivity is based on the clinical findings of nasal polyps, asthma, and significant exacerbation of CRS symptoms following use of aspirin or other NSAIDs. The pathogenesis is poorly understood but it is thought to be caused by a defect in the arachidonic acid cascade leading to overproduction of leukotrienes, especially cysteinyl leukotriene, which is a mediator of inflammation and is associated with increased survival of eosinophils.[3] There seems to be a genetic predisposition to aspirin sensitivity syndrome.[3,18–21]

PROGNOSIS

Aspirin sensitivity has a poor response to corticosteroids and a progressive clinical course with worsening of asthma and CRS.

SINONASAL TRACT INFECTIONS

BACTERIAL

Rhinoscleroma (Klebsiella rhinoscleromatis)

Introduction
Rhinoscleroma (RS) is a chronic, self-limited, granulomatous disease that involves the upper respiratory tract. The disease is caused by *Klebsiella rhinoscleromatis*, a gram-negative organism that is rare in the United States but is more commonly seen in Central America, Africa, India, and Indonesia.[22–26] The disease is contracted by direct

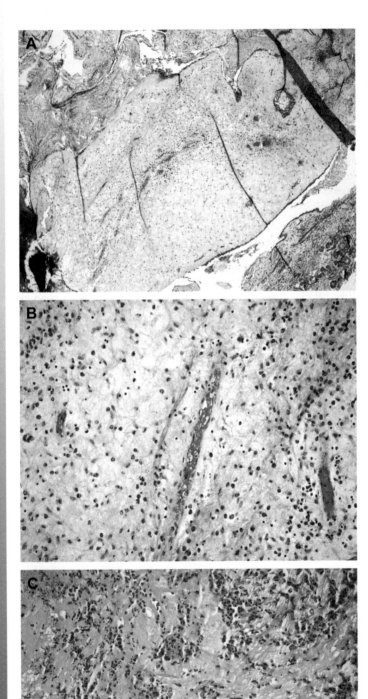

Fig. 3. Aspirin sensitivity syndrome. (A) Low-power view of sinonasal inflammatory polyp in a patient with aspirin sensitivity syndrome (Hematoxylin-eosin; original magnification ×50). (B) Higher power shows chronic inflammation with numerous eosinophils (hematoxylin-eosin; original magnification ×100). (C) Allergic mucin with Charcot-Leyden crystals in patient with aspirin sensitivity syndrome. Silver stains were negative for fungal organisms (hematoxylin-eosin; original magnification ×100).

inhalation and is associated with crowded conditions and poor hygiene. All cases of *K rhinoscleromatis* infection involve the nasal cavity, but other upper respiratory tract structures can also be infected. There is no gender predilection and disease can be seen at any age, although more commonly in those less than 30 years old. Patients most commonly present with rhinorrhea, epistaxis, and anosmia. Patients with long-standing, untreated infections may present with nasal deformities.

There are 3 stages of RS:

1. The catarrhal or atrophic stage, in which patients have a nonspecific rhinitis that develops into a purulent nasal discharge with mucosal crusting; this stage can last weeks to months
2. The granulomatous or hypertrophic stage, in which there is development of nasal polyps, bleeding, nasal enlargement, and nasal cartilage destruction
3. The sclerotic or fibrotic stage, in which the inflammatory changes undergo fibrosis; this can result in significant facial deformities

Gross features
Clinically, RS lesions are pale and the mucosa is thickened with polyp formation. The polyps most commonly involve the nasal septum and spare the sinuses.

Microscopic features
The most characteristic histopathology is seen in the granulomatous phase of the disease, in which there is a marked inflammatory infiltrate composed of lymphocytes and plasma cells (Fig. 4A). The most characteristic finding is the presence of groups of large vacuolated histiocytes (Mikulicz cells) that contain gram-negative organisms (Fig. 4B). Bacteria, when numerous, can occasionally be seen on hematoxylin-eosin (H and E) stain, but Gram stain, periodic acid Schiff (PAS), silver, or immunohistochemistry are often required to confirm the diagnosis. The end stage of the infection is characterized by significant fibrosis. Diagnostic cells may not be observed in this stage (Box 2).

Differential diagnosis
The differential diagnosis of RS includes other infectious granulomatous diseases caused by bacteria (leprosy, tuberculosis, and syphilis), fungi (histoplasmosis), and parasites (mucocutaneous leishmaniasis). Noninfectious processes to be considered include inflammatory conditions, such as Rosai-Dorfman disease (RDD); antineutrophil cytoplasmic antibody (ANCA)–associated vasculitides (granulomatosis with polyangiitis

[GPA]); eosinophilic GPA (EGPA; formerly known as Churg-Strauss syndrome); cocaine-induced midline destructive lesions (CIMDL); and neoplastic processes, particularly natural killer (NK) T-cell lymphoma.

Diagnosis
The diagnosis of RS can be made by culturing the organism from tissue samples; however, only 50% of cultured lesions are positive.[22] The diagnosis can also be made by cytologic examination of smears of nasal brushing material, which may show the characteristic large, vacuolated Mikulicz cells containing the bacterial organisms.[22–26] Tissue biopsies also reveal distinctive findings, as outlined earlier.

Although RS is caused by a bacterial infection, there have been reports of potential genetic predisposition with familial cases and the potential that the inflammatory reaction generated toward the organism may be related to a defect in immune regulation.[3,27] Recently developed mouse models suggest a potential for interleukin-10 to drive the production of the Mikulicz cells.[28]

Prognosis
The disease is treated by long-term antibiotic therapy, usually tetracycline or other tetracyclinelike compounds, followed by surgery to remove the affected tissue. With early treatment, the prognosis is excellent, although the recurrence rate is high. Patients in the sclerotic phase are at risk for airway obstruction, which can be life threatening and less responsive to antibiotic therapy.

Leprosy (Mycobacterium leprae)

Introduction
Infection by *Mycobacterium leprae* causes leprosy, an infection that is rare in the United States and fairly common in other parts of the world, such as Brazil, India, Madagascar, Mozambique, and Nepal.[22–24] The disease usually affects superficial peripheral nerves, skin, and mucous membranes. Disease manifestations are a result of the inflammatory reaction to the organism, leading to scarring and deformities. Involvement of the nasal cavity and paranasal sinuses may manifest before the skin lesions. Nasal mucosa is almost always involved, although involvement may be subclinical.[23,24] Leprosy is a spectrum of diseases ranging from a localized, self-limited process (tuberculoid leprosy [TL]) to systemic disease that, left untreated, may be fatal (lepromatous leprosy). The lepromatous form often shows nasal involvement, with the septum most commonly involved. Patients often present with rhinorrhea, purulent discharge, bleeding,

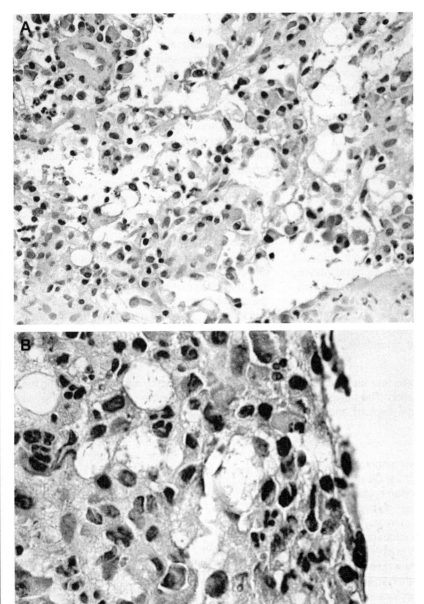

Fig. 4. Rhinoscleroma. (A) Mixed inflammatory infiltrate consisting of lymphocytes, plasma cells, and vacuolated histiocytes in patient with rhinoscleroma (hematoxylin-eosin; original magnification ×200). (B) High-power view of vacuolated histiocytes containing rod-shaped bacterial organisms in patient with rhinoscleroma (hematoxylin-eosin; original magnification ×500).

and anosmia. Like other chronic necrotizing infectious processes, septal perforation with saddle-nose deformity and nasal atrophy can be seen.

Gross findings

Grossly, early mucosal lesions may appear as pale, yellow plaques or thickening of the sinonasal mucosa. During later stages, the lesions may ulcerate and become more nodular. Late-stage lesions can present with necrotizing midline disease with nasal cartilage destruction and saddle-nose deformities.

Microscopic findings

Histologic findings vary according to the form of leprosy and the histology varies with the immune response to the infection. In TL there are submucosal noncaseating granulomas that destroy nerves, and organisms are difficult to identify (Fig. 5A). In lepromatous leprosy there is a diffuse

> **Box 2**
> **Key points for rhinoscleroma**
>
> Causative agent of RS is *K rhinoscleromatis*
>
> RS most commonly affects nasal cavity; may involve other upper respiratory tract structures
>
> Cultures are often negative
>
> Microscopic characteristic: lymphocytes, plasma cells, and histiocytes with organisms (Mikulicz cells)
>
> Characteristic histology is in the granulomatous/hypertrophic stage
>
> Organisms stain with Gram stain (gram negative)
>
> End stage is sclerotic and may result in respiratory compromise
>
> Treatment is long-term antibiotics

submucosal inflammatory reaction consisting of macrophages, foamy histiocytes (Virchow or leprae cells) (see **Fig. 5**B), and many intracellular organisms. Epithelioid cells and giant cells are not found. Inflammation is most prominent around blood vessels and nerves. There is a spectrum of disease types between TL and lepromatous leprosy, with the TL form of the disease able to progress to lepromatous forms (**Box 3**).

Differential diagnosis

The differential diagnosis of TL and lepromatous leprosy includes other causes of granulomatous disease, such as other infections (RS), GPA, and RDD.

Diagnosis

M leprae does not grow well in culture and diagnosis often relies on histopathologic diagnosis, serologic testing, or molecular testing.[29,30] The histologic finding of inflammation around nerves may be a clue to the disease. The organism often does not stain with routine stains for acid-fast bacilli (AFB) but modified acid-fast stains (Fite) show organisms within macrophages (see **Fig. 5**C). Organisms are often rare in the tuberculoid forms but are often numerous in the lepromatous forms. In situ hybridization can be used to speciate the organisms in tissue but is often difficult to perform and interpret.[31] Assays have been developed for demonstration of *M leprae*–specific DNA and ribosomal RNA (rRNA) sequences in various specimens, such as nasal smears, skin, and blood.[22,29,30] Polymerase chain reaction (PCR) for bacterial DNA is most sensitive and can detect fewer than 10 organisms.[32] Genetic factors are important for disease susceptibility, including the type of inflammatory response as well as the types of cells infected by the organism.[3] The genetics behind leprosy are complex, with polymorphisms in a variety of genes associated with different forms of the disease.[3,33]

Prognosis

Treatment of leprosy involves multiagent antibiotic therapy with at least rifampin and dapsone. Resolution of the infection may take years. With early diagnosis and treatment, progression of disease can be limited, but recovery of neuronal function is variable. Long-standing sinonasal leprosy can result in facial deformities.

OTHER SINONASAL BACTERIAL INFECTIONS

SYPHILIS

Another cause of necrotizing nasal lesions is infection by *Treponema pallidum*, the causal agent of syphilis.[22–24] Nasal disease secondary to *T pallidum* can occur at any age and may be seen in neonatal, primary, secondary, and tertiary disease, although the sinonasal tract is more commonly involved in tertiary disease. The necrotizing lesions can lead to bone and cartilage destruction with creation of midline deformity.

MYCOBACTERIUM TUBERCULOSIS

Mycobacterium tuberculosis should also be kept in mind when evaluating patients with a necrotizing granulomatous sinonasal lesions.[22–24] Sinonasal tuberculosis (TB) usually is a result of secondary involvement by pulmonary disease, but it may occur as a primary lesion. Ulceration and septal perforation may be seen. Usually granulomas are well formed and necrotizing, with the main differential diagnosis being sarcoidosis. The diagnosis is confirmed by AFB staining, culture, or molecular studies.

SINONASAL FUNGAL INFECTIONS

Fungal rhinosinusitis (FRS) comprises a spectrum of disease processes that vary in clinical presentation, histologic appearance, and biological

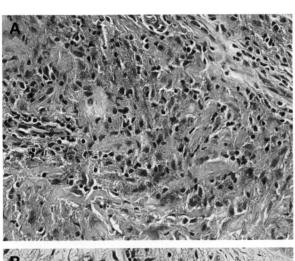

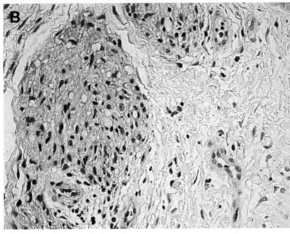

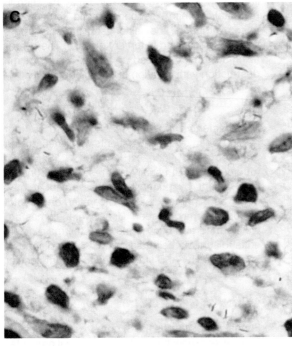

Fig. 5. Leprosy. (*A*) Granulomatous inflammatory reaction in patient with TL (hematoxylin-eosin; original magnification ×100). (*B*) Foamy/vacuolated cellular infiltrate in a patient with lepromatous leprosy (hematoxylin-eosin; original magnification ×100). (*C*) Scattered Fite-positive organisms in patient with lepromatous leprosy (Fite stain; original magnification ×500).

Box 3
Key points for leprosy

Caused by *M leprae*

M leprae infection causes a spectrum of disease from tuberculoid (granulomatous reaction) to lepromatous (nongranulomatous reaction)

Disease caused by inflammatory reaction to the organism

Nerves commonly involved

Nasal cavity common site of involvement

TL is characterized by granulomatous reaction

Lepromatous leprosy is characterized by histiocytic reaction with numerous intracellular organisms

Organisms stain with modified acid-fast stain (Fite)

Early diagnosis and treatment can stop disease progression (neuronal function may not recover)

Lepromatous leprosy can be fatal

---

significance.[34–38] FRS can be acute (aggressive; symptoms for <30 days), subacute (symptoms for 30–90 days), and chronic (indolent; symptoms for >90 days). FRS is most commonly classified as noninvasive or invasive based on whether fungi have invaded into tissue. Although FRS has been studied for several years, more recently terminology, classification, and pathogenesis have been better defined (**Table 1**).

NONINVASIVE FUNGAL RHINOSINUSITIS

ALLERGIC FUNGAL RHINOSINUSITIS

Introduction

AFRS does not represent a true infection but is considered to be an inflammatory reaction toward fungi that have inhabited the sinonasal tract.[38–41] AFRS occurs in immunocompetent, atopic patients who present with symptoms of CRS not

---

Table 1
Fungal rhinosinusitis classification

	Microscopic Features
Noninvasive FRS	
Fungus ball	Entangled mass of fungi with minimal surrounding inflammatory reaction or surrounding fibrinous necrotic exudate containing fungal forms; no tissue invasion or granulomatous reaction is present Cultures usually negative but when positive usually *Aspergillus* sp
AFRS	Presence of AM (mucinous material admixed with eosinophils, acute inflammatory cells, eosinophilic debris, and Charcot-Leyden crystals) with sparse fungal elements or positive fungal cultures; no tissue invasion present Cultures usually grow *Aspergillus* sp or dematiaceous fungi
Invasive FRS	
Acute	Invasion of fungal forms into submucosa with frequent angioinvasion and necrosis in a patient with symptoms of less than 1-mo duration Cultures usually grow *Aspergillus* sp or *Rhizopus* sp
Chronic	Invasion of fungal forms into submucosa often with surrounding chronic inflammation and fibrosis in patient with long-standing symptoms (>3-mo duration) Cultures usually grow *Aspergillus fumigatus*
Chronic granulomatous	Invasion of fungal forms into submucosa, often with surrounding chronic inflammation, fibrosis, and granuloma production in patient with long-standing symptoms (>3-mo duration) Cultures usually grow *Aspergillus flavus*

responsive to conservative (medical) therapy. AFRS occurs equally in male and female patients at any age, although it is most common in adolescents and young adults and is seen more commonly in warm, humid climates such as in the southern and southeastern United States, India, and the Middle East, although a high incidence has also been reported in large urban areas.[38–41] Patients present with headaches; obstruction; and rarely masslike lesions, which can produce proptosis. The fungi associated with AFRS depend on the geography but most commonly *Aspergillus* sp and dematiaceous fungi are implicated.

Gross Features

Grossly, the sinus contents (which may be abundant) from patients with AFRS are described as inspissated, claylike material that is green, brown, or grayish.

Microscopic Features

Histologic examination of the sinus contents from patients with AFRS often shows CRS with eosinophils.[37] The most characteristic feature is the presence of AM, which is histologically characterized by the presence of inspissated mucin admixed with sloughed epithelial cells, eosinophils, Charcot-Leyden crystals, eosinophilic and necrotic debris, and other inflammatory cells arranged in a layered pattern and associated with rare, scattered fungal hyphae, which, although they may be seen on H and E stain, are best highlighted by silver or PAS stains (**Fig. 6**). All of the material received from sinus contents of patients with suspected AFRS should be histologically examined because fungal hyphae are often scarce.

Differential Diagnosis

The differential diagnosis of AFRS includes other entities that can lead to the formation of AM, including aspirin sensitivity syndrome. Fungal stains and cultures may be helpful to distinguish between the two; however, fungi in AFRS can be sparse so a negative culture or fungal stain does not definitively exclude AFRS. Another entity included in the differential diagnosis of AFRS is fungal ball (FB; discussed later), which grossly can look similar and microscopically at low power can show a layered appearance similar to AM, but on higher power is composed predominantly of fungal elements sometimes admixed with necrotic/fibrinous debris.

Diagnosis

Several criteria for diagnosing AFRS have been developed but the most commonly used are those of Bent and Kuhn,[42] with major criteria including nasal polyposis, the presence of AM, the presence of fungi on histology or by culture, type 1 hypersensitivity to fungi by testing, and characteristic findings on computed tomography scan. However, a simplified approach includes a pathologic definition, which is the presence of AM with fungal organisms identified microscopically or by culture.[40]

Microscopically AM must be seen. Eosinophilic mucin is now the preferred term instead of AM because there is debate regarding whether the pathogenesis of AFRS is allergic.[8,38,39] AM has also been described in patients without evidence of fungal infection. Eosinophilic mucinous rhinosinusitis (EMRS) is a term to describe a patient population that shows AM but no histologic or culture evidence of fungus.[43] More recent studies have called into question EMRS as a separate entity stating that if more sensitive methods for evaluating for fungi in AM were used, such as protease digestion with trypsin before Grocott methenamine silver (GMS) stain, that detection of fungi may be improved[44] (**Box 4**).

Prognosis

The treatment of AFRS is often surgery with postoperative steroids. Recurrences are common. Antifungal therapy has not been proposed and, so far, studies that have used antifungals in AFRS, and in CRS in general, have been unsuccessful, although some investigators have questioned whether the correct antifungal regimens have been used.[45]

FUNGAL BALL

INTRODUCTION

A second form of noninvasive FRS is the fungal ball (FB), an extramucosal, entangled mass of fungi usually associated with minimal mucosal inflammation.[37,38,46,47] The most recent FRS guidelines consider FB to be the most appropriate term for this entity, as opposed to previously used terms such as mycetoma (a term used to describe a chronic, soft tissue granulomatous fungal infection) and aspergilloma (fungal organisms other than *Aspergillus* sp can cause an FB).[34,35] For unknown reasons, FBs are more commonly identified unilaterally in the maxillary sinus in middle-aged to

Fig. 6. AFRS. (*A*) Low-power view of AM showing eosinophilic mucin with a layered appearance mixed with inflammatory and sloughed epithelial cells. (hematoxylin-eosin; original magnification ×50). (*B*) AM with collections of eosinophils (hematoxylin-eosin; original magnification ×100). (*C*) AM showing rare fungal forms on hematoxylin-eosin staining. Cultures grew *Curvularia* sp (hematoxylin-eosin; original magnification ×200).

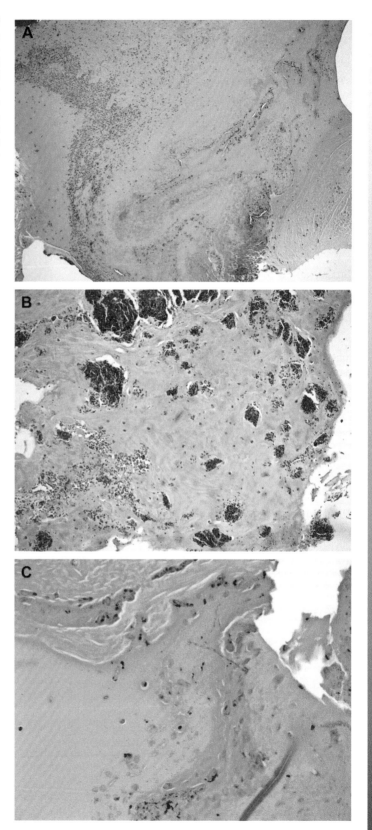

Box 4
Key points for allergic fungal rhinosinusitis

Not a true fungal infection but an inflammatory reaction to fungi

Patients often present with nasal polyps

Associated with AM containing sparse fungi

AM may be seen in other conditions associated with eosinophilic inflammation

Commonly associated with dematiaceous fungi (*Alternaria*, *Bipolaris*, *Curvularia*, and so forth) and *Aspergillus* sp

---

elderly women.[37,46,47] Most patients are immunocompetent, healthy, and nonatopic.

GROSS FINDINGS

Grossly an FB often is dark brown and friable. It may grossly resemble the AM seen in AFRS.

MICROSCOPIC FINDINGS

On histology, FBs are characterized by entangled masses of fungal organisms or masses of fungi embedded in fibrinous, necrotic exudate, with minimal mucosal inflammatory reaction (**Fig. 7**). By definition, no tissue invasion or granulomatous reaction should be identified in the surrounding tissue. If granulomas are present, the possibility of chronic invasive granulomatous FRS should be considered (**Box 5**).

DIFFERENTIAL DIAGNOSIS

The differential diagnosis of FB is AM, as explained earlier (characteristic of AFRS). If there is extensive necrotic material without visible fungi on H and E staining, a necrotic neoplasm may be considered. Specials stains for fungus usually highlight the numerous fungal organisms.

DIAGNOSIS

The diagnosis of FB is made by histopathologic examination of material removed during surgery. Fungal cultures are often negative; however, the most commonly isolated pathogen is *Aspergillus* sp. Prior surgery and prior dental procedures have been considered risk factors for FB development.[46,47] In addition, FBs may develop when there are blockages of the sinonasal passages, such as the presence of an obstructing neoplasm.

PROGNOSIS

Treatment consists of surgical removal of the fungal material without the need for antifungal therapy. The prognosis is excellent following surgery for removal of the lesion. Only rarely does FB recur following debridement.

INVASIVE FUNGAL RHINOSINUSITIS

Invasive sinonasal fungal disease (IFRS) may be acute or chronic depending on the duration of symptoms. Most IFRS cases are acute. Chronic forms of the disease are rare and have been characterized in more detail elsewhere.

ACUTE INVASIVE FUNGAL RHINOSINUSITIS

INTRODUCTION

Acute IFRS (AIFRS) is a severe form of sinonasal fungal disease that is characterized by rapid onset (<4 weeks' duration) and an aggressive clinical course, particularly if untreated.[37,38,48–51] AIFRS is seen in immunocompromised patients, particularly those with hematologic malignancies with low absolute neutrophil counts. The fungal organisms invade tissue and blood vessels, resulting in tissue necrosis and infarction.[38,48] Organisms can invade vital structures, including the brain and large arteries. AIFRS is serious and can be rapidly progressive, even fatal, if not clinically and pathologically recognized.

GROSS FINDINGS

Grossly, the mucosa appears pale and necrotic because of vascular thrombosis from fungal invasion.

MICROSCOPIC FINDINGS

On histology, the mucosa shows infarction vascular thrombosis and usually scant inflammatory cells. Close review shows angioinvasion of fungal forms, resulting in lumenal thrombosis. Although the fungi are usually seen on routine H and E stains, silver and PAS stains are often useful at highlighting the organisms, particularly in vessel

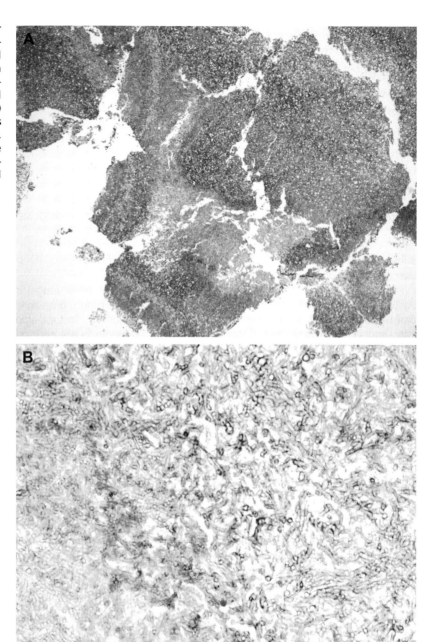

Fig. 7. FB. (*A*) Low-power view of FB showing entangled mass of fungal forms associated with necrotic debris (hematoxylin-eosin; original magnification ×50). (*B*) FB showing entangles mass of fungal forms. Cultures were negative for fungal organisms (hematoxylin-eosin; original magnification ×200).

walls and vascular space lumens, where they are often mixed with fibrin (**Box 6, Fig. 8**).

DIFFERENTIAL DIAGNOSIS

The differential diagnosis of AIFRS includes other causes of necrotizing sinonasal diseases, including infectious diseases and vasculitic processes. The clinical history as well as the identification of fungal forms aids in the diagnosis.

DIAGNOSIS

The diagnosis of AIFRS includes histopathologic identification of tissue-invasive fungal forms, which is often performed during intraoperative consultation. Frozen section is almost always required because this technique can be performed in a rapid fashion and provides surgeons with immediate results for treatment planning.[52,53] On histology, the mucosa shows infarction, vascular thrombosis, and little inflammation. Close review

> **Box 5**
> **Key points for fungal ball**
>
> Entangled mass of fungus without inflammatory reaction
>
> Not associated with allergic diseases
>
> Most commonly seen in elderly women
>
> Most common in maxillary sinus
>
> Often unilateral
>
> Cultures often negative but when positive grow *Aspergillus* sp
>
> Treatment is surgery
>
> Rare cases can progress to invasive disease in immunosuppressed individuals

shows angioinvasion of fungal forms resulting in vascular thrombosis. On permanent sections, silver and PAS stains are often useful for highlighting the organisms. Specific fungal agents can be identified by culture, immunohistochemistry, and in situ hybridization. Most cases grow either *Aspergillus* sp or *Rhizopus* sp in culture. In approximately 30% of patients with AIFRS, fungal cultures are negative.[53] Rapid in situ hybridization for rRNA targets has become a useful means of identifying fungal species in patients with AIFRS.[54]

PROGNOSIS

The treatment of AIFRS is usually debridement surgery followed by intravenous antifungals. Rapid diagnosis is critical because fungal forms may grow into vital structures, including the orbit and cranial cavity, and patients with involvement of these structures have a significantly high morbidity and mortality. Treatment with antifungal agents varies depending on the pathogen isolated.

OTHER FUNGAL INFECTIONS

Several other fungal infections may also cause necrotizing, granulomatous sinonasal lesions, including histoplasmosis, coccidioidomycosis, blastomycosis, and cryptococcosis. Most of these result from dissemination of pulmonary disease.[22]

PROTOZOAL INFECTIONS

Leishmaniasis

Introduction
Leishmaniasis is caused by the obligate intracellular protozoal parasite *Leishmania* spp, transmitted by the female sandfly.[22–24] There are many species, and the spectrum of disease is broad. In the United States, the disease is uncommon but more than 1 million cases of leishmaniasis are diagnosed annually in countries where sandflies are common. There are 3 forms of disease: (1) cutaneous (most common), (2) visceral, and (3) mucocutaneous (rarest form of disease). Mucosal leishmaniasis is caused predominantly

> **Box 6**
> **Key points for acute invasive fungal rhinosinusitis**
>
> Most common in immunosuppressed patients with absolute neutropenia
>
> Rapid onset of symptoms
>
> Critical diagnosis; often assessed initially by frozen section
>
> Fungi show invasion into tissue and blood vessels with thrombosis
>
> Tissue shows infarction, hemorrhage, and necrosis with minimal inflammatory infiltrate (patients are neutropenic)
>
> Organisms can invade vital structures such as large arteries, central nervous system, and orbit
>
> Most commonly associated with *Aspergillus* sp or *Rhizopus* sp
>
> Treatment is surgery followed by antifungal therapy
>
> Prognosis is poor (even with treatment)

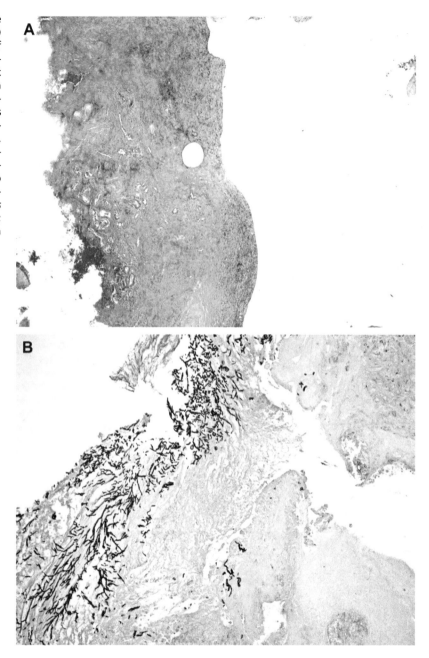

Fig. 8. Acute invasive fungal rhinosinusitis. (*A*) Low-power view of infarcted sinonasal mucosa without significant inflammatory reaction in patient with acute invasive fungal rhinosinusitis (hematoxylin-eosin; original magnification ×50). (*B*) Silver stain highlighting fungal organisms invading into sinonasal mucosa. Cultures grew *Aspergillus fumigatus* (silver stain; original magnification ×100).

by *Leishmania braziliensis* and *Leishmania panamensis*. Mucosal involvement alone is rare and the nasal cavity is the most frequent site of involvement.[22–24,55–57] Mucosal lesions may develop as a result of disseminated disease or direct contact with skin lesions. Patients with sinonasal involvement present with epistaxis, rhinorrhea, obstruction, necrosis, and midline destruction.

Gross features

Sinonasal leishmaniasis presents with destructive ulcerated lesions. The infected mucosa grossly shows edema, redness, ulceration, bleeding, obstruction, and necrosis. Long-standing disease can lead to septal cartilage destruction and facial deformity.

Microscopic features

On histology, infection is characterized by ulceration with marked lymphocytic and plasmacytic inflammation and granulation tissue. Rarely the inflammation can be granulomatous. The organisms are found in the cytoplasm of histiocytes; are small, round, and measure 1 to 3 μm; and can be seen on H and E stain (Fig. 9). Organisms tend to be located in the periphery of the histiocyte cytoplasm and their nucleoli stain with Giemsa stain, but this is best appreciated on smears taken from lesions as opposed to tissue sections. In tissue sections, the organisms may be highlighted with Brown and Hopps modified Gram stain.

Differential diagnosis

The differential diagnosis of Leishmania is Histoplasma capsulatum, which are also 1 to 3 μm in size and identified within histiocytes in infected individuals; however, Histoplasma are encapsulated organisms, whereas Leishmania are not. The inflammatory reaction to the organisms may lead to a very broad differential diagnosis, including other infections, vasculitis, and neoplasms (lymphoma).

Diagnosis

Diagnosis is usually made by identification of organisms in tissue or cytologic specimens, with material taken from the ulcer base having the

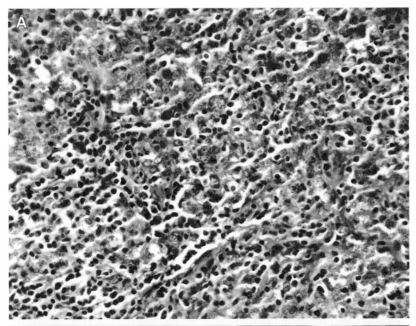

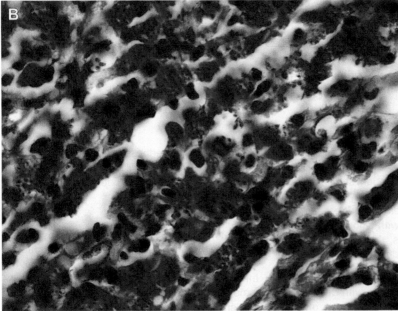

Fig. 9. Leishmaniasis. (A) Biopsy from patient with leishmaniasis showing a mixed infiltrate consisting of lymphocytes, plasma cells, and histiocytes. (B) High-power view of leishmaniasis with the presence of organisms within the cytoplasm of histiocytes (hematoxylin-eosin; original magnification ×500).

highest yield.[22,57,58] Detection by PCR is the most sensitive method for the disease diagnosis.[22,57,58] Immunohistochemistry and in situ hybridization have also been used to identify the organisms in tissue.[59] In countries where tests are not available, the diagnosis is made on a clinical basis.

Prognosis

With early treatment, most patients are cured, but untreated cases can be fatal. The complications of mucosal leishmaniasis include secondary bacterial infection of ulcerated lesions and bleeding. If sinonasal disease is left untreated, there may be erosion of the nasal septum and the palate, resulting in disfigurement.

There have been documented familial clusters of leishmaniasis but it is unknown whether there are caused by contamination from family members being in close proximity, or by the host immune response to the organism having a genetic component[3,60] (**Box 7**).

OTHER RARE INFECTIONS

RHINOSPORIDIOSIS

Introduction

Rhinosporidiosis is a chronic sinonasal infection caused by *Rhinosporidium seeberi*, an organism infrequently encountered in the United States but endemic to India, Sri Lanka, South America, and Africa.[22–24,61] The organism is a eukaryotic parasite, once considered fungal but now classified with other parasitic microorganisms (class Mesomycetozoea).[22–24,61] *R seeberi* most commonly infects the nasal mucosa, although patients may present with cutaneous disease and, rarely, involvement of the lacrimal sac and parotid duct. Disease is often localized but may (rarely) be disseminated. Most patients present with nasal obstruction or bleeding.

Gross Features

Grossly, the lesions present as a soft, friable, hemorrhagic polyp (strawberrylike) that grossly resembles a sinonasal inflammatory polyp and that may show cystic changes on cut section.

Microscopic Features

On histology, the sinonasal mucosa is nonulcerated, but the epithelium is hyperplastic, hypervascular, and may show pseudoepitheliomatous hyperplasia. The organisms are observed in cysts up to 300 μm within the mucosa and submucosa, and there is an associated submucosal inflammatory cell infiltrate composed of neutrophils, lymphocytes, plasma cells, multinucleated giant cells, and scattered granulomas.

Differential Diagnosis

The main differential diagnosis for *R seeberi* infection is coccidioidomycosis; however, *R seeberi* is much larger and stains for mucicarmine, whereas *Coccidioides immitis* does not. At low power, rhinosporidiosis may be confused with the cystic changes seen in cylindrical cell papilloma (oncocytic schneiderian papilloma); however, the cysts seen in cylindrical cell papillomas are intramucosal only, not submucosal as in rhinosporidiosis.

Diagnosis

The organism does not grow in culture. The diagnosis of rhinosporidiosis can be made by biopsy, and organisms can be seen on routine H and E stain, silver stains, PAS stains, and mucicarmine. Diagnosis can also be made by fine-needle aspiration cytology of mass lesions.[61] The histology of the organisms is distinctive and additional special studies are often not warranted, although multiplex PCR methods have been developed to help distinguish *R seeberi* from other organisms.[62]

Prognosis

Treatment involves surgical excision of the lesions. The prognosis is excellent, except in patients with disseminated disease.

VASCULITIDES

ANTINEUTROPHIL CYTOPLASMIC ANTIBODY–ASSOCIATED VASCULITIDES IN THE SINONASAL TRACT

Necrotizing vasculitides associated with ANCAs include GPA (formerly known as Wegener granulomatosis) and EGPA. Both of these entities may involve the sinonasal tract, although GPA does so more commonly.

GRANULOMATOSIS WITH POLYANGIITIS (FORMERLY KNOWN AS WEGENER GRANULOMATOSIS)

INTRODUCTION

GPA is a necrotizing vasculitic process associated with cytoplasmic ANCA (c-ANCA).[23,24,48,63–66] It is a systemic disease that is most commonly associated with necrotizing granulomatous vasculitis of small vessels of the upper and lower respiratory tract and kidneys; however, the disease can be localized to a single site. Patients with GPA have autoantibodies to proteinase 3, a protein found in neutrophilic granules, although not all GPA is related to ANCA. Although GPA is of unknown

> **Box 7**
> **Key features of granulomatosis with polyangiitis (formerly known as Wegener granulomatosis)**
>
> Small vessel vasculitis associated with c-ANCA (proteinase 3)
>
> Likely has autoimmune, infectious, environmental, and genetic components
>
> Affects upper and lower respiratory tract and kidney
>
> Most patients (85%) initially present with sinonasal symptoms
>
> Histology shows basophilic necrosis, granulomatous inflammation, and necrotizing vasculitis (<20% of cases have all 3 findings)
>
> Multiple biopsies may be needed to make diagnosis
>
> Differential diagnosis is infections, other vasculitides, NK/T-cell lymphoma, cocaine-induced midline destructive disease, idiopathic midline destructive disease

cause, the pathogenesis is thought to be multifactorial, with a combination of environmental, toxins, genetic, and likely infectious factors involved.[3,23,24,48,63–66] Men and women are equally affected and the disease can be seen at any age, although most patients are more than 45 years old. Clinically, more than 85% of patients present with sinonasal symptoms ranging from mild obstruction to nasal cartilage destruction.

GROSS FINDINGS

Grossly the sinonasal mucosa shows diffuse ulceration and crusting. Long-standing cases can present with cartilage destruction and midline deformities.

MICROSCOPIC FINDINGS

On histology, necrotizing vasculitis and inflammation consisting of histiocytes, lymphocytes, plasma cells, and multinucleated giant cells surrounding geographic areas of basophilic necrosis are characteristic (**Fig. 10, Table 2**).

DIFFERENTIAL DIAGNOSIS

The differential diagnosis of GPA is broad and includes infection, other types of vasculitides, idiopathic midline destructive diseases, CIMDL, and NK T-cell lymphoma.

DIAGNOSIS

The diagnosis of GPA is often suspected based on clinical findings and the presence of the characteristic c-ANCA, which is identified in most patients, although a negative c-ANCA does not preclude a diagnosis of GPA. The diagnosis of GPA is often one of exclusion. Tissue biopsy with the presence of granulomatous vasculitis is often required to confirm the diagnosis. A

diagnosis of GPA is difficult to make on nasal biopsies and usually multiple biopsies are necessary before a definitive diagnosis can be rendered. Microscopically, with the presence of necrosis and granulomatous inflammation, the exclusion of infectious diseases, including bacterial and fungal diseases, is necessary. Gram, GMS, AFB, and Fite stains often should be performed to exclude bacterial, fungal, and mycobacterial diseases. Care must be taken to not miss intracellular microorganisms. Other granulomatous diseases need to be excluded. Although granulomas are seen in GPA, they are usually not well formed, which should aid in excluding infection and sarcoidosis. Other causes of ANCA-associated vasculitis, such as EGPA, should also be excluded. EGPA is a rare ANCA-associated vasculitis (usually perinuclear ANCA) syndrome characterized by bronchial asthma, systemic necrotizing vasculitis, and peripheral eosinophilia. Although uncommon, the disease may present with sinonasal involvement.[67] Sinonasal tract involvement consists of sinonasal polyps and chronic sinusitis with eosinophils (early) and rarely diagnostic necrotizing vasculitis (late in the disease process) (**Fig. 11**). EGPA has less lung and renal involvement and more cutaneous involvement than GPA. CIMDL often shares histologic similarities to GPA and they may be impossible to distinguish from each other histologically because both may present with necrotizing vasculitis.[48,68–71] However, although both entities may have ANCA, GPA targets P3, whereas CIMDL targets another antigen. Distinction from lymphoma may be difficult, particularly with extensive necrosis, but an NK T-cell lymphoma diagnosis is usually associated with the presence of Epstein-Barr virus (EBV)–positive, cytologically atypical lymphocytes.[48]

Fig. 10. (*A*) GPA showing granulomatous inflammation and geographic necrosis (hematoxylin-eosin; original magnification ×100). (*B*) Medium-sized blood vessel with granulomatous vasculitis in a patient with GPA (hematoxylin-eosin; original magnification ×100).

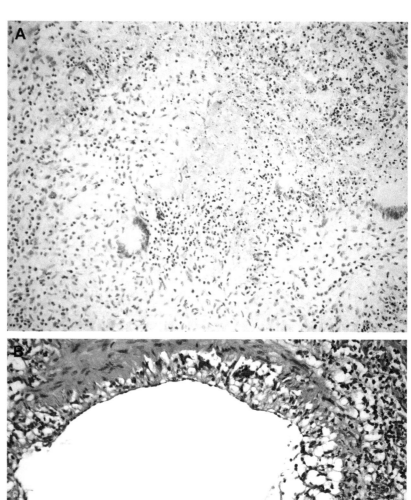

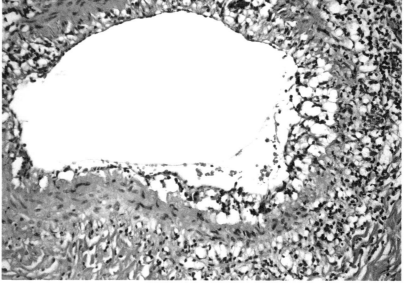

COCAINE-INDUCED MIDLINE DESTRUCTIVE LESIONS

Cocaine abuse has been associated with the development of CIMDL in the sinonasal area. Short-term cocaine use can lead to mucosal ulceration and necrosis.[24,48,68–71] Long-term use has been associated with ischemia of not only the mucosal tissue but cartilage and bone, resulting in midline deformity and septal/palatal perforations.

MICROSCOPIC FINDINGS

On histology, significant granulomatous inflammation, infarction, necrosis, and giant cell reaction can be seen (**Fig. 12**). Necrotizing vasculitis may be evident. Polarizable foreign material may be evident in the giant cells.

DIFFERENTIAL DIAGNOSIS

CIMDL shows clinical and histopathologic overlap with other midline destructive lesions, particularly

Table 2
Nonneoplastic necrotizing sinonasal lesions

Cause	Specific Causes	Diagnostic Studies	Characteristic Histology
Bacterial	Rhinoscleroma	H and E; Gram stain, Warthin-Starry, Brown-Hopps	Foamy histiocytes with gram-negative organisms (Mikulicz cells) admixed with plasma cells/lymphocytes
	Mycobacterial: leprosy	Fite stain	Spectrum of disease with granulomas (tuberculoid) with sparse organisms to foamy histiocytic reaction with numerous organisms and no granulomas
Fungal	Acute invasive disease: *Aspergillus*; Zygomycetes	Frozen section; H and E; silver or PAS stain, ISH, culture	Angioinvasion of organisms with vascular thrombosis, infarction, and necrosis with minimal inflammatory reaction
Parasitic	Leishmaniasis	H and E; Brown-Hopps; Giemsa; PCR; ISH or immunostain	Lymphoplasmacytic inflammation with 1–3 μ peripherally located intrahistiocytic organisms
	Rhinosporidiosis	H and E; mucicarmine	Intramucosal and submucosal cysts filled with organisms
Autoimmune	GPA	H and E; elastic stain; c-ANCA, p-ANCA, rule out other causes	GPA: basophilic necrosis, granulomatous inflammation with giant cells (without well-formed granulomas), vasculitis; all 3 seen in <20% of cases
	EGPA		EGPA: chronic sinusitis with polyps; eosinophils (most common); necrotizing eosinophilic vasculitis (uncommon)
Other	Cocaine-induced midline destructive lesion	Polarizer to visualize foreign body; clinical history	Similar to findings seen in GPA

Abbreviation: ISH, in situ hybridization.

GPA. Infection and neoplasia need to be excluded as described for GPA.

DIAGNOSIS

The diagnosis of CIMDL may be difficult, particularly because the clinical history of cocaine abuse may be lacking to both the pathologist as well as the clinician. CIMDL can be associated with the presence of ANCA overlapping vasculitic syndromes. The cause of CIMDL is not clear. It is thought that ANCA development may be related to bacterial superinfection of mucosal ulcers. In addition, CIMDL may be autoimmune in origin, which likely explains why CIMDL is a rare entity compared with the number of individuals thought to abuse cocaine. The ANCA in CIMDL is often p-ANCA, targets human neutrophil elastase, but patients can also have c-ANCA targeting P3 and therefore the distinction from GPA can be difficult. The pathogenesis of cocaine in the development of CIMDL likely involves vasoconstriction, resulting in ischemia and mucosal and bone/cartilage necrosis, but recent evidence also implicates the possibility of levamisole (which is a known contaminant in cocaine) playing a role in CIMDL. Most importantly, although CIMDL may be associated with the presence of ANCA, CIMDL does not respond to immunosuppressive therapy like GPA. It is highly recommended that clinicians perform urine or serum drug testing in patients with midline destructive disease either at initial presentation or if the patient fails initial treatment (see **Table 2**).

PROGNOSIS

CIMDL does not respond to immunosuppressive therapy. The best therapy is to halt the cocaine use, plus surgery to repair any midline destructive lesions if possible.

IDIOPATHIC MIDLINE DESTRUCTIVE DISEASE

Despite extensive work-up, in some cases the cause of midline destructive disease remains

Fig. 11. EGPA. (*A*) Sinonasal mucosa from a patient with EGPA showing marked chronic inflammation with a significant eosinophilic reaction (hematoxylin-eosin; original magnification ×50). (*B*) Sinonasal mucosa from a patient with EGPA showing granulomatous inflammation with eosinophilic abscess (hematoxylin-eosin; original magnification ×100). (*C*) Sinonasal mucosa from a patient with EGPA showing necrotizing vasculitis (hematoxylin-eosin; original magnification ×100).

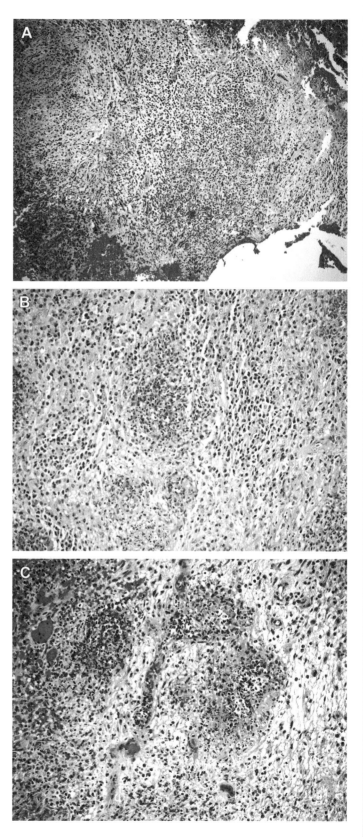

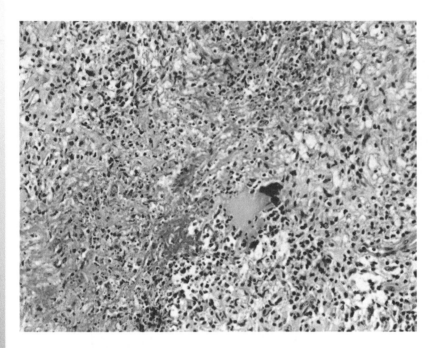

Fig. 12. Sinonasal mucosa with necrotizing inflammation with giant cell reaction in a patient with cocaine-induced midline destructive lesion. On histology this lesion mimics that seen in GPA (hematoxylin-eosin; original magnification ×100).

unknown. However, recent investigators have identified additional entities associated with development of midline sinonasal destruction, such as immunoglobulin (Ig) G4–related diseases and Rag-1 mutations.[48,72,73]

EXTRANODAL SINUS HISTIOCYTOSIS WITH MASSIVE LYMPHADENOPATHY (ROSAI-DORFMAN DISEASE)

INTRODUCTION

RDD is a rare disorder of unknown cause characterized by a histiocytic proliferation most commonly involving lymph nodes but that can also involve extranodal sites, in particular the nasal cavity and paranasal sinuses.[74] About 10% of cases involve the sinonasal tract and about 20% of those cases do not show evidence of nodal disease.[74] Patients with sinonasal RDD present with bleeding; obstruction; and, in late stages, nasal deformity. The cause of RDD is unknown but it is thought to be an aberrant immunologic response to some infectious agent. Potential proposed pathogens include viruses (EBV, parvovirus B19, human herpes viruses) or bacteria (*Klebsiella*, *Brucella*). In addition, a relationship between IgG4 disease has been proposed.[74–77]

GROSS FINDINGS

The gross findings are nonspecific but include mucosal thickening and the formation of polyps

of varying sizes. Bone destruction is not usually seen.

MICROSCOPIC FINDINGS

On histology, sinonasal RDD shows submucosal fibrosis and lymphoid aggregates (without germinal center formation) alternating with a mixed population of histiocytes, lymphocytes, and plasma cells (**Fig. 13**). The histiocytes are often numerous with abundant clear to granular cytoplasm and may show a nested appearance, but this may be less than is seen in nodal disease. Emperipolesis (the engulfment of inflammatory cells) is often not as prominent as in nodal disease. Granulomas are not seen.

DIFFERENTIAL DIAGNOSIS

The differential diagnosis includes inflammatory sinonasal polyps, which also can rarely contain RDD-type histiocytes[4]; infectious diseases, particularly lepromatous leprosy and rhinoscleroma; Langerhans cell histiocytoses; ANCA-associated vasculitides; and hematolymphoid malignancies.

DIAGNOSIS

The diagnosis is based on the histologic findings as well as exclusion of everything in the differential diagnosis described earlier. Special stains (Gram, GMS, AFB, and Fite) to exclude infection should be performed. The histiocytes in RDD stain for S100 but they are negative for CD1a, excluding

Fig. 13. RDD. (*A*) Extranodal RDD involving the sinonasal mucosa. There is fibrosis, lymphocytes, and plasma cell as well as eosinophilic histiocytes with granular cytoplasm (hematoxylin-eosin; original magnification ×50). (*B*) Higher power shows the eosinophilic histiocytes with granular cytoplasm (hematoxylin-eosin; original magnification ×100). (*C*) S100 stain highlights the histiocytes in RDD (these cells are negative for CD1a, ruling out Langerhans cell histiocytosis) (diaminobenzidine hematoxylin counterstain; original magnification ×200).

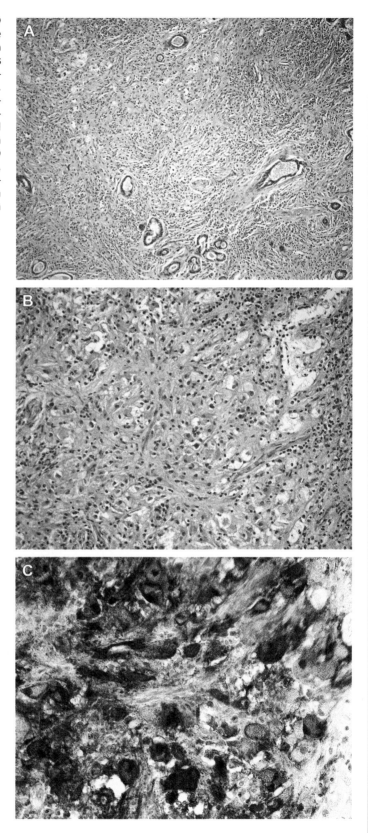

Langerhans cell histiocytosis. The marking of cells as histiocytes should help exclude lymphoid malignancies, although subsequent lymphoid malignancies have been reported in patients diagnosed with RDD.[74]

PROGNOSIS

The clinical course of RDD is indolent but the disease rarely goes into remission and recurrence is common. Treatment is on a case-by-case basis and is supportive.

SARCOIDOSIS

INTRODUCTION

Sarcoidosis is a chronic systemic disease of unknown cause characterized by nonnecrotizing granulomas that may involve multiple sites,

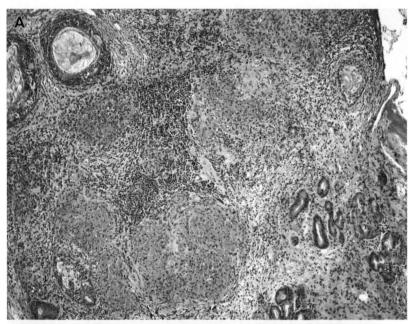

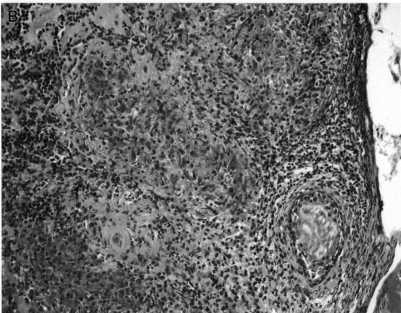

Fig. 14. Sarcoid. (*A, B*) Nonnecrotizing granulomas in a patient with a history of sarcoidosis and symptoms of severe CRS.

including the sinonasal tract in approximately 1% of patients.[23,24,78–82] The disease can occur at any age but most commonly occurs in young adults. Sarcoidosis of the sinonasal tract is often asymptomatic but patients may present with nonspecific symptoms such as nasal crusting, anosmia, and obstruction.[23,24,78–82]

GROSS DESCRIPTION

Patients may present with nasal mucosal hypertrophy, polyps, and rarely septal perforation. Grossly, sinonasal mucosal lesions are friable and crusted. In addition, submucosal nodules, formed by fibrosis and granulomatous inflammation, may be present, and extensive cartilage destruction may be seen.

MICROSCOPIC DESCRIPTION

On histology, well-formed epithelioid granulomas without necrosis are characteristic (**Fig. 14**). Occasionally central necrosis is seen in rare granulomas. Long-standing cases may show significant fibrosis.

DIFFERENTIAL DIAGNOSIS

Infection and other causes of granulomatous inflammation (eg, bacterial, mycobacterial, and fungal infections; prior surgical intervention; vasculitis; and autoimmune diseases) need to be excluded before making a diagnosis of sinonasal sarcoidosis.

DIAGNOSIS

Sarcoidosis is often a diagnosis of exclusion. Other causes of granulomatous disease, particularly infection, need to be excluded with special stains and culture if needed. Vasculitic diseases such as GPA or EGPA may be in the differential diagnosis, but granulomas in those entities are usually not well formed.

The pathogenesis of sarcoidosis, although unknown, is considered multifactorial with genetic, environmental, and possibly infectious factors likely.[3,83] Familial cases of sarcoidosis are well known.[3,83]

PROGNOSIS

Treatment with corticosteroids is recommended as well as surgical management to alleviate sinonasal symptoms. Most patients experience remission of their sinonasal symptoms with treatment. Disease may be persistent and progress systemically in some patients.

SUMMARY

The sinonasal tract is frequently affected by inflammatory lesions that arise through complex interactions of environmental, infectious, and genetic factors. Although the differential diagnoses often overlap, the use of histochemical, immunohistochemical, and molecular studies can often help in the differential diagnosis.

REFERENCES

1. Fokkens WJ, Lund VJ, Mullol J, et al. European position paper on rhinosinusitis and nasal polyps 2012. Rhinology 2012;50(Suppl 23):1–298.
2. Wood AJ, Douglas RG. Pathogenesis and treatment of chronic rhinosinusitis. Postgrad Med J 2010;86:359–64.
3. Montone KT. The molecular genetics of inflammatory, autoimmune, and infectious diseases of the sinonasal tract: a review. Arch Pathol Lab Med 2014;138(6):745–53.
4. Wilsher MJ, Bonar F. Rosai-Dorfman-type histiocytes occur in eosinophilic chronic rhinosinusitis and potentially play a role in disease initiation and resistance. Histopathology 2016;69(4):655–66.
5. Fakhri S, Frenkiel S, Hamid QA. Current views of the molecular biology of chronic sinusitis. J Otolaryngol 2002;31(Suppl 1):S2–9.
6. Brook I. Chronic sinusitis in children and adults: role of bacteria and antimicrobial management. Curr Allergy Asthma Rep 2005;5(6):482–90.
7. Stephenson MF, Mfuna L, Dowd SE, et al. Molecular characterization of the polymicrobial flora in chronic rhinosinusitis. J Otolaryngol Head Neck Surg 2010; 39(2):182–7.
8. Ponikau JU, Sherris DA, Kern EB, et al. The diagnosis and incidence of allergic fungal sinusitis. Mayo Clin Proc 1999;74:877–84.
9. Tewfik MA, Bosse Y, Al-Shemari H. Desrosiers: genetics of chronic rhinosinusitis: a primer. J Otolaryngol Head Neck Surg 2010;39(1):62–8.
10. Mfuna-Endam L, Zhang Y, Desrosiers MY. Genetics of rhinosinusitis. Curr Allergy Asthma Rep 2011; 11(3):236–46.
11. Wang X, Moylan B, Leopold DA, et al. Mutation in the gene responsible for cystic fibrosis and predisposition to chronic rhinosinusitis in the general population. JAMA 2000;284:1814–9.
12. Bernstein JM, Anon JB, Rontal M, et al. Genetic polymorphisms in chronic hyperplastic sinusitis with nasal polyposis. Laryngoscope 2009;119(7):1258–64.
13. Polzehl D, Moeller P, Riechelmann H, et al. Distinct features of chronic rhinosinusitis with and without nasal polyps. Allergy 2006;61:1280–9.
14. Rostowska-Nadolska B, Karpal M, Fraczek M, et al. A microarray study of gene expression profiles in nasal polyps. Auris Nasus Larynx 2011;38:58–64.

15. Fritz SB, Terrell JE, Conner ER, et al. Nasal mucosal gene expression in patients with allergic rhinitis with and without nasal polyps. J Allergy Clin Immunol 2003;112:1057–63.

16. Farooque SP, Lee TH. Aspirin-sensitive respiratory disease. Annu Rev Physiol 2009;71:465–87.

17. Ramadan HH, Quraishi HA. Allergic mucin without fungus. Am J Rhinol 1997;11(2):145–7.

18. Dekker JW, Nizankowska E, Schmitz-Schumann M, et al. Aspirin-induced asthma and HLA-DRB1 and HLA-DPB1 genotypes. Clin Exp Allergy 1997;27(5):574–7.

19. Palikhe NS, Kim SH, Cho BY, et al. IL-13 gene polymorphisms are associated with rhinosinusitis and eosinophilic inflammation in aspirin intolerant asthma. Allergy Asthma Immunol Res 2010;2(2):134–40.

20. Jinnai N, Sakagami T, Sekigawa T, et al. Polymorphisms in the prostaglandin E2 receptor subtype 2 gene confer susceptibility to aspirin-intolerant asthma: a candidate gene approach. Hum Mol Genet 2004;13(24):3203–17.

21. Sekigawa T, Tajima A, Hasegawa T, et al. Gene expression profiles in human nasal polyp tissues and identification of genetic susceptibility in aspirin-intolerant asthma. Clin Exp Allergy 2009;39(7):972–81.

22. Montone KT. Infectious diseases of the head and neck: a review. Am J Clin Pathol 2007;128(1):35–67.

23. Nwawka OK, Nadgir R, Fujita A, et al. Granulomatous disease in the head and neck: developing a differential diagnosis. Radiographics 2014;34:1240–56.

24. Laudien M. Orphan diseases of the nose and paranasal sinuses: pathogenesis-clinic-therapy. GMS Curr Top Otorhinolaryngol Head Neck Surg 2015;14:1–18.

25. de Pontual L, Ovetchkine P, Rodriguez D, et al. Rhinoscleroma: a French national retrospective study of epidemiologic and clinical features. Clin Infect Dis 2008;47:1396–402.

26. Mukara BK, Munyarugamba P, Dazert S, et al. Rhinoscleroma: a case series report and review of the literature. Eur Arch Otorhinolaryngol 2014;271(7):1851–6.

27. Sanchez-Marin LA, Bross-Soriano D, Arrieta J, et al. Association of HLA-DQA1*03011-DQB1*0301 haplotype with the development of respiratory scleroma. Otolaryngol Head Neck Surg 2006;136:481–3.

28. Fevre C, Almeida AS, Taront S, et al. A novel murine model of rhinoscleroma identifies Mikulicz cells, the disease signature, as IL-10 dependent derivatives of inflammatory monocytes. EMBO Mol Med 2013;5(4):516–30.

29. Moschella SL. An update on the diagnosis and treatment of leprosy. J Am Acad Dermatol 2004;51(3):417–26.

30. Katoch VM. Advances in the diagnosis and treatment of leprosy. Indian J Lepr 2002;2002:1–14.

31. Natrajan M, Katoch K, Katoch VM, et al. In situ hybridization in the histological diagnosis of early and clinically suspect leprosy. Int J Lepr Other Mycobact Dis 2004;72(3):296–305.

32. Scollard DM, Gillis TP, Williams DL. Polymerase chain reaction assay for the detection and identification of Mycobacterium leprae in patients in the United States. Am J Clin Pathol 1998;109(5):642–6.

33. Fitness J, Tosh K, Hill AVS. Genetics and susceptibility to leprosy. Genes Immun 2002;3:441–53.

34. Chakrabarti A, Das A, Panda NK. Controversies surrounding the categorization of fungal sinusitis. Med Mycol 2009;47(Suppl 1):S299–308.

35. Chakrabarti A, Denning DW, Ferguson BJ, et al. Fungal rhinosinusitis: a categorization and definitional scheme addressing current controversies. Laryngoscope 2009;119:1809–18.

36. Das A, Bal A, Chakrabarti A, et al. Spectrum of fungal rhinosinusitis; histopathologist's perspective. Histopathology 2009;54:854–9.

37. Montone KT, Livolsi VA, Feldman MD, et al. Fungal rhinosinusitis: a report of 400 patients at a single university medical center. Int J Otolaryngol 2012;2012:684835.

38. Montone K. Recent considerations in the classification and pathogenesis of fungal rhinosinusitis in pathobiology of human disease: a dynamic encyclopedia of disease mechanisms. 2014. p. 1432–44.

39. Montone K. Role of fungi in the pathophysiology of chronic rhinosinusitis: an update. Curr Allergy Asthma Rep 2013;13(2):224–8.

40. Schubert MS. Allergic fungal sinusitis: pathophysiology, diagnosis and management. Med Mycol 2009;47(Suppl 1):S324–30.

41. Laury AM, Wise SK. Allergic fungal rhinosinusitis. Am J Rhinol 2013;27:S26–7.

42. Bent JP, Kuhn F. Diagnosis of allergic fungal sinusitis. Otolaryngol Head Neck Surg 1994;111:580–8.

43. Ferguson BJ. Eosinophilic mucin rhinosinusitis: a distinct clinicopathological entity. Laryngoscope 2000;110(5):799–813.

44. Guo C, Ghaderoshi S, Kephart GM, et al. Improving the detection of fungi in eosinophilic mucin: seeing what we could not see before. Otolaryngol Head Neck Surg 2012;147(5):943–9.

45. Sacks PL, Harvey RJ, Gallagher RM, et al. Antifungal therapy in the treatment of chronic rhinosinusitis: a meta-analysis. Am J Rhinol Allergy 2012;26:141–7.

46. Dufour X, Kauffman-Lacroix C, Ferrie JC, et al. Paranasal sinus fungal ball epidemiology, clinical features, and diagnosis. A retrospective analysis of 173 cases from a single center in France 1989-2002. Med Mycol 2006;44:61–7.

47. Nicolai P, Lombardi D, Tomenzoli D, et al. Fungus ball of the paranasal sinuses: experience in 160 patients treated with endoscopic surgery. Laryngoscope 2009;119(11):2275–9.

48. Montone KT. Differential diagnosis of necrotizing sinonasal diseases. Arch Pathol Lab Med 2015; 139(12):1508–14.

49. Duggal P, Wise SK. Invasive fungal rhinosinusitis. Am J Rhinol Allergy 2013;27:S28–30.

50. Süslü AE, Oğretmenoğlu O, Süslü N, et al. Acute invasive fungal rhinosinusitis: our experience with 19 patients. Eur Arch Otorhinolaryngol 2009;266(1):77–82.

51. Monroe MM, McLean M, Sautter N, et al. Invasive fungal rhinosinusitis: a 15 year experience with 29 patients. Laryngoscope 2013;123:1583–7.

52. Taxy JB, El-Zayaty S, Langerman A. Acute fungal sinusitis: natural history and the role of frozen section. Am J Clin Pathol 2009;132(1):86–93.

53. Ghadiali MT, Deckard NA, Farooq U, et al. Frozen-section biopsy analysis for acute invasive fungal rhinosinusitis. Otolaryngol Head Neck Surg 2007;136(5):714–9.

54. Montone KT, LiVolsi VA, Lanza DC, et al. In situ hybridization for specific fungal organisms in acute invasive fungal rhinosinusitis. Am J Clin Pathol 2011;135(2):190–9.

55. Crovetto-Martínez R, Aguirre-Urizar JM, Orte-Aldea C, et al. Mucocutaneous leishmaniasis must be included in the differential diagnosis of midline destructive disease: two case reports. Oral Surg Oral Med Oral Pathol Oral Radiol 2015;119(1):e20–6.

56. Lessa MM, Lessa HA, Castro TWN, et al. Mucosal leishmaniasis: epidemiological and clinical aspects. Braz J Otorhinolaryngol 2007;73(6):843–7.

57. Daneshbod Y, Oryan A, Davarmanesh M, et al. Clinical, histopathologic, and cytologic diagnosis of mucosal leishmaniasis and literature review. Arch Pathol Lab Med 2011;135(4):478–82.

58. Guerreiro JB, Cruz AA, Barral A, et al. Mucosal leishmaniasis: quantitative nasal cytology as a marker of disease activity and indicator of healing. Ann Otol Rhinol Laryngol 2000;109(1):89–94.

59. van Eys GJ, Schoone GJ, Ligthart GS, et al. Detection of *Leishmania* parasites by DNA in situ hybridization with non-radioactive probes. Parasitol Res 1987;73(3):199–202.

60. Campin S, Kwiatkowski D, Dessein A. Mendelian and complex genetics of susceptibility and resistance to parasitic infections. Semin Immunol 2006; 18:411–22.

61. Das S, Kashyap B, Barua M, et al. Nasal rhinosporidiosis in humans: new interpretations and a review of the literature of this enigmatic disease. Med Mycol 2011;49(3):311–5.

62. Saha S, Mondal D, Khetawat D, et al. A molecular approach (multiplex polymerase chain reaction) for diagnosis of rhinosporidiosis. Indian J Otolaryngol Head Neck Surg 2002;54(4):264–7.

63. Kallenberg CGM. Advances in pathogenesis and treatment of ANCA-associated vasculitis. 2014. Available at: www.discoverymedicine.com. Accessed October 11, 2014.

64. Tarabishy AB, Schulte M, Papaliodis GN, et al. Wegener's granulomatosis: clinical manifestations, differential diagnosis, and management of ocular and systemic disease. Surv Ophthalmol 2010;55(5): 429–44.

65. Lutalo PMK, D'Cruz DP. Diagnosis and classification of granulomatosis with polyangiitis (aka Wegener's granulomatosis). J Autoimmun 2014;48-49:94–8.

66. Trimarchi M, Sinico RA, Teggi R, et al. Otorhinolaryngological manifestations in granulomatosis with polyangiitis (Wegener's). Autoimmun Rev 2013;12:501–5.

67. Bacciu A, Bacciu S, Mercante G, et al. Ear, nose and throat manifestations of Churg-Strauss syndrome. Acta Otolaryngol 2006;126(5):503–9.

68. Trimarchi M, Bussi M, Sinico RA, et al. Cocaine-induced midline destructive lesions – An autoimmune disease? Autoimmun Rev 2013;12(4): 496–501.

69. Alamino RP, Espinosa LR. Vasculitis mimics: cocaine-induced midline destructive lesions. Am J Med Sci 2013;346(5):430–1.

70. Jimenez-Gallo D, Albarran-Planelles C, Linares-Barrios M, et al. Pyoderma gangrenosum and Wegener granulomatosis-like syndrome induced by cocaine. Clin Exp Dermatol 2013;38(8):878–82.

71. Zwang NA, van Wagner LB, Rose S. A case of levamisole-induced vasculitis and cocaine-induced midline destructive lesion: a case report. J Clin Rheumatol 2011;17(4):197–200.

72. Della-Torre E, Mattoo H, Mahajan VS, et al. IgG4-related midline destructive lesion. Ann Rheum Dis 2014;73:1434–6.

73. De Ravin SS, Cowen EW, Zarember KA, et al. Hypomorphic Rag mutations can cause destructive midline granulomatous disease. Blood 2010; 116(8):1263–71.

74. Kreisel FH. Hematolymphoid lesions of the sinonasal tract. Head Neck Pathol 2016;10:109–17.

75. Menon MP, Evbuomwan MO, Rosai J, et al. A subset of Rosai-Dorfman disease cases exhibit increased IgG4 positive plasma cells: another red herring or a true association with IgG4 related disease. Histopathology 2014;64:655–9.

76. Zhang X, Hyjek E, Vardiman J. A subset of Rosai-Dorfman disease exhibits features of IgG4-related disease. Am J Clin Pathol 2013;139:622–32.

77. Liu L, Perry AM, Cao W, et al. Relationship between Rosai-Dorfman disease and IgG4-related disease. Study of 32 cases. Am J Clin Pathol 2013;140: 395–402.

78. Kohanski MA, Reh DD. Granulomatous disease and chronic sinusitis. Am J Rhinol Allergy 2013;27(3): S39–41.

79. Kirsten AM, Watz H, Kirsten D. Sarcoidosis with involvement of the paranasal sinuses – a retrospective analysis of 12 biopsy-proven cases. BMC Pulm Med 2013;13:59.

80. Reed J, deShazo RD, Houle TT, et al. Clinical features of sarcoid rhinosinusitis. Am J Med 2010;123(9):856–62.

81. Aubart FC, Ouayoun M, Brauner M, et al. Sinonasal involvement in sarcoidosis: a case-control study of 20 patients. Medicine 2006;85(6):365–71.

82. Braun JJ, Gentine A, Pauli G. Sinonasal sarcoidosis: review and report of fifteen cases. Laryngoscope 2004;114(11):1960–3.

83. Iannuzzi MC. Genetics of sarcoidosis. Semin Respir Crit Care Med 2007;28(1):15–21.

Salivary Gland Tumors
Current Concepts and Controversies

Raja R. Seethala, MD

KEYWORDS

• Salivary gland • Translocations • Molecular • Correlative • Neoplasia • Classification

---

Key points

- Biphasic salivary gland tumors are a common category of tumors with morphologic overlap between entities; combined morphologic and immunohistochemical approaches are often needed to resolve diagnostic considerations.

- Mammary analogue secretory carcinoma is a new and distinctive entity characterized by an ETV6-NTRK3 translocation; differential diagnosis is varied but includes acinic cell carcinoma and low-grade intraductal carcinoma.

- Polymorphous low-grade adenocarcinoma and cribriform adenocarcinoma of (minor) salivary gland origin are related entities with differing clinicopathologic profiles despite overlap; they are the subject of an ongoing taxonomic debate.

ABSTRACT

This current review focuses on current concepts and controversies for select key salivary gland epithelial neoplasms. Rather than the traditional organization of benign and malignant tumors, this review is structured around select key topics: biphasic tumors, mammary analogue secretory carcinoma, and the controversy surrounding polymorphous low-grade adenocarcinoma and cribriform adenocarcinoma of (minor) salivary gland origin.

OVERVIEW

Despite their diversity, salivary gland tumors are rare, with fewer than 15 cases per 100,000 individuals annually.[1] Most (75%–85%)[2–4] are benign; salivary carcinomas comprise less than 0.5% of all cancers, and only ∼6% of head and neck cancers. Each salivary gland entity has distinctive clinical, morphologic, and immunophenotypic characteristics necessitating accurate classification. The histologic overlap between many entities, including both benign and malignant neoplasms, adds considerably to the diagnostic challenge for surgical pathologists. However, morphologic characterization of both old and novel salivary gland tumors has been refined over the past several years. In addition, immunohistochemical markers, which have the historical reputation of adding more confusion to salivary tumor diagnosis, have evolved into highly useful supplementary aides to visualization of cell compartments and cell populations, thus benefitting salivary gland tumor taxonomy. Immunohistochemistry also has an expanding role as a surrogate marker of molecular alterations. Still evolving is the role of molecular diagnostics and theranostics in salivary gland tumors. Many monomorphic salivary gland tumors are now known to harbor defining balanced translocations, some of which are readily testable on paraffin-embedded materials either by fluorescence in situ hybridization (FISH), reverse transcription polymerase chain reaction (RT-PCR), or next-generation sequencing. In contrast, pleomorphic salivary gland tumors often show complex molecular alterations that are now beginning to have therapeutic implications. The advent

---

Disclosures: None.
Department of Pathology and Laboratory Medicine, University of Pittsburgh, A614.X Presbyterian University Hospital, 200 Lothrop Street, Pittsburgh, PA 15213, USA
E-mail address: seethalarr@upmc.edu

Surgical Pathology 10 (2017) 155–176
http://dx.doi.org/10.1016/j.path.2016.11.004
1875-9181/17/© 2016 Elsevier Inc. All rights reserved.

surgpath.theclinics.com

of molecular testing in salivary gland tumors has not only improved classification overall but has enabled refinements of morphologic criteria used to ensure purity in a given category. However, it has been a source of controversy for some tumor types. The basic and comprehensive clinicopathologic characteristics of salivary gland tumors have been well detailed in the prior iteration of this issue.[5,6] This article focuses on key diagnostic issues.

BIPHASIC SALIVARY GLAND TUMORS

Biphasic salivary gland tumors are tumors composed of luminal ductal cells and abluminal basal/myoepithelial cells. Integral to these tumors is a bilayered arrangement of these components, although they may vary in proportion. This bilayered appearance is readily noticeable on light microscopy, and can be accentuated by immunostains (summarized in **Table 1**). Low-molecular-weight keratin immunostains highlight luminal ductal cells intensely and show variable to negative staining in the abluminal myoepithelial components. High-molecular-weight keratins show an opposite profile with preferential staining of myoepithelial components. p63 and ΔNp63 (p40) highlight basal/myoepithelial cells. Muscle markers are restricted to purely to myoepithelial cell types. Markers of intercalated/terminal duct phenotype, such as S100 and SOX10, highlight both ductal and myoepithelial cell types to varying degrees. DOG1 is more variable but may stain both cell types as well. The prototypical biphasic tumors include pleomorphic adenoma, basal cell adenoma/adenocarcinoma, epithelial-myoepithelial carcinoma (EMCA), adenoid cystic carcinoma, and Warthin tumor, which are not discussed here.

PLEOMORPHIC ADENOMA (BENIGN MIXED TUMOR)

INTRODUCTION

Pleomorphic adenoma (PA) remains the most common salivary gland epithelial tumor, in both adults and children, and comprises one-half to two-thirds of all benign salivary gland tumors.[2,4] It predominates in the parotid (~80%), but can be seen at any salivary site. Tumors usually occur in the fourth to fifth decade with a small female predilection. Little is known about the cause of PA. The notable risk factor is a prior history of radiation exposure.[7] PAs show translocations involving 12q13-15[8] or 8q12[9] in 40% to 70% of PAs involving *HMGA2* (12q13-15) and *PLAG1*

Table 1
Basic immunohistochemical staining profile for biphasic tumors

Immunomarkers	Staining Pattern
Low-molecular-weight cytokeratins	Luminal ductal cells: strongly positive Abluminal myoepithelial/basal cells: variable to negative
High-molecular-weight cytokeratins	Luminal ductal cells: variable to negative Abluminal myoepithelial/basal cells: strongly positive
p63	Luminal ductal cells: variable to negative Abluminal myoepithelial/basal cells: strongly positive
ΔNp63	Luminal ductal cells: negative Abluminal myoepithelial/basal cells: strongly positive
Muscle markers (calponin, smooth muscle actin, smooth muscle myosin heavy chain)	Luminal ductal cells: negative Abluminal myoepithelial/basal cells: positive only in myoepithelial cells
S100	Luminal ductal cells: variable in intercalated duct type cells, otherwise negative Abluminal myoepithelial/basal cells: variably positive
SOX10	Luminal ductal cells: positive Abluminal myoepithelial/basal cells: positive Acini: positive
DOG1	Luminal ductal cells: weakly to moderately positive, intercalated duct type cells only, apical luminal pattern Abluminal myoepithelial/basal cells: variable Acini: strongly positive apical, complete membranous staining in acinic cell carcinoma

(8q12). Translocation-positive pleomorphic adenomas tend to have more of a classic morphology and occur in younger individuals.[9] Familial PA is rare,[10] as are multifocal/bilateral PA, which comprise only 6% of multifocal/bilateral parotid tumors.[11] Pleomorphic adenomas typically present as painless masses. Palatal tumors may show ulceration.

GROSS FEATURES

Most palatal and superficial parotid PA are less than 3 cm, but deep lobe parapharyngeal PA may average more than 5 cm.[12–14] PA is characteristically well circumscribed and shows a lobular gray appearance reminiscent of cartilage. Myxoid tumors are more gelatinous, whereas cellular tumors are more firm and may appear tan-white. Cystic or pseudocystic change may be noted, particularly following fine-needle aspiration. Fibrosis and hemorrhage may occur, particularly in large tumors, but this should raise concern for malignant transformation.

MICROSCOPIC FEATURES

Basic Features

PAs derive their name from the broad diversity of morphologic patterns but, fundamentally, they are biphasic tumors, defined by an integral dual luminal ductal and abluminal myoepithelial component of varying proportions. Most PAs are encapsulated, but minor salivary gland PAs are more likely to be only partially or completely unencapsulated. About half are classic with a fairly even admixture of cellular and stromal elements, with a quarter classified as cellular with little stroma, or myxoid with stromal predominance. Myoepithelial cells characteristically stream off from tubules into a myxoid stroma, and range from ovoid to plasmacytoid to spindled.[14,15] Stroma is typically a pale blue fibromyxoid appearance with embedded transformed stellate myoepithelial cells. At least half of PAs show true chondroid elements. Up to one-quarter of PAs may show squamous metaplasia.[14,15] Oncocytic and clear cell change, sebaceous elements, mucous cells, luminal psammoma bodies, and tyrosine crystals are uncommon overall (<10%) but well documented.[15]

PA are biphasic tumors. As such they display the basic biphasic immunoprofile defined earlier. p63 and ΔNp63 (p40) also highlight areas of squamous metaplasia. Glial fibrillary acidic protein may highlight myoepithelial cells as well as stromal elements. PLAG1 immunohistochemistry may serve as a surrogate for *PLAG1* translocations.

Special Features/Variants

Cytonuclear atypia

Cytonuclear atypia in PA encompasses a spectrum of changes ranging from reactive/degenerative to precancerous, but is not well stratified. Indistinct, smudgy chromatin without evidence of cell turnover (ie, mitoses, apoptotic bodies) is typically considered degenerative, and often is preferentially seen in myoepithelial components. Ductal cells in PA may undergo apocrine change (underreported, likely considered to be oncocytic change) and show random nuclear size variation and occasional prominent nucleoli common to apocrine glands elsewhere. As these apocrine foci become more proliferative, they begin to overlap with intracapsular carcinoma ex PA (discussed later). Apocrine change can be highlighted by GCDFP-15 and androgen receptor (AR).

Infiltration, pseudopodia, satellite nodules

Perhaps the most common special feature in PA is focal infiltration or capsular discontinuity designated as pseudopodia (Fig. 1). The prevalence of this feature increases with extent of sampling and almost half of PAs show pseudopodia.[15,16] About 10% to 15% show separate satellite nodules even without a history of recurrence. Pseudopodia tend to be paucicellular and composed of myxoid stroma seemingly leaking into the adjacent adipose tissue. This condition does not indicate malignancy.

Vascular invasion

Vascular invasion is present in up to 1% to 3% of all PAs (Fig. 2). Presumed mechanisms for this in an otherwise benign neoplasm is prior mechanical disruption, including secondary changes from fine-needle aspiration. These deposits often show degenerative change and background hemorrhage, hemosiderin, and macrophages. Despite the concerns that may be raised, this is not considered a malignant feature.

Metastases

Metastasizing PA is exceptionally rare despite the noticeable proportion of tumors that may involve vessels. Even of the cases reported, it is conjectured that some are likely to be carcinoma ex PA with a maturing stromal component. Presumed pathogenesis is similar to that of vascular invasion, but here the mechanical disruption is more pronounced and repeated; that is, multiple surgical procedures for recurrence. Even if the term metastasizing PA is used, it should not be preceded by the term benign because these behave aggressively (discussed later).

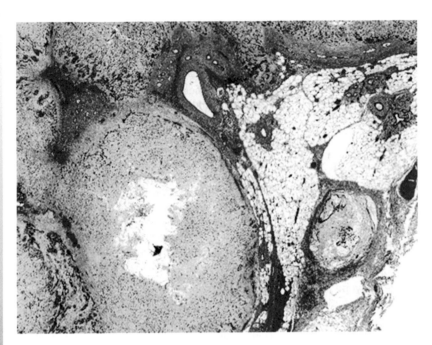

Fig. 1. PA showing a pseudopod (H&E, ×20).

Skin adnexal type differentiation

Some PAs show skin adnexal–type differentiation beyond simply isolated sebaceous nests or squamous metaplasia. These tumors predominate in the palate, but can be seen in other sites. This morphology consists of various components of folliculosebaceous units, including infundibulocystic structures, and epidermoid squamous features (**Fig. 3**). Basaloid germinative-type features may be noted as well.

Mucoepidermoid or squamoglandular metaplasia

A special form of squamous and mucous cell metaplasia is a combination reminiscent of mucoepidermoid carcinoma. Immature predominantly nonkeratinizing squamous metaplasia shows interspersed mucous cells in these foci. They are shown to be negative for *MAML2* translocations that characterize mucoepidermoid carcinoma (discussed later).

Fig. 2. Cellular PA (H&E, ×100) showing a tumor deposit in vessel (*inset* [H&E, ×200]).

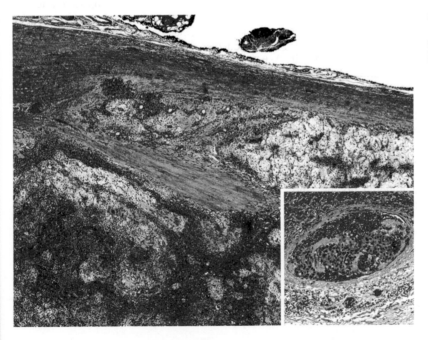

Stromal metaplasias

PA may show a variety of stromal metaplastic changes, including osseous metaplasia, Schwann-type stroma, and lipomatous metaplasia. Lipomatous metaplasia often accompanies skin adnexal–type differentiation.

TREATMENT AND PROGNOSIS

PA is treated surgically and has a very low recurrence rate in modern cohorts (0%–5%), with incomplete resection being the main risk for recurrence. For parotid tumors, pseudopodia pose a theoretic risk for recurrence with narrow resections. If untreated, up to 15% of PAs are estimated to undergo malignant transformation, justifying resection. Metastasizing PA is fairly aggressive and as many as 40% of patients die with disease.[17]

Key Features
PLEOMORPHIC ADENOMA

- PA is the most common salivary gland neoplasm and a large proportion harbor translocations associated with *PLAG1* or *HMGA2*.

- PA shows a broad diversity of architectural, stromal, and cytonuclear features, but is a fundamentally biphasic tumor.

- Random atypia without overgrowth, mitoses, apoptosis, or necrosis is insufficient to designate as intracapsular carcinoma.

- Unusual features such as atypia, pseudopodia, and vascular invasion may raise concern for malignancy, but are still acceptable for PA.

- Metaplasias in PA may overlap with other salivary tumor types.

BASAL CELL ADENOMA AND ADENOCARCINOMA

INTRODUCTION

Basal cell adenoma (BCA) and basal cell adenocarcinoma (BCAC) are rare and almost always arise in the parotid. BCAs have a female predilection of 2:1, occurring in the fourth to fifth decades, whereas BCACs have an even sex distribution and tend to occur 1 decade later. A subset are multifocal and occur within the setting of multiple cylindromatosis and trichoepitheliomas (Brooke-Spiegler syndrome).[18] Biologically, 2 major subgroups exist: those with *CYLD1* mutations (including syndromic variants), and those with *CTTNB1* mutations.

GROSS FEATURES

BCA and BCAC do not have distinctive gross features and show a uniform tan cut surface. BCAs are uninodular and encapsulated, whereas BCACs show a multinodular pattern of permeation with fibrosis. Syndromic BCA and BCAC may show multiple lesions.

MICROSCOPIC FEATURES

BCA and BCAC can be divided into tubulotrabecular, cribriform, membranous, and solid growth patterns (**Fig. 4**). BCAs are more likely to be tubulotrabecular, whereas BCACs are more often membranous or solid. Integral to all types are a biphasic basaloid epithelial proliferation with peripheral palisading of the outermost abluminal cell layer. The abluminal basal cells can be subdivided into outer dark palisaded cells and inner pale basal cells with vesicular nuclei and squamoid features, arguably meriting the term triphasic tumor, most evident in the tubulotrabecular pattern. The cribriform pattern is similar but also manifests cribriform pseudoglandular spaces with matrix reminiscent of adenoid cystic carcinoma. The membranous pattern is essentially the salivary counterpart of dermal eccrine cylindroma, showing a jigsawlike configuration of tumor nests with central hyaline droplets of matrix. The solid pattern may simply be an overgrowth of any of the prior patterns, and may show minimal ductal elements. Mature squamous and sebaceous elements may be present in all patterns. Many tubulotrabecular BCAs and some BCACs show a distinctive spindled myoepithelial cell–derived stroma surrounding the epithelial components. BCACs are typically low grade and are delineated more by their infiltration than by the level of cytonuclear atypia. Perineural invasion is present in one-third of cases. Mitoses are often more than 4 per 10 high-power fields.

BCA and BCAC show variable biphasic immunostaining depending on growth pattern. In addition, the abluminal cells can be substratified, resulting in a triphasic profile (**Fig. 5**): the peripheral palisaded dark cell layer is myoepithelial, and positive for muscle markers as well as high-molecular-weight keratins and p63/p40. The overlying pale abluminal cell layer is only

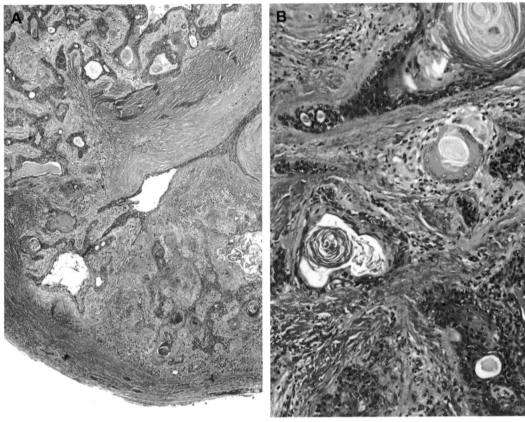

Fig. 3. PA with skin adnexal differentiation. (*A*) The tumor shows cystic change and squamous metaplasia. (H&E, ×40). (*B*) Basaloid nests and infundibulocystic structures are juxtaposed to bilayered tubules. (H&E, ×200).

positive for p63/p40 and high-molecular-weight keratins. When myoepithelial-derived stroma is present, it is intensely positive for S100 (**Fig. 6**A).[19] The tubulotrabecular pattern correlates with *CTTNB1* mutations, which may manifest as nuclear beta-catenin (see **Fig. 6**B), and/or coactivator Lymphoid enhancer-binding factor 1 (LEF-1) staining (see **Fig. 6**C), usually in the dark cell layer and myoepithelial-derived stroma.[20] The membranous pattern, which associates with *CYLD1* alterations, is less likely to show these changes.[18] Ki-67 level may be increased in (>5%) in BCACs compared with BCA.[21]

TREATMENT AND PROGNOSIS

BCAs have a low recurrence rate of ~2%, although the membranous variant, given its propensity for multifocality, may have a recurrence rate as high as 25%. BCACs usually show an indolent behavior, but may be locally aggressive, with about one-third recurring. Regional and distant metastatic rates are ~8% to 12% and ~2% to 4% respectively.[22,23] BCA is treated surgically. BCAC is primarily treated surgically with

regional lymph node dissection as needed. High-stage tumors are treated with radiotherapy, which may improve outcome compared with surgery alone.[23]

Key Features
BASAL CELL ADENOMA AND BASAL CELL ADENOCARCINOMA

- BCA and BCAC are rare parotid gland tumors occurring almost exclusively in the parotid, and a subset are associated with multiple cylindromatosis (Brooke-Spiegler syndrome).

- Tumors show a variety of patterns and the abluminal cells can be further substratified morphologically and immunohistochemically, imparting a triphasic appearance.

- *CTTNB1* and *CYLD1* alterations divide tumors into at least 2 subgroups: the CTTNB1 phenotype (thus showing nuclear beta-catenin) tends to be tubulotrabecular, whereas the CYLD1 phenotype tends to be membranous.

- BCACs are low grade, distinguished from BCAs mainly by infiltration.

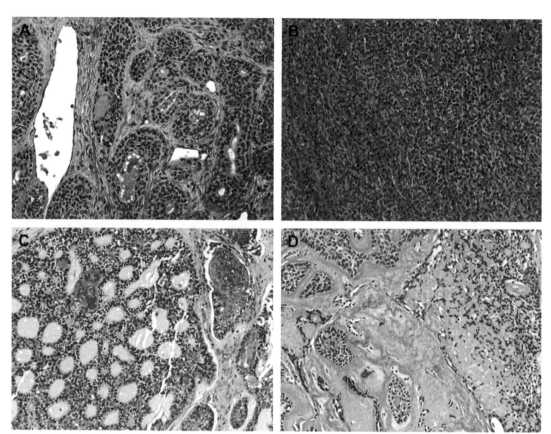

Fig. 4. BCA and BCAC growth patterns. (H&E, ×200). (*A*) Tubulotrabecular, (*B*) solid, (*C*) cribriform with squamous metaplasia, (*D*) membranous.

EPITHELIAL-MYOEPITHELIAL CARCINOMA

INTRODUCTION

EMCA is a biphasic salivary gland malignancy that can occur at any site that contains salivary or seromucinous glands but most frequently occurs in parotid gland (60%–80%) with a peak incidence in the sixth decade. There is a female predilection of 3:2.[24] *RAS* mutations are noted in 20% to 25% of tumors, with *HRAS* codon 61 mutations being among the most common.[25]

GROSS FEATURES

EMCAs characteristically show a homogeneous, multinodular, tan-white cut surface with nodules separated by variable fibrosis. Almost 30% of tumors show varying levels of encapsulation, which may be deceptive. Necrosis and hemorrhage are largely restricted to high-grade tumors.

MICROSCOPIC FEATURES

As the name implies, EMCA is a prototypically biphasic tumor (**Fig. 7**), composed of eosinophilic luminal ductal cells and typically clear, polygonal, abluminal myoepithelial cells that predominate in a ~2:1 to 3:1 proportion to ductal cells. Given the partial encapsulation and rounded border of tumor nodules, limited sampling may be deceiving, imparting the appearance of a benign tumor. Numerous variants are described, most notably oncocytic, apocrine, and high-grade transformed (**Fig. 8**). Oncocytic EMCA has a propensity for papillary growth and sebaceous metaplasia, and apocrine EMCA often shows ductal overgrowth.[26] EMCA with high-grade transformation (HGT) consists of a progression of ductal and/or myoepithelial elements in EMCA to a high-grade carcinoma.[27] Immunohistochemically, as expected, these tumors show a biphasic staining profile noted earlier (**Fig. 9**). Apocrine EMCA also shows AR and GCDFP-15 staining in the ductal components. In EMCA-HGT, the biphasic staining profile may be lost.

TREATMENT AND PROGNOSIS

EMCA is typically a low-grade tumor with a 5-year disease-specific survival of 90% to 95% and

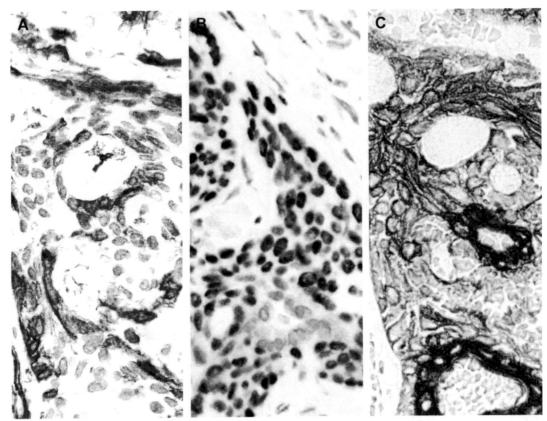

Fig. 5. Triphasic staining in BCA/BCAC. (original magnification, ×200). (*A*) Actin stains the outermost palisaded dark cell layers. (*B*) p63 stains both the outer dark and intermediate pale cells. (*C*) Cytokeratin is strongly positive in ducts but only weakly positive in the abluminal dark and pale cell layers.

10-year disease-specific survival of 80% to 90%.[24,28] Although recurrence rates are about one-third,[24] they are often late, with a median disease-free survival of about 11 years. Regional and distant metastases are uncommon overall (2%–5%).[28] Main prognostic features in EMCA include margin status, vascular invasion, necrosis, and high-grade features, particularly in the

myoepithelial components.[24] EMCA is primarily treated surgically with no discernable value to additional treatment with radiotherapy.[24,28] Data are limited on EMCA-HGT but seem to point to an aggressive course.[27]

ADENOID CYSTIC CARCINOMA

INTRODUCTION

Adenoid cystic carcinoma (ACC) is a morphologically bland but highly infiltrative and aggressive biphasic basaloid tumor whose basic clinicopathologic features are well characterized. ACC is more common at minor salivary sites; however, parotid gland is still the most common single site.[29] Age distribution is wide, with a peak incidence between the fifth and sixth decades, and there is a slight female predilection. The most significant advance in the understanding of ACC is the discovery and characterization of MYB and activation of its downstream targets in this tumor.[30] Specifically, an *MYB-NFIB* translocation [t(6;9)(q22-23;p23-24)] is the main mechanism

---

Key Features
EPITHELIAL-MYOEPITHELIAL CARCINOMA

- EMCAs are low-grade prototypically biphasic malignancies with key variant morphologies including oncocytic, apocrine, and EMCA with HGT.

- About one-quarter show *RAS* mutations, typically *HRAS* codon 61.

- EMCAs show a deceptively bland multinodular growth pattern and may be partially encapsulated.

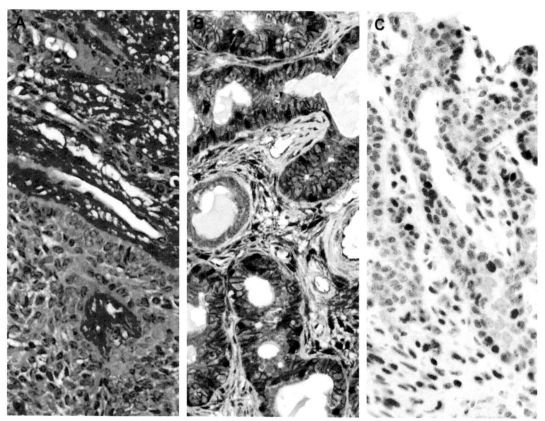

Fig. 6. Additional markers in BCA/BCAC (original magnification, ×200). (*A*) S100 (*red*) highlights myoepithelial-derived stroma. (*B*) Beta-catenin and (*C*) LEF-1 show nuclear staining in the palisaded dark layers and myoepithelial-derived stroma.

for this. Translocation of *MYB* proto-oncogene (typically with transcription factor *NFIB*) has been shown by break-apart or fusion FISH or fusion transcript RT-PCR in 30% to 80% of cases.[31–33] A subset (approximately one-third) of MYB-negative tumors have an alternate translocation, *MYBL1-NFIB*.[34]

GROSS FEATURES

ACC is highly infiltrative and thus gross assessment of disease extent is particularly challenging, especially in the intraoperative setting. ACC usually shows an ill-defined, homogeneous, tan-white cut surface. Bone involvement is typical of sinonasal ACC.

MICROSCOPIC FEATURES

ACC consists of a characteristic infiltrative proliferation of luminal ducts and abluminal myoepithelial cells arranged in tubular, cribriform, or solid growth patterns (**Fig. 10**). Perineural invasion is almost invariably present with adequate sampling. Tumor cells are embedded in a myxo-hyaline stroma that forms cylinders in cribriform

areas. Both ductal and myoepithelial components consist of monomorphic, angulated, hyper-chromatic nuclei with scant cytoplasm. A distinctive feature of ACC is the clefting of tumor nests from the stroma. A rare sclerosing variant of ACC shows tumor cells compressed by abundant hyaline stroma (**Fig. 11**A).[35] As with EMCA and many other tumors, ACC may undergo HGT (see **Fig. 11**B). ACC-HGT is typically an overgrowth of the ductal component into a pleomorphic high-grade or undifferentiated adenocarcinoma.[36]

Immunohistochemically, ACC shows a biphasic staining profile. In addition, CD117 or c-kit is often strongly positive, mainly in the ductal component. Furthermore, MYB protein overexpression can be seen in 60% to 80% of ACCs, including a large proportion of fusion-negative cases.[31–33]

TREATMENT AND PROGNOSIS

ACC shows a slow but relentless progression. Five-year survival is as high as 90%, but 15-year survival is less than 70%,[37] and this decreases sharply afterward.[38] Growth pattern and stage

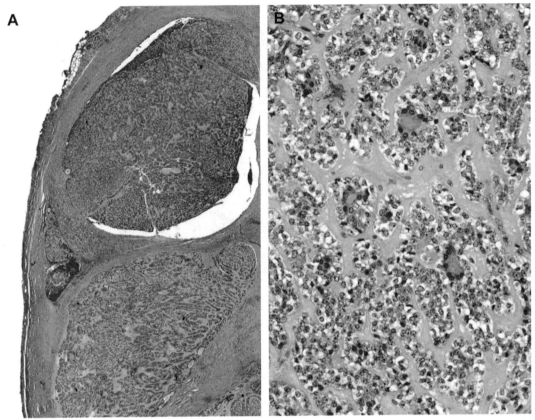

Fig. 7. EMCA. (*A*) Multinodular growth pattern with sclerosis and partial encapsulation. (H&E, ×20). (*B*) Prototypical biphasic tubular growth with pale abluminal myoepithelial cells and eosinophilic luminal ductal cells. (H&E, ×100).

are major prognosticators. In general, solid growth of more than 30% correlates with adverse outcome.[39] ACC is unusual in that the risk for regional spread is low (~5%–20%) in relation to its propensity for local recurrence.[39] About 10% to 15% of patients show distant metastases, typically to lungs, bone, and brain.[37,39] Treatment includes surgery as well as radiation. Resection of metastases, particularly those of lung, may prolong survival, although the overall benefit is not well established.[40] In contrast, ACC-HGT is rapidly aggressive, with median survival of 12 to 36 months.[36] Unlike its conventional counterpart, nodal disease is frequent.

Key Features
ADENOID CYSTIC CARCINOMA

- ACC is a well-characterized, slow-growing, but relentless salivary gland malignancy with favorable 5-year survival but poor long-term outcomes.

- Tumors are now defined by *MYB* alterations, typically a *MYB-NFIB* translocation, although *MYBL1* alterations are now described as well.

- The tumor is typically highly infiltrative and is a biphasic tumor composed of a mixture of tubular, cribriform, and solid growth of angulated hyperchromatic cells with scant cytoplasm.

- The myxohyaline stroma is characteristic, as is the clefting of tumor nests from this stroma.

- HGT is typically a progression of the ductal component to an undifferentiated carcinoma or poorly differentiated adenocarcinoma. ACC-HGT has a more aggressive outcome and rapid course.

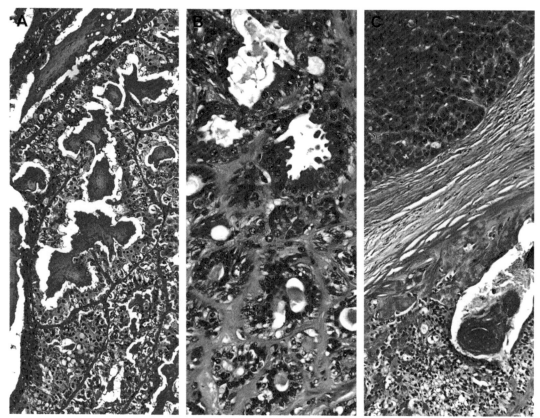

Fig. 8. EMCA variants (H&E, ×200) (*A*) Oncocytic EMCA showing large-caliber tubules and abortive papillae. (*B*) Apocrine EMCA (*top*) transitioning from conventional component. (*C*) EMCA with high-grade transformation of myoepithelial component (*top*).

DIFFERENTIAL DIAGNOSIS

The key features of the aforementioned biphasic tumors are summarized in Table 2.

Tumor border is useful in the distinction because PA and BCA have an encapsulated, well-demarcated border; EMCA and BCAC have a multinodular, infiltrative growth with variable sclerosis; and ACC is frankly infiltrative. One caveat is that membranous BCA may be multifocal and can simulate malignancy, although these multiple foci do not have as much stromal reaction and are not confluent, as expected for BCAC. However, tumor border may not be apparent on small biopsies. Thus, without tumor normal interface, it may be prudent to defer final diagnosis to resection. Intervening stroma may be a useful diagnostic feature as well. PA shows characteristic myxoid stroma containing spindled to stellate myoepithelial cells that stream from the tubules. BCA may show a peculiar myxoid myoepithelial-derived stroma, but this stroma is uniform and distinct from the tubulotrabecular elements. All biphasic tumors may show cylinders of matrix

that mimic the appearance of ACC, thus other features must be taken into consideration. Peripheral palisading and triphasic morphology/immunophenotype are useful discriminators of BCA and BCAC from other biphasic tumors. ACCs are distinct from the other tumors in their starkly angulated hyperchromatic nuclei and clefting of tumor nests from the stroma. In addition, ACC tends to be a pure tumor with an exceptionally low frequency of metaplasias. EMCAs typically show polygonal clear cell morphology in their abluminal myoepithelial components. Useful ancillary markers are summarized in Table 2. Although c-kit is commonly overexpressed in ACC, it is also noted in EMCA and BCAC and is thus not particularly useful here.[24]

PAs also have other distinctive diagnostic considerations. Aside from biphasic tumors, stroma-rich PAs may overlap with nodular fasciitis, schwannomas, and chondroid lesions such as synovial chondromatosis. Additional sections and levels in a stroma-rich lesion to identify ductal elements are key first steps to distinguish myxoid PA from a true mesenchymal lesion.

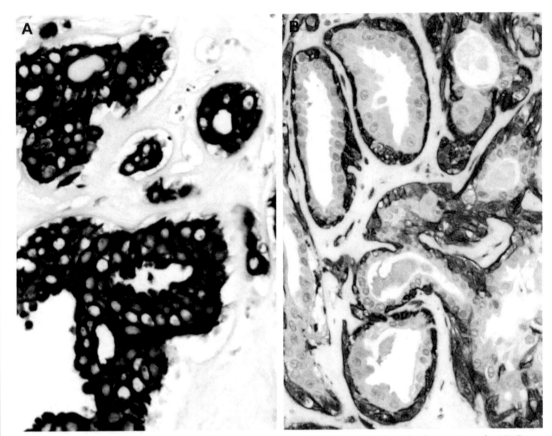

Fig. 9. Biphasic profile in EMCA. (original magnification, ×400). (*A*) Luminal ductal cells are strongly AE1/3 positive. (*B*) Actin (*black*)-p63 (*red*) double stain highlights the abluminal myoepithelial cells.

However, immunohistochemical markers may be needed as well to highlight the myoepithelial components. Pseudopodia and vascular invasion may raise concern for malignancy. Atypia, particularly when random and unaccompanied by other features such as overgrowth and high cell turnover, is not sufficient alone to designate as intracapsular carcinoma. Unlike truly invasive malignant tumors, these areas are devoid of sclerosis/desmoplasia and are fairly paucicellular with myxoid stroma. Regarding metaplasias, the key to distinguishing these from their mimics (ie, mucoepidermoid metaplasia in PA vs mucoepidermoid carcinoma) is to recognize the PA components, which may necessitate levels, additional sections, or immunohistochemical staining to document myoepithelial phenotypes.

MAMMARY ANALOGUE SECRETORY CARCINOMA

INTRODUCTION

Mammary analogue secretory carcinoma (MASC) is a salivary gland malignancy that was recognized based on distinctive morphologic and molecular features.[41,42] It is named for its recapitulation of (juvenile) secretory carcinoma of breast, along with its shared molecular phenotype. Most MASCs were historically designated as acinic cell carcinoma or adenocarcinoma not otherwise specified. Although parotid is still the most common site, in contrast with acinic cell carcinoma, minor salivary sites are more frequently involved than acinic cell carcinoma.[41,43] MASC typically occurs in the fifth to sixth decades with an even sex predilection, in contrast with the female predominance in acinic cell carcinoma.

Like secretory carcinoma of breast, and other tumors such as infantile fibrosarcoma, mesoblastic nephroma, and a subgroup of leukemias and papillary thyroid carcinomas, MASCs usually harbor a t(12;15)(p13;q25), resulting in an *ETV6-NTRK3*.[42] A subset of MASCs show *ETV6* rearrangements with as-yet unknown partner.[44]

GROSS FEATURES

Most MASCs are less than 2 cm.[45] Grossly they range from a solid tan-brown to cystic.

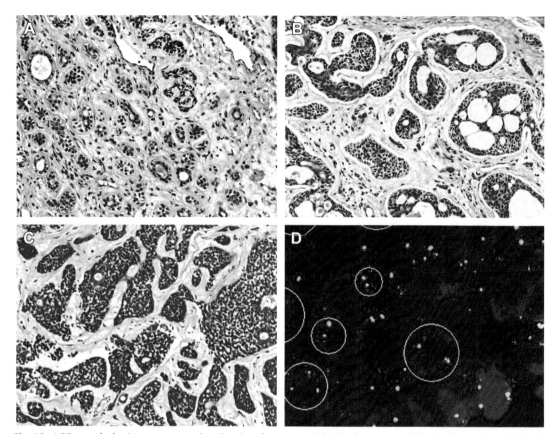

Fig. 10. ACC morphologic spectrum and molecular phenotype. (*A*) Tubular pattern, (*B*) cribriform, (*C*) solid. (H&E, ×100). (*D*) Fusion FISH for *MYB-NFIB* translocation (*circled cells* show a *fused yellow signal*).

MICROSCOPIC FEATURES

MASCs share the growth patterns of acinic cell carcinoma, but instead are characterized by the multivacuolated eosinophilic cytoplasm, often with luminal and intracytoplasmic mucin and no true zymogen granules (**Fig. 12**A). Papillary cystic architecture is now considered rare in true acinic cell carcinoma and is far more common in MASC. Both MASCs show globular rather than granular staining. MASCs are S100 (see **Fig. 12**B) and mammaglobin positive, and typically negative for DOG1.[46] SOX-10, a marker of intercalated duct and acinar cells, is positive as well.

Tumors with *ETV6* and an unknown partner tend to be more infiltrative and sclerotic. MASC with HGT can occur.

TREATMENT AND PROGNOSIS

Outcome data are limited, but MASC is typically indolent, like acinic cell carcinoma. It may show a slightly higher lymph node metastatic rate (up to 25%) than true acinic cell carcinoma.[45] Treatment is mainly surgical. Adverse prognostic features include stage and HGT.[47] With the

development of selective tyrosine kinase inhibitors, recognition of MASC for advanced-stage cases may eventually have direct therapeutic relevance.[48]

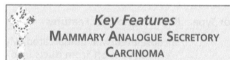

Key Features
MAMMARY ANALOGUE SECRETORY CARCINOMA

- MASC is a new entity identified from a subset of acinic cell carcinomas and adenocarcinomas not otherwise specified, based on its resemblance to breast secretory carcinoma.

- MASC is characterized by growth patterns similar to those of acinic cell carcinoma, but distinguished by the vacuolated eosinophilic cytoplasm and luminal secretions.

- MASC is typically S100 and mammaglobin positive.

- MASC is characterized by an *ETV6-NTRK3* translocation, with some sclerotic infiltrative tumors showing *ETV6* translocations with an unknown partner.

- MASCs are typically indolent; MASC-HGT exist but are rare.

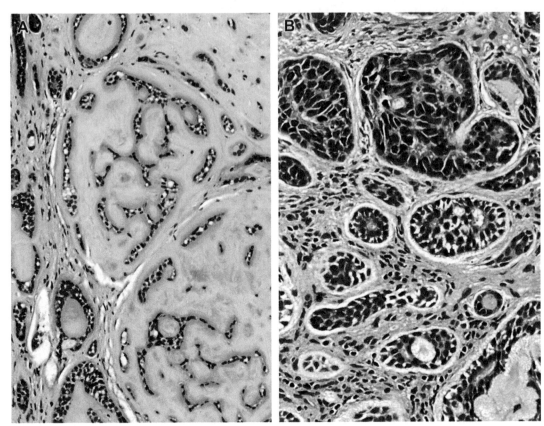

Fig. 11. ACC variants. (H&E, ×200). (*A*) Sclerosing ACC with scant compressed cellular elements. (*B*) ACC-HGT with progression to a pleomorphic adenocarcinoma (*top*).

Table 2
Biphasic tumor diagnostic features

Tumor Type	Key Morphologic Features	Key Ancillary Studies
PA	Encapsulated/well demarcated. Myoepithelial cells stream off from ducts into a chondromyxoid stroma	GFAP staining of stroma. PLAG immunostaining *PLAG1* or *HMGA2* rearrangements
BCA	Encapsulated/well demarcated. Peripheral palisading with outer dark basal layer, intermediate pale basal layer and luminal ductal layer (triphasic). Intervening myoepithelial-derived spindled stroma is distinct from tubules and trabeculae. Squamous and sebaceous elements	Triphasic immunophenotype Tubulotrabecular tumors: LEF1 and nuclear beta-catenin Membranous tumors: *CYLD1* alterations
BCAC	Multinodular to infiltrative; otherwise similar to BCA	Similar to BCA; mitoses often >4 per 10 HPF; Ki-67 often >5%
EMCA	Multinodular with sclerosis Polygonal, often clear abluminal myoepithelial cells	*HRAS* codon 61 mutations in a subset
ACC	Highly infiltrative, angulated, hyperchromatic tumor cells clefting from stroma. Metaplastic features (squamous, oncocytic, sebaceous) are exceptionally rare	MYB or MYBL1 alterations

Abbreviation: HPF, high-power field.

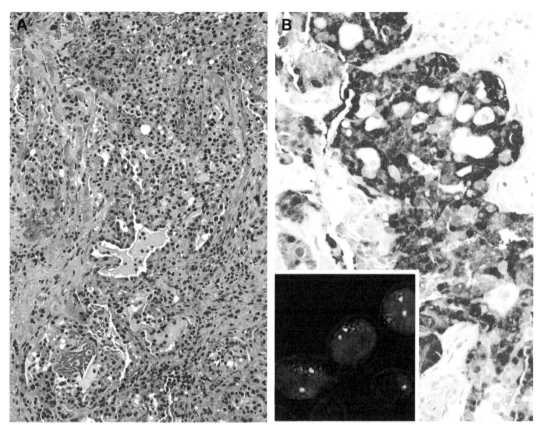

Fig. 12. MASC morphology and phenotype. (*A*) Solid to follicular growth with numerous secretions; the tumor cells are eosinophilic and vacuolated. (H&E, ×100). (*B*) S100 is strongly positive. (original magnification, ×200). (*Inset*) ETV6 break-apart FISH showing a translocation denoted by a split red green signal, with the intact copy being yellow.

DIFFERENTIAL DIAGNOSIS

Testing for the *ETV6* gene rearrangements is the definitive diagnostic test to confirm MASC, but other considerations should be ruled in or ruled out by morphology and immunostains to limit unnecessary testing. The key differential diagnostic considerations for MASC are summarized in **Table 3**. The main diagnostic considerations include acinic cell carcinoma, and low-grade intraductal carcinoma (ie, low-grade cribriform cystadenocarcinoma or low-grade salivary duct carcinoma).

Acinic cell carcinoma is mainly distinguished by cytomorphologic features because it shares growth patterns with MASC. Acinic cell carcinoma shows true basophilic zymogen granules (**Fig. 13**A), although oncocytic, clear cell, and vacuolar change occasionally obfuscate this feature. Tumor cells tend to be more monomorphic than those of MASC. Aside from the granular periodic acid–Schiff staining after diastase in acinic cell carcinoma, the other useful marker is DOG1, which shows a strong membranous and apical staining pattern (see **Fig. 13**B).[46] Low-grade intraductal carcinoma

(low-grade cribriform cystadenocarcinoma) can mimic the appearance of MASC (see **Fig. 13**C), particularly if it is oncocyte papillary pattern–rich.[49] In addition, this tumor may also show S100 and mammaglobin staining.[50] However, morphologically, areas consisting of monomorphic cuboidal cells with scant eosinophilic cytoplasm reminiscent of low-grade ductal carcinoma in situ of breast are useful discriminatory features. In addition, a p63 immunostain shows a purely, or at least predominantly, intraductal growth pattern (see **Fig. 13**D). Intraductal growth, when present in MASC, is focal.[45,51] It is important to distinguish low-grade intraductal carcinoma from MASC, because the course for the former is essentially benign.

Other less common but still important diagnostic considerations for MASC include mucoepidermoid carcinoma, salivary duct carcinoma, and mucin-producing signet ring adenocarcinoma (ie, secretory myoepithelial carcinoma).[45] Mucoepidermoid carcinomas with adequate sampling show epidermoid and intermediate cell components and are usually S100 negative. Mucin-producing signet

Table 3
Key differential diagnoses for mammary analogue secretory carcinoma

	MASC	Acinic Cell Carcinoma	Intraductal Carcinoma
Site distribution	Major and minor salivary	Major salivary, minor extremely rare	Major salivary (parotid), minor extremely rare
Growth patterns	Solid, follicular, microcystic, papillary cystic	Solid, follicular, microcystic, papillary cystic is extremely rare	Solid, cribriform, cystic, papillary, micropapillary
Lymphoid stroma	Yes	Yes	Yes (rare)
Cell morphology	Eosinophilic vacuolated cells with globular luminal and intracytoplasmic secretions	Granular basophilic cells; oncocytic, clear cell, and vacuolar change less prominent	Scant lightly eosinophilic cytoplasm; oncocytic papillary change fairly common
Nuclei	Fairly monomorphic, slight size variation	Usually monomorphic	Monomorphic and evenly spaced
Immunophenotype	S100, mammaglobin positive, DOG1 weak to negative, p63 only occasional intraductal foci	S100 weak to negative, mammaglobin negative, DOG1 membranous and apical, p63 negative	S100, mammaglobin positive, DOG1 weak to negative, p63 almost entirely intraductal

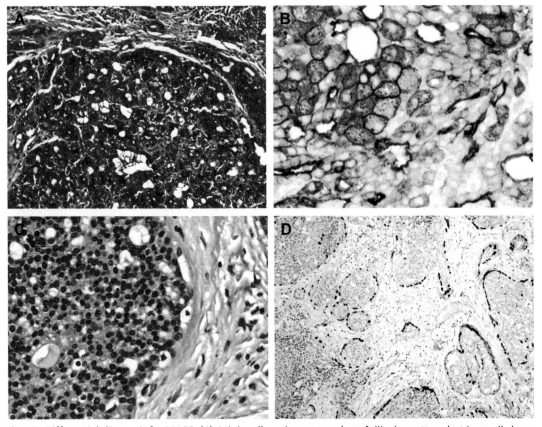

Fig. 13. Differential diagnosis for MASC. (*A*) Acinic cell carcinoma can show follicular pattern but is usually basophilic secondary to zymogen granules. (H&E, ×100). (*B*) DOG1 shows intense membranous and apical staining (H&E, ×400). (*C*) Low-grade intraductal carcinoma can resemble MASC but consists of more monomorphic evenly spaced cells with scanter cytoplasm reminiscent of breast low-grade ductal carcinoma in situ (H&E, ×400). (*D*) Staining with p63 highlights the intraductal nature of the tumor (original magnification, ×100).

ring adenocarcinoma shows univacuolated rather than multivacuolated cells and may show muscle marker expression, in contrast with MASC. Salivary duct carcinoma is an apocrine tumor and is AR positive and S100 negative; this can be confused with MASC-HGT in particular. Rarely, polymorphous low-grade adenocarcinoma/cribriform adenocarcinoma of (minor) salivary gland origin (CAMSG) enters the differential diagnosis, mainly secondary to immunophenotypic overlap. However, the nuclear features are characteristically ovoid and vesicular to clear with scant, less vacuolated cytoplasm than is seen in MASC.

POLYMORPHOUS LOW-GRADE ADENOCARCINOMA AND CRIBRIFORM ADENOCARCINOMA OF (MINOR) SALIVARY GLAND

(CLASSIC) POLYMORPHOUS LOW-GRADE ADENOCARCINOMA

Introduction

Polymorphous low-grade adenocarcinoma (PLGA) has been the most contentious entity over the past decade. The term PLGA was first used in 1984 by Evans and Batsakis[52] to describe an infiltrative salivary tumor with a variety of growth patterns but bland nuclei. The growth pattern and stromal characteristics mimic those of ACC and historically have been diagnostically challenging to differentiate. However, the importance of distinction lies in the much more indolent behavior of PLGA compared with ACC. PLGAs almost exclusively occur in minor salivary sites, with the palate being the most frequent. They predominate in the fifth decade and show a female predilection of 2:1.[53–55]

Recent studies indicate that classic PLGA frequently (~75%) shows *PRKD1* E710D mutations,[56,57] and less than 10% show *PRKD1, PRKD12,* or *PRKD13* translocations.[58]

Gross Features

PLGA consists of an ill-defined, homogeneous, tan cut surface. For palatal tumors, bone involvement is common.[55]

Microscopic Features

PLGA shows a spectrum of tubular, fascicular, cribriform, papillary, or solid architecture. Classically they are infiltrative and show a targetoid appearance with perineural invasion (**Fig. 14**A, B). Despite their diverse growth patterns, they fundamentally consist of 1 cell type with a (terminal) ductal phenotype, consisting of uniform ovoid vesicular nuclei and scant to moderate lightly eosinophilic cytoplasm. S100 is diffusely strongly positive in these tumors,[53,55] but they do not have a prominent basal or myoepithelial component. Nonetheless, they are often p63 positive in a random rather than patterned fashion, but the more myoepithelial cell–specific ΔNp63 antibody, p40, is still negative.[59]

Tumors in general are low grade, hence the name; however, tumors with mitotic rates greater than 3 per 10 high-power fields, nuclear size variation, and even necrosis exist,[55,60] which has led some investigators to suggest ceasing to use the term low grade in the name of the tumor. Overt HGT has been described as well.[61]

CRIBRIFORM ADENOCARCINOMA OF (MINOR) SALIVARY GLAND ORIGIN

Introduction

At base-of-tongue sites, a distinctive cribriform architecture was noted along with more overtly cleared (papillary thyroid carcinoma–like) nuclei, initiating the proposal for reclassification of this subset of tumors as cribriform adenocarcinoma of tongue, and subsequently CAMSG.[62] CAMSG, as suggested by the name, predominate at minor salivary sites, frequently base of tongue and other extrapalatal sites.[60] Age and gender distributions are similar to those of classic PLGA.

Gross Features

CAMSG is grossly similar to PLGA, although often more friable and cystic. It is also roughly 1 cm larger on average.[60,62]

Microscopic Features

Despite the presence of "cribriform" in the proposed name for this tumor, the growth pattern is more characteristically papillary glomeruloid. CAMSG morphology tends to show more cytonuclear atypia than classic PLGA and shows prominent vesicular, clear, ovoid nuclei with membrane irregularities reminiscent of those seen in papillary thyroid carcinoma (see **Fig. 14**C, D). The growth pattern is infiltrative but not as neurotropic as in classic PLGA, and these tumors have a higher propensity for lymphatic invasion.

Treatment and Prognosis: Polymorphous Low-Grade Adenocarcinoma and Cribriform Adenocarcinoma of (Minor) Salivary Gland Origin

Most tumors are indolent but with local recurrence rates of 10% to 30% and regional metastases of about 15%. Distant metastases and death from disease are exceptionally rare.[53–55,60,62,63] CAMSGs have a higher rate of regional and

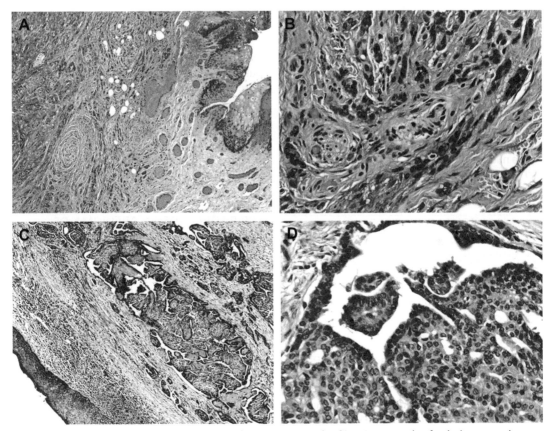

Fig. 14. PLGA versus CAMSG. (*A*) Classic PLGA shows a targetoid infiltrative growth of tubules around nerves (H&E, ×40). (*B*) Tumor cells around the nerves show ovoid vesicular nuclei (H&E, ×200). (*C*) CAMSG shows a papillary glomeruloid architecture (H&E, ×40). (*D*) Cribriform and papillary areas show ovoid vesicular to clear papillary thyroid carcinoma–like nuclei (H&E, ×200).

possibly distant spread. However, histologic designation of CAMSG versus PLGA recently only showed slight differences in outcome, with papillary architecture greater than 10% and cribriform architecture greater than 30% being more important, regardless of histologic designation.[60] HGT is not well characterized clinically because it has rarely been reported.[61]

Key Features
POLYMORPHOUS LOW-GRADE ADENOCARCINOMA AND CRIBRIFORM ADENOCARCINOMA OF (MINOR) SALIVARY GLAND ORIGIN

- PLGA is a low-grade infiltrative malignancy with a mixture of tubular, cribriform, papillary, and solid growth, arranged in fascicles with targetoid neurotropism, predominating in palate and other minor salivary sites and historically mistaken for ACC.

- CAMSG is a tumor with distinctive cribriform/papillary glomeruloid morphologic and highly vesicular papillary thyroid carcinoma–like nuclei predominating in base of tongue and other minor salivary sites.

- PLGA is phenotypically ductal, and strongly S100 positive, but may show p63 immunoreactivity in a nonpatterned fashion; however, p40 is negative.

- PLGAs are characterized by *PRKD1* E710D mutations, whereas CAMSGs are characterized by *PRKD1-3* translocations; however, molecular overlap exists.

- CAMSGs have a higher capacity for nodal spread; cribriform and papillary growth alone are stronger adverse prognosticators than classification as PLGA versus CAMSG.

Differential Diagnosis and Controversies

The main controversy surrounding PLGA centers on CAMSG, and is one of speciation. Based on clinical, morphologic, and molecular differences, many clinicians advocate for separation of CAMSG into a distinct entity. The counterargument is that there is still morphologic and molecular overlap between these entities. In addition, tumors with indeterminate designation have been described as well, further indicating that morphologic features are not entirely distinct between these entities.[56,58,60] Justification of separating CAMSG is more tenuous than for other entities, notably MASC. In stark contrast, MASC has a specific (at least in the context of salivary tumors) defining molecular alteration, uniformly distinctive morphology compared with acinic cell carcinoma, far more easily justifying separation. Thus the ultimate decision on separation of CAMSG and PLGA may require additional studies, but likely will still be subjective.

A minor controversy is the retention of "low grade" in the diagnosis of PLGA. Although most tumors are still low grade, intermediate-grade and even high-grade variants have been described.[55,60,61] Retaining the term low grade may preclude recognition of a higher-grade spectrum within this category of tumors. Removing the term low grade would necessitate enumerating criteria to separate intermediate-grade and high-grade tumors.

In addition, a common but overrated diagnostic dilemma is between PLGA/CAMSG (more frequently classic PLGA) and ACC. Both tumors share growth patterns, but have fundamental differences. Most importantly, PLGA is a monophasic ductal tumor with minimal to no myoepithelial elements. ACC is a biphasic tumor. Recognition of this distinction trivializes this dilemma with adequate sampling (it may still be difficult on biopsies) and allows for a proper framework in using immunohistochemical stains. Furthermore, ACC shows angulated hyperchromatic nuclei and PLGA (and especially CAMSG) show vesicular ovoid cleared nuclei. PLGA does not show the biphasic pattern of muscle marker expression as noted earlier. Both ACC and PLGA may show p63 staining, but ACC shows an abluminal pattern, whereas PLGA staining is diffuse or random and variable. However, with limited sampling, p40, the more specific myoepithelial marker, can be useful because it is retained in ACC abluminal cells, and negative in PLGA.[59] In contrast, S100 is intensely positive in PLGA, and weak to negative in ACC. C-kit is more frequently positive in ACC, but PLGA may also show focal expression. MYB immunostains are generally specific for ACC. The distinction between PLGA, CAMSG, and ACC is summarized in **Table 4**.

Table 4
Comparison of polymorphous low-grade adenocarcinoma, cribriform adenocarcinoma of (minor) salivary gland origin, and adenoid cystic carcinoma

	PLGA	CAMSG	ACC
Site	Minor salivary (palate predominant)	Minor salivary (base of tongue predominant)	Major and minor salivary
Growth	Tubular, cribriform, papillary and solid, targetoid	Cribriform, papillary-glomeruloid	Tubular, cribriform, solid
Phenotype	Monophasic (terminal) ductal	Monophasic (terminal) ductal	Biphasic
Nuclear features	Vesicular and ovoid nuclei	Exaggerated vesicular (papillary thyroid carcinoma–like) nuclei	Angulated hyperchromatic nuclei
Immunophenotype	p63: nonpatterned S100: strongly positive Muscle marker and p40: negative	p63: nonpatterned S100: strongly positive Muscle marker and p40: negative	Biphasic staining S100: weak to negative
Key molecular alterations	PRKD1 E710D mutations	PRKD1-3 translocations	MYB, MYB-L1 alterations

REFERENCES

1. Ellis GL, Auclair PL, Gnepp DR. Salivary gland neoplasms: general considerations. . Surgical pathology of the salivary glands. Philadelpia: Saunders; 1991. p. 135–64.
2. Spiro RH. Salivary neoplasms: overview of a 35-year experience with 2,807 patients. Head Neck Surg 1986;8(3):177–84.
3. Zhan KY, Khaja SF, Flack AB, et al. Benign parotid tumors. Otolaryngol Clin North Am 2016;49(2):327–42.
4. Bradley PJ, McGurk M. Incidence of salivary gland neoplasms in a defined UK population. Br J Oral Maxillofac Surg 2013;51(5):399–403.
5. Seethala RR, Barnes EL. Rare malignant and benign salivary gland epithelial tumors. Surg Pathol Clin 2011;4(4):1217–72.
6. Seethala RR, Barnes EL. Common malignant salivary gland epithelial tumors. Surg Pathol Clin 2011;4(4):1177–215.
7. Takeichi N, Hirose F, Yamamoto H, et al. Salivary gland tumors in atomic bomb survivors, Hiroshima, Japan. II. Pathologic study and supplementary epidemiologic observations. Cancer 1983;52(2):377–85.
8. Bullerdiek J, Hutter KJ, Brandt G, et al. Cytogenetic investigations on a cell line derived from a carcinoma arising in a salivary gland pleomorphic adenoma. Cancer Genet Cytogenet 1990;44(2):253–62.
9. Bullerdiek J, Wobst G, Meyer-Bolte K, et al. Cytogenetic subtyping of 220 salivary gland pleomorphic adenomas: correlation to occurrence, histological subtype, and in vitro cellular behavior. Cancer Genet Cytogenet 1993;65(1):27–31.
10. Ahn MS, Hayashi GM, Hilsinger RL Jr, et al. Familial mixed tumors of the parotid gland. Head Neck 1999;21(8):772–5.
11. Yu GY, Ma DQ, Zhang Y, et al. Multiple primary tumours of the parotid gland. Int J Oral Maxillofac Surg 2004;33(6):531–4.
12. Kadletz L, Grasl S, Grasl MC, et al. Extracapsular dissection versus superficial parotidectomy in benign parotid gland tumors: the Vienna Medical School experience. Head Neck 2016, [Epub ahead of print].
13. Kato H, Kanematsu M, Mizuta K, et al. Imaging findings of parapharyngeal space pleomorphic adenoma in comparison with parotid gland pleomorphic adenoma. Jpn J Radiol 2013;31(11):724–30.
14. Wu YC, Wang YP, Cheng SJ, et al. Clinicopathological study of 74 palatal pleomorphic adenomas. J Formos Med Assoc 2016;115(1):25–30.
15. Lopes ML, Barroso KM, Henriques AC, et al. Pleomorphic adenomas of the salivary glands: retrospective multicentric study of 130 cases with emphasis on histopathological features. Eur Arch Otorhinolaryngol 2016, [Epub ahead of print].
16. Zbaren P, Stauffer E. Pleomorphic adenoma of the parotid gland: histopathologic analysis of the capsular characteristics of 218 tumors. Head Neck 2007;29(8):751–7.
17. Bradley PJ. 'Metastasizing pleomorphic salivary adenoma' should now be considered a low-grade malignancy with a lethal potential. Curr Opin Otolaryngol Head Neck Surg 2005;13(2):123–6.
18. Kazakov DV, Schaller J, Vanecek T, et al. Brooke-Spiegler syndrome: report of a case with a novel mutation in the CYLD gene and different types of somatic mutations in benign and malignant tumors. J Cutan Pathol 2010;37(8):886–90.
19. Dardick I, Daley TD, van Nostrand AW. Basal cell adenoma with myoepithelial cell-derived "stroma": a new major salivary gland tumor entity. Head Neck Surg 1986;8(4):257–67.
20. Bilodeau EA, Acquafondata M, Barnes EL, et al. A comparative analysis of LEF-1 in odontogenic and salivary tumors. Hum Pathol 2015;46(2):255–9.
21. Nagao T, Sugano I, Ishida Y, et al. Basal cell adenocarcinoma of the salivary glands: comparison with basal cell adenoma through assessment of cell proliferation, apoptosis, and expression of p53 and bcl-2. Cancer 1998;82(3):439–47.
22. Muller S, Barnes L. Basal cell adenocarcinoma of the salivary glands. Report of seven cases and review of the literature. Cancer 1996;78(12):2471–7.
23. Zhan KY, Lentsch EJ. Basal cell adenocarcinoma of the major salivary glands: a population-level study of 509 cases. Laryngoscope 2016;126(5):1086–90.
24. Seethala RR, Barnes EL, Hunt JL. Epithelial-myoepithelial carcinoma: a review of the clinicopathologic spectrum and immunophenotypic characteristics in 61 tumors of the salivary glands and upper aerodigestive tract. Am J Surg Pathol 2007;31(1):44–57.
25. Chiosea SI, Miller M, Seethala RR. HRAS mutations in epithelial-myoepithelial carcinoma. Head Neck Pathol 2014;8(2):146–50.
26. Seethala RR. Oncocytic and apocrine epithelial myoepithelial carcinoma: novel variants of a challenging tumor. Head Neck Pathol 2013;7(Suppl 1):S77–84.
27. Roy P, Bullock MJ, Perez-Ordonez B, et al. Epithelial-myoepithelial carcinoma with high grade transformation. Am J Surg Pathol 2010;34(9):1258–65.
28. Vazquez A, Patel TD, D'Aguillo CM, et al. Epithelial-myoepithelial carcinoma of the salivary glands: an analysis of 246 cases. Otolaryngol Head Neck Surg 2015;153(4):569–74.
29. Li N, Xu L, Zhao H, et al. A comparison of the demographics, clinical features, and survival of patients with adenoid cystic carcinoma of major and minor salivary glands versus less common sites within the Surveillance, Epidemiology, and End Results registry. Cancer 2012;118(16):3945–53.

30. Persson M, Andren Y, Mark J, et al. Recurrent fusion of MYB and NFIB transcription factor genes in carcinomas of the breast and head and neck. Proc Natl Acad Sci U S A 2009;106(44):18740–4.

31. Brill LB 2nd, Kanner WA, Fehr A, et al. Analysis of MYB expression and MYB-NFIB gene fusions in adenoid cystic carcinoma and other salivary neoplasms. Mod Pathol 2011;24(9):1169–76.

32. West RB, Kong C, Clarke N, et al. MYB expression and translocation in adenoid cystic carcinomas and other salivary gland tumors with clinicopathologic correlation. Am J Surg Pathol 2011;35(1):92–9.

33. Mitani Y, Li J, Rao PH, et al. Comprehensive analysis of the MYB-NFIB gene fusion in salivary adenoid cystic carcinoma: incidence, variability, and clinicopathologic significance. Clin Cancer Res 2010; 16(19):4722–31.

34. Mitani Y, Liu B, Rao PH, et al. Novel MYBL1 gene rearrangements with recurrent MYBL1-NFIB fusions in salivary adenoid cystic carcinomas lacking t(6;9) translocations. Clin Cancer Res 2016; 22(3):725–33.

35. Albores-Saavedra J, Wu J, Uribe-Uribe N. The sclerosing variant of adenoid cystic carcinoma: a previously unrecognized neoplasm of major salivary glands. Ann Diagn Pathol 2006;10(1):1–7.

36. Seethala RR, Hunt JL, Baloch ZW, et al. Adenoid cystic carcinoma with high-grade transformation: a report of 11 cases and a review of the literature. Am J Surg Pathol 2007;31(11):1683–94.

37. Ellington CL, Goodman M, Kono SA, et al. Adenoid cystic carcinoma of the head and neck: incidence and survival trends based on 1973-2007 surveillance, epidemiology, and end results data. Cancer 2012;118(18):4444–51.

38. Spiro RH, Huvos AG, Strong EW. Adenoid cystic carcinoma of salivary origin. A clinicopathologic study of 242 cases. Am J Surg 1974;128(4):512–20.

39. Seethala RR. Histologic grading and prognostic biomarkers in salivary gland carcinomas. Adv Anat Pathol 2011;18(1):29–45.

40. Bobbio A, Copelli C, Ampollini L, et al. Lung metastasis resection of adenoid cystic carcinoma of salivary glands. Eur J Cardiothorac Surg 2008;33(5): 790–3.

41. Chiosea SI, Griffith C, Assaad A, et al. The profile of acinic cell carcinoma after recognition of mammary analog secretory carcinoma. Am J Surg Pathol 2012;36(3):343–50.

42. Skalova A, Vanecek T, Sima R, et al. Mammary analogue secretory carcinoma of salivary glands, containing the ETV6-NTRK3 fusion gene: a hitherto undescribed salivary gland tumor entity. Am J Surg Pathol 2010;34(5):599–608.

43. Bishop JA, Yonescu R, Batista D, et al. Most nonparotid "acinic cell carcinomas" represent mammary analog secretory carcinomas. Am J Surg Pathol 2013;37(7):1053–7.

44. Skalova A, Vanecek T, Simpson RH, et al. Mammary analogue secretory carcinoma of salivary glands: molecular analysis of 25 ETV6 gene rearranged tumors with lack of detection of classical ETV6-NTRK3 fusion transcript by standard RT-PCR: report of 4 cases harboring ETV6-X gene fusion. Am J Surg Pathol 2016;40(1):3–13.

45. Chiosea SI, Griffith C, Assaad A, et al. Clinicopathological characterization of mammary analogue secretory carcinoma of salivary glands. Histopathology 2012;61(3):387–94.

46. Chenevert J, Duvvuri U, Chiosea S, et al. DOG1: a novel marker of salivary acinar and intercalated duct differentiation. Mod Pathol 2012;25(7):919–29.

47. Skalova A, Vanecek T, Majewska H, et al. Mammary analogue secretory carcinoma of salivary glands with high-grade transformation: report of 3 cases with the ETV6-NTRK3 gene fusion and analysis of TP53, beta-catenin, EGFR, and CCND1 genes. Am J Surg Pathol 2014;38(1):23–33.

48. Drilon A, Li G, Dogan S, et al. What hides behind the MASC: clinical response and acquired resistance to entrectinib after ETV6-NTRK3 identification in a mammary analogue secretory carcinoma (MASC). Ann Oncol 2016;27(5):920–6.

49. Brandwein-Gensler MS, Gnepp DR. Low grade cribriform cystadenocarcinoma. In: Barnes L, Eveson JW, Reichart P, et al, editors. World Health Organization classification of tumours: pathology and genetics of head and neck tumours. Lyon (France): IARC; 2005. p. 233.

50. Stevens TM, Kovalovsky AO, Velosa C, et al. Mammary analog secretory carcinoma, low-grade salivary duct carcinoma, and mimickers: a comparative study. Mod Pathol 2015;28(8):1084–100.

51. Connor A, Perez-Ordonez B, Shago M, et al. Mammary analog secretory carcinoma of salivary gland origin with the ETV6 gene rearrangement by FISH: expanded morphologic and immunohistochemical spectrum of a recently described entity. Am J Surg Pathol 2012;36(1):27–34.

52. Evans HL, Batsakis JG. Polymorphous low-grade adenocarcinoma of minor salivary glands. A study of 14 cases of a distinctive neoplasm. Cancer 1984; 53(4):935–42.

53. Castle JT, Thompson LD, Frommelt RA, et al. Polymorphous low grade adenocarcinoma: a clinicopathologic study of 164 cases. Cancer 1999;86(2): 207–19.

54. Evans HL, Luna MA. Polymorphous low-grade adenocarcinoma: a study of 40 cases with long-term follow up and an evaluation of the importance of papillary areas. Am J Surg Pathol 2000;24(10): 1319–28.

55. Seethala RR, Johnson JT, Barnes EL, et al. Polymor-
    phous low-grade adenocarcinoma: the University of
    Pittsburgh experience. Arch Otolaryngol Head Neck
    Surg 2010;136(4):385–92.
56. Weinreb I, Piscuoglio S, Martelotto LG, et al. Hotspot
    activating PRKD1 somatic mutations in polymor-
    phous low-grade adenocarcinomas of the salivary
    glands. Nat Genet 2014;46(11):1166–9.
57. Weinreb I, Chiosea SI, Seethala RR, et al. Genotypic
    and phenotypic comparison of polymorphous and
    cribriform adenocarcinomas of salivary gland. Mod
    Pathol 2015;28(S2):333.
58. Weinreb I, Zhang L, Tirunagari LM, et al. Novel
    PRKD gene rearrangements and variant fusions
    in cribriform adenocarcinoma of salivary gland
    origin. Genes Chromosomes Cancer 2014;53(10):
    845–56.
59. Rooper L, Sharma R, Bishop JA. Polymorphous
    low grade adenocarcinoma has a consistent
    p63+/p40- immunophenotype that helps distin-
    guish it from adenoid cystic carcinoma and cellular
    pleomorphic adenoma. Head Neck Pathol 2015;
    9(1):79–84.
60. Xu B, Aneja A, Ghossein R, et al. Predictors of
    Outcome in the Phenotypic Spectrum of Polymor-
    phous Low-grade Adenocarcinoma (PLGA) and Crib-
    riform Adenocarcinoma of Salivary Gland (CASG): a
    retrospective study of 69 patients. Am J Surg Pathol
    2016;40(11):1526–37.
61. Simpson RH, Pereira EM, Ribeiro AC, et al. Polymor-
    phous low-grade adenocarcinoma of the salivary
    glands with transformation to high-grade carcinoma.
    Histopathology 2002;41(3):250–9.
62. Skalova A, Sima R, Kaspirkova-Nemcova J, et al. Crib-
    riform adenocarcinoma of minor salivary gland origin
    principally affecting the tongue: characterization of
    new entity. Am J Surg Pathol 2011;35(8):1168–76.
63. Michal M, Skalova A, Simpson RH, et al. Cribriform
    adenocarcinoma of the tongue: a hitherto unrecog-
    nized type of adenocarcinoma characteristically
    occurring in the tongue. Histopathology 1999;35(6):
    495–501.

Odontogenic Cysts and Neoplasms

Elizabeth Ann Bilodeau, DMD, MD, MSEd[a],*, Bobby M. Collins, DDS, MS[b]

KEYWORDS

- Odontogenic cysts • Gnathic • Odontoma • Keratocystic odontogenic tumor • Ameloblastoma
- Calcifying epithelial odontogenic tumor • Clear cell odontogenic carcinoma

ABSTRACT

This article reviews a myriad of common and uncommon odontogenic cysts and tumors. The clinical presentation, gross and microscopic features, differential diagnosis, prognosis, and diagnostic pitfalls are addressed for inflammatory cysts (periapical cyst, mandibular infected buccal cyst/paradental cyst), developmental cysts (dentigerous, lateral periodontal, glandular odontogenic, orthokeratinized odontogenic cyst), benign tumors (keratocystic odontogenic tumor, ameloblastoma, adenomatoid odontogenic tumor, calcifying epithelial odontogenic tumor, ameloblastic fibroma and fibroodontoma, odontoma, squamous odontogenic tumor, calcifying cystic odontogenic tumor, primordial odontogenic tumor, central odontogenic fibroma, and odontogenic myxomas), and malignant tumors (clear cell odontogenic carcinoma, ameloblastic carcinoma, ameloblastic fibrosarcoma).

OVERVIEW

In considering all gnathic cysts, embryologic process fusion, epithelial enclavement, and epithelial invagination put epithelium in the jaws, but the odontogenic entities rely solely on invagination from the thickened "horseshoe" band of epithelium overlying the maxillary and mandibular ridges where teeth will develop and subsequent enclavement by alveolar bone. The thickened surface epithelium sends an epithelial cord (dental lamina) into the underlying ectomesenchyme to form the dental organ.[1]

The epithelial extension stops well above the basal bone. The downward epithelial migration, formation of the dental organ, and the ectomesenchyme immediately surrounding it (dental follicle) provides the impetus for formation of alveolar bone (and also the periodontal ligament periradicularly) that envelops and encases the dental organ. Thus, odontogenic epithelium is embedded in bone. The dental lamina leaves behind a canal through which future tooth eruption is guided (gubernacular canal).

The subsequent breakdown of dental lamina (Rests of Serres), Hertwig's epithelial root sheath (which guides root development and dissolves to leave Rests of Malassez) and postfunctional ameloblasts, and other entities (reduced enamel epithelium) leave residual epithelium in the jaws. Cellular characteristics of the embryologic odontogenic epithelium provide presumptive origin of the cysts and tumors (ie, cytoplasmic clearing owing to glycogen accumulation, suggests their origin as from residual dental lamina).[2,3]

There are inflammatory and developmental cysts (Table 1). Some odontogenic tumors may have a cystic morphology clinically and grossly. Inflammation and associated growth factors stimulate epithelial hyperplasia of apical periodontal ligament retained rests of Malassez and provide a "loop and arcade" hyperplasia or spherical enlargement of the epithelial remnants that outgrows its blood supply, causing central necrosis. The osmotic gradient that pulls fluid (plasma) from surrounding tissue to enhance cystic enlargement.

The odontogenic epithelium entrapped in the bone and in the periodontal ligament that gives rise to both developmental and inflammatory cysts can undergo neoplastic transformation as well. Neoplastic transformation of any of the elements of the dental organ and the aforementioned cysts

[a] Department of Diagnostic Sciences, University of Pittsburgh School of Dental Medicine, G-135 Salk Hall, 3501 Terrace Street, Pittsburgh, PA 15261, USA; [b] Department of Surgical Science, East Carolina University School of Dental Medicine, 1851 MacGregor Downs Road, Greenville, NC 27834, USA
* Corresponding author.
E-mail address: Elizabeth.bilodeau@dental.pitt.edu

Surgical Pathology 10 (2017) 177–222
http://dx.doi.org/10.1016/j.path.2016.10.006
1875-9181/17/© 2016 Elsevier Inc. All rights reserved.

Table 1
Odontogenic cyst classification schema

Developmental Odontogenic Cysts	Inflammatory Odontogenic Cysts	Odontogenic Cystic Neoplasms
Dentigerous cyst	Periapical (radicular) cyst	Keratocystic odontogenic tumor
Lateral periodontal cyst	Residual cyst	Calcifying cystic odontogenic tumor
Glandular odontogenic cyst	Paradental cyst	
Orthokeratinized odontogenic cyst		

From Robinson R, Vincent S. Tumors and cysts of the jaws. In: Silverberg S, editor. 4th edition. Silver Spring (MD): ARP Press; 2012. p. 11–37.

is possible. Therefore, odontogenic tumors can be purely epithelial, purely mesenchymal, or mixtures thereof. Furthermore, the capacity for these tumors to produce tooth structure add to the already broad morphologic diversity. The odontogenic epithelium has a pluripotential character, so nonodontogenic tumors such as mucoepidermoid carcinoma and primary intraosseous carcinoma can occur within the jaws.

With completion of tooth development (**Fig. 1**), postfunctional odontogenic epithelium (reduced enamel epithelium) overlying the crown of the tooth merges with the surface mucosa during eruption. As the tooth perforates the oral epithelium, this reduced enamel epithelium is attached at the cemento–enamel junction and becomes the junctional epithelium of the gingival sulcus, and epithelial attachment to the tooth and part of the periodontium. The periodontal ligament is the fibrous connective tissue subjacent to junctional epithelium

that supports the tooth in its alveolar bone housing. This mesenchymal tissue is contiguous with the pulpal tissue of the tooth at the apical foramen and at various other foramina of lateral and accessory canals within tooth roots.

PERIAPICAL (RADICULAR) CYST

Periapical (radicular) cysts are inflammatory odontogenic cysts, and overall are the most common cyst of the jaws. They must be associated with the apex of a nonvital tooth (**Fig. 2**).[4] Clinically, the tooth may be carious or have a past history of trauma. Periapical cysts arise from expansion of residual epithelial remnants from tooth development. The epithelial proliferation in precursor inflamed granulation tissue at the apex, termed a periapical granuloma, incurs increasing osmotic pressure leads to cyst formation and expansion. Radiographically, a well-demarcated radiolucency

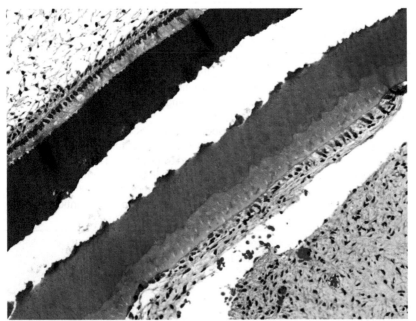

Fig. 1. Developing tooth with loose stellate reticulum adjacent to the ameloblastic layer that is secreting basophilic enamel. The enamel layer is juxtaposed (here, artifactually separated) against eosinophilic dentin with prominent tubules rimmed by odontoblasts. Note that ameloblastic epithelium is prominent in ameloblastoma, recapitulating odontogenesis.

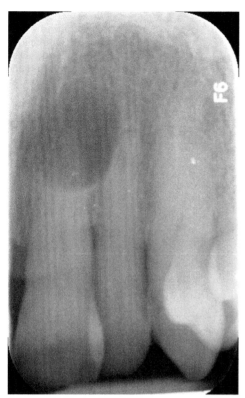

Fig. 2. Periapical radiograph of a clinically nonvital tooth with a large, well-defined periapical radiolucency.

is present and associated with the apex of the tooth. A presumptive clinicoradiographic impression of a periapical cyst is made when the radiolucency has a diameter of greater than 20 mm.[5] Because lateral or accessory root canals may be present, lesions may not be centered at the apex of the root. Typically, lesions are well-defined, unilocular radiolucencies that are less than 1.0 cm in diameter; however, lesions can continue to expand if left untreated. As surgical pathologists, this clinical information and lesional location relative to a tooth may be lacking.

The periodontal ligament will contain spheres, rosettes, or rests of odontogenic epithelium and will become inflamed owing to pulpal necrosis, and bacterial infection of the gingival sulcus. The inflammation at the periapical region of the tooth eventuates into granulation tissue from the wounding afforded by pulpal inflammation. This inflamed granulation tissue has been referred to historically as a periapical granuloma. This is a misnomer, because it is not granulomatous inflammation, but merely inflamed granulation tissue and should be more correctly referred to as periapical periodontitis. The periapical granuloma immediately precedes the periapical cyst, which derives from

inflammatory stimulation of those previously mentioned residual epithelial rests. Endodontic therapy results in subsequent bone healing in approximately 66% of cases and periapical surgery heals in approximately 95% of cases. Persistent radiolucencies after therapy may represent periapical scars (dense fibrous connective tissue).[6]

GROSS FEATURES

If the lesion is submitted with an extracted tooth, adherent tissue may be seen in the periapical region with or without resorption of the underlying tooth structure. More commonly, after curettage of the lesion, friable soft tissue fragments are submitted.

MICROSCOPIC FEATURES

Periapical cysts are lined by a thin, 1 to 2 cell layered, commonly nonkeratinized stratified squamous epithelium surrounded by an inflamed connective tissue wall (**Fig. 3**). Inflammatory hyperplasia of luminal epithelium produces a "loop and arcade" array. Bacteria, hemosiderin, and cholesterol clefts are frequent findings. Lesions associated with endodontically treated teeth (teeth treated with a root canal) often have brown or black pigmented, granular, or crystalline foreign material within the connective tissue and sometimes a foreign body cell reaction (**Fig. 4**). If a radiograph is provided, the origin of the foreign/restorative material is evident.

Within the periapical granuloma and periapical cyst, abundant plasma cells, "Russell bodies", and pyronine bodies are noted as part of a mixed or purely chronic inflammatory cell infiltrate. Rarely, giant cell hyaline angiopathy may be encountered, which is an inflammatory reaction that may be seen when vegetable matter embedded in mesenchymal tissue through food mastication and open access to periapical connective tissue (see **Fig. 4**). This lightly eosinophilic secretion represents inflammatory exudate (extravasated serum) and may surround vegetable material and be concomitant with foreign body giant cells and vascular inflammation.[7–10] This is not specific to periapical cysts, but may be seen in other inflammatory cysts, such as the paradental cyst.

DIFFERENTIAL DIAGNOSIS

The differential diagnosis may include other inflamed odontogenic cysts (**Table 2**). To discriminate between periapical and residual cysts, correlation with the clinical and radiographic findings is necessary. Residual cysts are similar

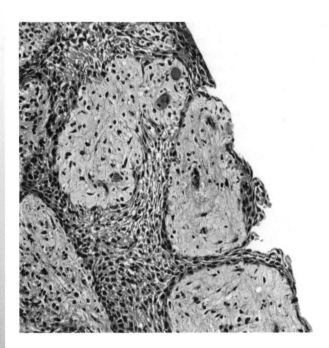

Fig. 3. Periapical cyst. Nonkeratinized stratified squamous epithelium in a "loop and arcade" pattern with inflammation noted in the adjacent stroma.

microscopically to periapical cysts, but are persistent lesions after exodontia. The periapical cyst must be associated with a tooth present within the jaws, whereas the residual cyst has no existing tooth association. Correlation with the clinical and radiographic findings is important in determining the relationship of the lesion to a tooth and is required to discriminate these entities.

PROGNOSIS

Treatment is conventional root canal therapy or enucleation of the cyst/granuloma, often at the time of extraction or during an apicoectomy (an endodontic procedure that removes the lesion and tooth apex). Extraction of a tooth, with inadequate curettage, may result in a persistent lesion termed a residual cyst.

Key Points
PERIAPICAL CYST

Most common cyst of the jaws, an inflammatory odontogenic cyst

Expansion of residual epithelium from tooth development

Uniform, unilocular radiolucency, apex of nonviable tooth

Inflammatory hyperplasia of luminal epithelial produces a "loop and arcade array"

BUCCAL BIFURCATION CYST/PARADENTAL CYST

Another inflammatory odontogenic cyst, rarer than the periapical cyst, has been variously referred to as a mandibular infected buccal cyst, a buccal bifurcation cyst, and a paradental cyst. The cyst results from inflammation of the junctional epithelium that forms the gingival sulcus around the erupted tooth. These cysts have the histopathologic features of the periapical cysts, but anatomically they are pericoronal, at least at the sulcus of the crown. Causality such as enamel projections into the furcation of mandibular first and second molar teeth (mandibular infected buccal cyst) resulting in more apically directed epithelial attachment and posteruptive inflammatory expansion of the reduced enamel epithelium (paradental cyst) has been proposed.[11,12]

DIFFERENTIAL DIAGNOSIS

The distinction from a periapical cyst and even an inflamed dentigerous cyst is problematic and requires appropriate history and radiographs.

DENTIGEROUS CYST

Dentigerous cysts are associated with the crown of an impacted tooth or partially erupted tooth, connecting at the cervical portion of the tooth (the cemento-enamel junction) (**Fig. 5**). These cysts represent the second most common cyst

Fig. 4. Giant cell hyaline angiopathy. (*A*) Amorphous eosinophilic hyaline rings with concomitant foreign body giant cells. (*B*) Under polarized light, crystalline foreign material is brightly refractile.

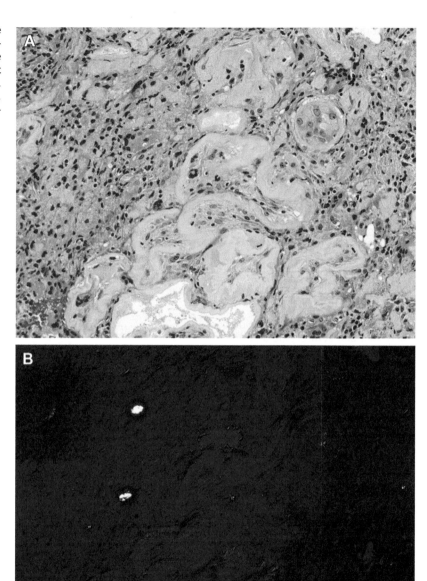

of the jaws and the most common developmental cysts.[13] Permanent third molars and maxillary canines are the teeth most likely to fail to erupt and consequently are associated most frequently with dentigerous cysts. Usually asymptomatic, unless inflamed, these cysts are often detected when a tooth fails to erupt and a radiograph is taken. A follicular space of greater than 3 mm is considered to be abnormal, although there is overlap between the appearance of enlarged or hyperplastic dental follicles and dentigerous cysts.[14] Lesions may become quite large, several centimeters in size, displacing teeth. The radiographic features are not specific, presenting as a well-circumscribed, corticated, unilocular radiolucency associated with the crown of an impacted or partially impacted tooth. Radiographically, this appearance can be mimicked by an ameloblastoma or a keratocystic odontogenic tumor. When the tooth is impacted partially, with a portion exposed to the oral cavity and subsequent pericoronitis, cystic expansion of the remaining follicle and inflammation of the junctional epithelium can form a paradental cyst that extends in bone to the buccal or distal aspect of a partially erupted mandibular molar tooth.[11,15]

Key Points
DENTIGEROUS CYST

Developmental cyst can be several centimeters in size and can move teeth.

Dentigerous cyst is a unilocular radiolucency that must involve the crown of unerupted tooth, often third molars.

Luminal epithelium attaches at the cervical aspect of the tooth.

Radiographic appearance is not unique; ameloblastoma and keratocystic odontogenic tumor can mimic dentigerous cysts.

They are the second most common cyst of the jaws.

Inflamed dentigerous cysts can resemble periapical cyst histologically.

Ameloblastomatous and carcinomatous transformation can rarely occur.

GROSS FEATURES

Grossly, if the cyst is received intact, the crown of the tooth will be enveloped by the cyst with attachment at the cervical of the tooth (Fig. 6). More frequently, the lesion is removed via curettage, resulting in a fragmented lesion.

MICROSCOPIC FEATURES

An uninflamed dentigerous cyst is lined by nonkeratinized stratified squamous epithelium with a relatively flat interface with the adjacent connective tissue (Fig. 7). With inflammation, epithelial hyperplasia may be seen, making the discrimination between a periapical cyst and a paradental cyst challenging.[16] Surrounding the cyst is a fibrovascular connective tissue wall that may contain odontogenic rests. Within the surrounding connective tissue, inflamed cysts may exhibit cholesterol clefts with associated giant cells. Amorphous eosinophilic curvilinear Rushton bodies may be seen, although these are nonspecific and may be present in other odontogenic cysts (Fig. 8). Mucous cells have been found in more than 20% of dentigerous cysts, with concurrent cilia in 11%, and sebaceous cells may be present, reflecting the pluripotent nature of he odontogenic epithelium.[17] When ciliated epithelium is noted in a cyst from the maxillary arch, a comment should be included warning of a potential exposure of the maxillary sinus.

DIFFERENTIAL DIAGNOSIS

Other nonkeratinizing inflammatory cysts (periapical cysts or residual cysts) are similar microscopically to inflamed dentigerous cysts, including the paradental cyst. Correlation with the clinical and radiographic findings is important in determining the relationship of the lesion to a tooth and is required to discriminate these entities. A hyperplastic dental follicle may have overlapping histologic features with dentigerous cysts, but is usually associated with a plump, cuboidal to columnar, eosinophilic lining, generally occurring in younger patients (Fig. 9). For small dentigerous cysts, significant overlap with hyperplastic follicles is seen histologically; thus, the intraoperative impression of a cystic lesion is often relied on.[14] The pluripotentiality of the epithelial lining of dentigerous cysts, including the potential of cilia, mucous cells, and sebaceous cells, may make differentiation from a diagnosis of glandular odontogenic cysts (GOCs) challenging. However, additional features are required for the diagnosis of a GOC.[18] Other pathologies may be found arising in a dentigerous cyst, including but not limited to ameloblastomas and squamous cell carcinoma.[19–22]

Table 2
Comparison chart: Periapical cyst, residual cyst, and dentigerous cyst

Diagnosis	Periapical Cyst	Residual Cyst	Dentigerous Cyst
Clinical/radiographic features	Associated with the apex nonvital tooth (tooth may be grossly carious or have a past history of trauma)	Intraosseous radiolucency, persisting after exodontia	Associated with the crown of an impacted tooth, connecting at the cemento–enamel junction

Fig. 5. Dentigerous cyst, cropped panoramic radiograph. A well-defined, finely corticated radiolucency surrounding an impacted mandibular right third molar. Histologically, this was a dentigerous cyst.

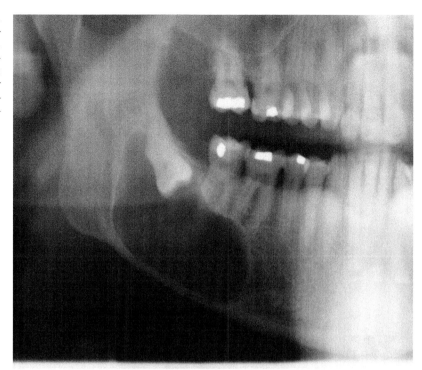

PROGNOSIS

Dentigerous cysts are treated by extraction of the associated tooth with curettage/enucleation, and with little incidence of recurrence.

LATERAL PERIODONTAL CYST/GINGIVAL CYST OF THE ADULT

Lateral periodontal cysts (LPCs) are developmental cysts thought to arise from rests of the dental

Fig. 6. Dentigerous cyst, gross appearance. Friable soft tissue connects with a formerly impacted tooth at the area of the cemento–enamel junction.

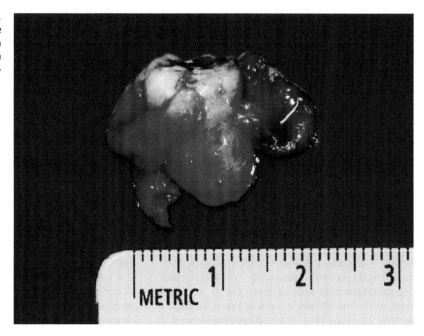

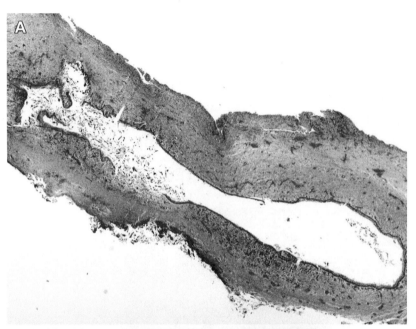

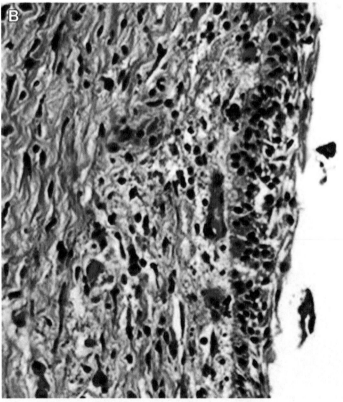

Fig. 7. Dentigerous cyst. (*A*) Low-power view of a dentigerous cyst. Cystic stratified Luminal squamous epithelium with inflammatory cells scattered within the underlying fibrous connective tissue wall. (*B*) Higher power view of squamous lining exhibiting some spongiosis secondary to inflammation.

lamina. Clinically, these are often incidental findings, usually presenting as well-demarcated uniloc-ular radiolucencies seen between the roots of vital teeth in the mandibular canine to premolar region in 70% of cases (Fig. 10).[23] When they occur in the maxilla, they are seen the canine–lateral region. The less common botryoid variant presents as a multilocular radiolucency. The gingival cyst of the adult is the soft tissue counterpart of the LPC and histologically it is quite similar.[24]

Fig. 8. Inflamed dentigerous cyst exhibiting cholesterol clefts, Rushton bodies, and underlying inflammation (*A*). Higher power view, exhibiting prominent eosinophilic polygonal Rushton bodies undergoing calcification (*B*).

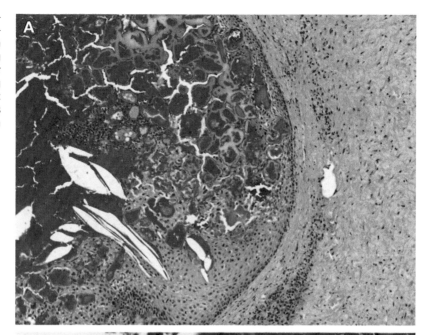

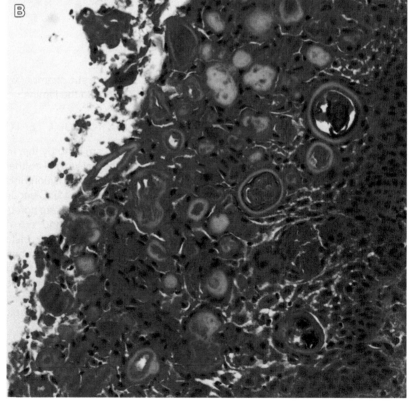

GROSS FEATURES

When received intact after being surgically enucleated, the red/brown lobular soft tissue is serum filled, compressible, and, when bisected, a smooth inner surface with focal luminal thickenings is noted. The botryoid variant is multilobular or grapelike and multichambered when bisected.

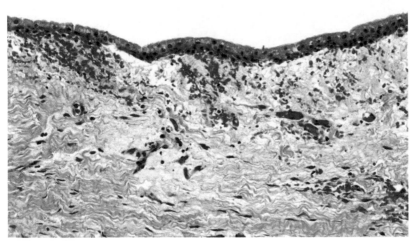

Fig. 9. Hyperplastic follicle. Eosinophilic cuboidal to columnar epithelium consistent with reduced enamel epithelium lines the follicle.

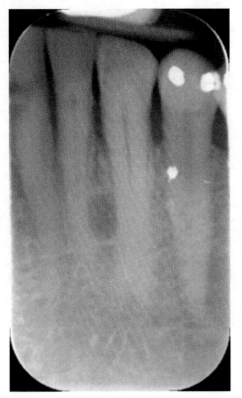

Fig. 10. Periapical radiograph of a lateral periodontal cyst. A small, well-defined radiolucency is seen between the roots of vital teeth.

Each cystic chamber will show the scattered thickenings in the lumina.

MICROSCOPIC FEATURES

LPC are lined by thin nonkeratinized squamous or cuboidal luminal epithelium that is 3 to 8 cell layers thick and transitions into focal plaquelike thickened areas (**Fig. 11**). Clear cells resulting from glycogen accumulation are noted in the plaquelike or nodular thickenings and are not uncommon.[25] Gingival cysts are similar histologically, but the cyst is surrounded by connective tissue and normal overlying epithelium may be seen. The botryoid odontogenic cyst is the multilocular variant of the LPC and the loculations are lined by thick and thin nonkeratinized epithelial lumina.[26,27]

DIFFERENTIAL DIAGNOSIS

LPC are intraosseous lesions, whereas in the gingival cyst, normal overlying stratified squamous epithelium may be seen. The botryoid odontogenic cyst, the multilocular variant of the LPC, may be confused with a GOC. However, additional features are required for the diagnosis of GOC (eg, microcysts or ductlike structures, mucous cells, apocrine snouting). LPCs may be mimicked radiographically by other odontogenic cysts/tumors such as a periapical cyst arising from an accessory

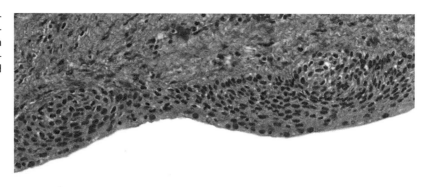

Fig. 11. Lateral periodontal cyst. Bland stratified squamous epithelium with plaquelike thickenings exhibiting a whorled morphology.

canal (lateral radicular cyst), keratocystic odontogenic tumor, or an ameloblastoma.

PROGNOSIS

Enucleation is curative, with a low recurrence rate.

GLANDULAR ODONTOGENIC CYST

GOC presents as either a unilocular or multilocular, well-defined lesion within the mandible in 70% of cases.[28,29] They are somewhat aggressive lesions, often causing cortical perforation and, less commonly, root displacement or resorption (**Fig. 12**).[29] The tooth root resorptive pattern is similar to that seen in ameloblastoma, that is a "straight edge" or "knife edge" character that degrades root length. They occur across a wide age range, with the mean age of presentation of 45.7 years, and a 1.3:1 male to female ratio.[28]

GROSS FEATURES

Grossly, lesions are cystic, and focal thickenings may be present within the lumina (**Fig. 13**).

MICROSCOPIC FEATURES

At low power, an epithelial lined cyst with a highly variable lining is evident. The major

histologic criteria of GOCs include (1) hobnailing or surface eosinophilic cells, (2) intraepithelial microcysts or duct-like structures, (3) apocrine snouting or decapitation secretions, (4) clear or vacuolated cells in the basal or parabasal layers, (5) marked variable thickening of the cyst lining, (6) papillary thickening or tufting, (7) mucous or goblet cells, (8) epithelial spheres or plaquelike thickenings, which may exhibit swirling, (9) cilia, and (10) multicystic architecture (**Fig. 14**).[18,30]

DIFFERENTIAL DIAGNOSIS

The differential diagnosis of GOC includes a dentigerous cyst with GOC-like features (ie, mucous and cilia prosoplasia), botryoid odontogenic cyst, and central mucoepidermoid carcinoma. In differentiating a GOC from a dentigerous cyst with GOC-like features, the presence of 7 or more features was highly predictive of a GOC whereas if 5 or fewer features were present, this was predictive of a non-GOC.[18] Furthermore, the presence of microcysts, clear cells, and plaquelike thickenings were the most useful features for this discrimination. GOCs are negative by fluorescent in situ hybridization for the t(11;19)(q21;p13) translocation, which results in a *MECT1-MAML2* fusion, which is often present

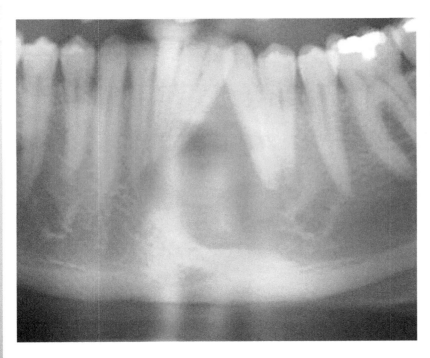

Fig. 12. Glandular odontogenic cyst, cropped panoramic radiograph. A large unilocular radiolucency is seen in the anterior mandible, displacing the left mandibular canine and lateral incisor.

in central mucoepidermoid carcinoma.[31,32] The multicystic variant of the LPC, the botryoid odontogenic cyst, may contain plaquelike thickenings; however, intraepithelial microcysts or ductlike structures are not present.

PROGNOSIS

GOCs are reported as having a recurrence rate of between 20% and 30%.[18,28] However, conservative therapy is the most common surgical

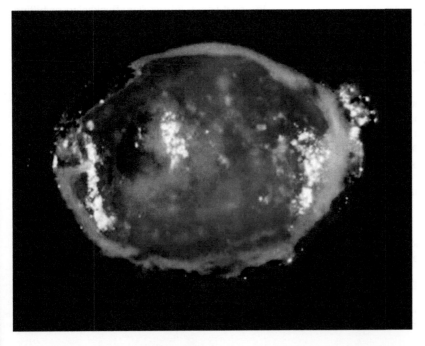

Fig. 13. Glandular odontogenic cyst, gross appearance. A bisected cyst demonstrates a thin translucent lining with focal thickenings.

management undertaken, including enucleation and curettage.[30,33]

Pitfalls
GLANDULAR ODONTOGENIC CYST

! On biopsy, a GOC may exhibit numerous mucous cells, whereas the other histologic features may be less obvious, leading to a misdiagnosis of a central mucoepidermoid carcinoma. GOC should be negative for *MAML2* rearrangement.

! Dentigerous cysts may exhibit mucous cell prosoplasia and cilia.

! Mucous cells and plaquelike thickenings are seen in LPCs.

Key Points
GLANDULAR ODONTOGENIC CYST

Aggressive developmental cyst, frequently recurs, common in anterior jaws

Resorbs tooth roots, like ameloblastoma

Histologically mucus goblet cells, respiratory epithelium and ductlike structures are noted

Luminal epithelium shows plaquelike thickenings as seen in LPC

Can resemble a central, low-grade mucoepidermoid carcinoma

ODONTOMA (COMPLEX AND COMPOUND TYPES)

Odontomas are the most common odontogenic tumor, more common than all others combined. Some prefer the designation of hamartoma for odontoma. Frequently, these pediatric tumors are detected radiographically by dentists during routine imaging or on investigation of a tooth failing to erupt. Blocking the eruption of a normal tooth, these tumors can be associated with a dentigerous cyst or hyperplastic follicle. Radiographically, these tissue are very radiodense, with a density comparable with normal tooth structure, and have a distinct radiolucent rim separating the lesion from adjacent bone (Fig. 15).

GROSS FEATURES

Compound odontomas are composed of numerous small abnormally formed teeth and the gross appearance is highly distinctive (Fig. 16). Complex odontomas are composed of hard and soft tissue that do not resemble normal teeth morphologically.

MICROSCOPIC FEATURES

Microscopically, compound odontomas are composed of small abnormally formed teeth (Fig. 17A). The enamel is mostly lost during the decalcification process. Complex odontomas are composed of a haphazard arrangement of dentin and enamel with admixed soft tissue (Fig. 17B). Less commonly, ghost cells may be seen in odontomas (Fig. 17C).[34]

DIFFERENTIAL DIAGNOSIS

Obtaining radiographs can assist in the diagnosis and correct subclassification of odontomas. The differential diagnosis can include a supernumerary tooth, ameloblastic fibroodontoma (AFO), an odontoma with ghost cells, and odontoma associated calcifying cystic odontogenic tumor (CCOT). When more than 2 teeth are contained in a dental sac, albeit arbitrary, the classification of a compound odontoma is used. Ghost cells are seen occasionally in odontomas. Odontoma-like structures can be associated with the cyst wall of a CCOT and are best classified as a CCOT-associated odontoma.[34] It should be noted that their behavior will be more consistent with that of an odontoma. Distinguishing an AFO from an immature odontoma can be challenging. AFO are more likely to be radiographically irregular with scattered opacities whereas odontomas have a central area of radiopacity. Treated by simple enucleation, the prognosis of odontomas is excellent, with a very low recurrence rate.

KERATOCYSTIC ODONTOGENIC TUMOR (ODONTOGENIC KERATOCYST)

Keratocystic odontogenic tumors (KCOTs) present as smooth bordered unilocular, unilocular with a scalloped border, or multilocular radiolucencies of the jaw with a strong predilection for the mandible (approximately 75%), and the most frequent subsite is the region of the angle and ramus. Lesions can become quite large with a propensity for anterior and posterior growth with little clinically evident buccolingual expansion of the cortices (Fig. 18). KCOTs may be seen in areas where a tooth fails to develop (primordial cyst). There is a very wide reported age distribution (8–82 years), but the mean age of presentation is in the third decade of life.[35,36] When KCOTs are diagnosed at a young age (<20 years) or multiple KCOTs are seen in a patient, a comment should be inserted to advise the clinician to evaluate the patient for nevoid basal cell carcinoma syndrome (**Box 1**).[37] Both sporadic and syndrome associated tumors may be associated with a *PTCH* gene mutation 9q22.3-q31.[38,39]

> ## Key Points
> ### KERATOCYSTIC ODONTOGENIC TUMOR (ODONTOGENIC KERATOCYST)
>
> Unilocular, scalloped, or multilocular radiolucency of posterior jaws
>
> Propensity to expand/grow in an anterior posterior direction
>
> Can be associated with impacted teeth, or LPC location
>
> May develop in place of a tooth (primordial cyst)
>
> Developmental cyst with a high recurrence rate
>
> Increased expression of proliferative markers
>
> Sporadic and syndromic occurrence (nevoid basal cell carcinoma syndrome)
>
> Characteristic histopathology of palisading, hyperchromatic basal layer of cuboidal to columnar cells
>
> Epithelium is 6 to 10 cell layers thick
>
> Flat epithelial/connective tissue interface in noninflamed cyst
>
> "Wavy" or "corrugated" parakeratotic luminal surface

GROSS FEATURES

Grossly, these lesions are thin walled and cystic. A characteristic "cheesy" material represents parakeratin produced by the luminal epithelium (**Fig. 19**). The epithelium may strip away from the connective tissue in these cysts, and close examination of the biopsy container for material is recommended.[40]

MICROSCOPIC FEATURES

KCOTs are lined by an approximately 6 to 10 cell layer parakeratinized stratified squamous epithelium of uniform thickness that exhibits a wavy, corrugated surface with a prominent, hyperchromatic, palisaded basal cell layer (**Fig. 20**). The

epithelium has a flat interface with the adjacent connective tissue.[41] Epithelium maybe seen floating freely at lower power. Satellite (daughter) cysts can be found in the connective tissue wall. Inflammation may obscure the classic histologic features of a KCOT, resulting in loss of parakeratinization and increased thickness of the epithelial lining and loss of the characteristic basal cell layer.[42] Treatment with marsupialization ("decompression or cystotomy") also results in the loss of classic features, with the lining becoming reminiscent of the normal adjacent mucosa. Tumors are positive for high-molecular-weight keratins, p53, and Ki-67 staining is increased, with mitoses present above the basal cell layer.[43–45]

DIFFERENTIAL DIAGNOSIS

The differential diagnosis may include orthokeratinized odontogenic cysts (OOC) or, when inflamed, a dentigerous cyst. Pitfalls on frozen section include sampling errors, insufficient epithelium, and inflammation, which may result in added challenges.[41,46]

PROGNOSIS

Features such as the existence of satellite (daughter) cysts, the propensity for subepithelial splitting, subepithelial hyaline deposition, and mitotic figure location have been associated with recurrence.[46,47] Treatment includes enucleation (with or without peripheral ostectomy, treatment with Carnoy solution, or cryotherapy), marsupialization, or resection. Carnoy solution is a mixture of chloroform, absolute ethanol, glacial acetic acid, and ferric chloride (originally a fixative that is now used as an intraoperative treatment of lesions such as KCOT, which have a high recurrence rate).[48] Recurrence rates of approximately 30% have been reported when treatment involves simple enucleation, but the adjunctive technique of chemical cauterization with Carnoy solution is associated with reduced recurrence rates (approximately 8%).[35,49] Significantly higher rates of recurrence (50%) are seen with KCOTs in patients with nevoid basal cell carcinoma syndrome.[35]

ORTHOKERATINIZED ODONTOGENIC CYST

OOC were considered initially as a variant of KCOT, but now are considered a discrete entity. The OOC is an uncommon cyst that histologically resembles an epithelial inclusion cyst and has no known association with a syndrome. The origin is likely the previously mentioned epithelial rests of the dental lamina. The OOC is found in adults as

Fig. 14. Glandular odontogenic cyst. Cilia, duct-like structures (*A*), and abundant mucous cells and luminal decapitation secretions or apocrine snouting (*B*) are seen.

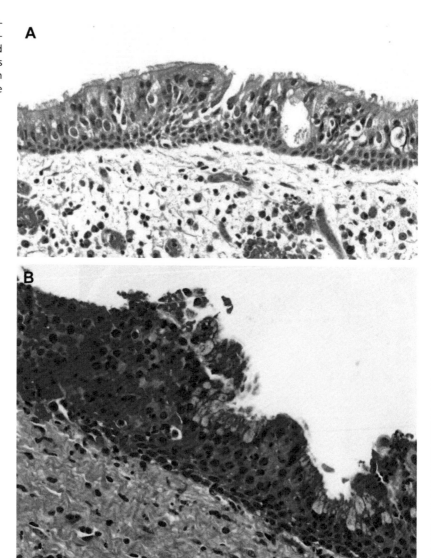

a unilocular radiolucency in the posterior mandible molar–ramus region. The cysts are more common in males, about 3:1 over females.[50] It is commonly associated with an impacted tooth, as are several of the cysts and tumors in this article. The radiographic appearance is a well-corticated, unilocular radiolucency that are often associated with an impacted or unerupted tooth, approximately 50% to 75% are indistinguishable from a dentigerous cyst.[50,51]

GROSS FEATURES

Grossly, OOCs are cystic with keratinaceous material in the lumen.

MICROSCOPIC FEATURES

The luminal epithelium is 5 to 15 cell layers in thickness and laminated orthokeratin is shed from a prominent granular layer. In some cases, "chevroning" of the laminated keratin is apparent. The basal layer does not have a palisaded appearance, the basal cells are not hyperchromatic, and there is a flat interface with the connective tissue wall when the cyst is not inflamed (**Fig. 21**).[50,51]

DIFFERENTIAL DIAGNOSIS

Discriminating OOC from KCOT is the most important differential diagnosis. As a caveat, if *any*

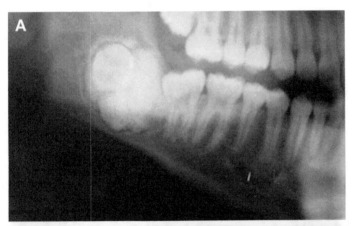

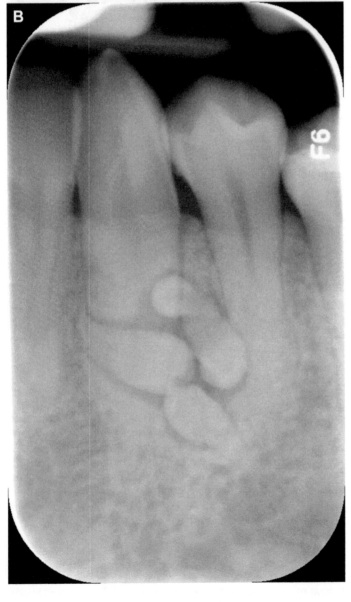

Fig. 15. Radiographic appearance of odontomas. (*A*) Complex odontoma exhibiting a mixed density lesion above an impacted right third molar. A well-defined radiolucent rim is present around the lesion, a characteristic radiographic feature of odontomas. (*B*) Compound odontoma exhibiting multiple malformed miniature teeth, each surrounded by a well-defined radiolucent rim. (*Courtesy of* Dr Anitha Potluri, Pittsburgh, PA.)

Fig. 16. Compound odontoma, gross appearance. Many small tooth-forms are present grossly.

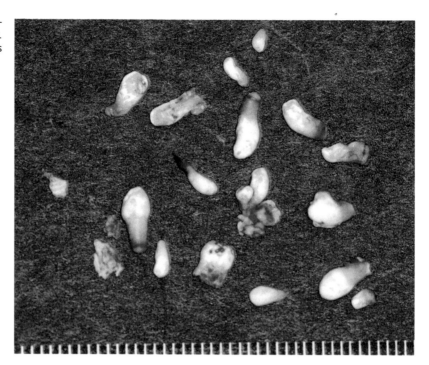

parakeratin is evident, the diagnosis is KCOT. Multiple OOCs have been reported in the literature.[51]

PROGNOSIS

Treatment is surgical excision or curettage. The lesions "shell out" as predicted from their well-demarcated radiographic appearance.

AMELOBLASTOMA

Ameloblastomas are common and potentially aggressive odontogenic tumors. They can be sub-classified as solid–multicystic (SMA), desmoplastic, unicystic (UA), or peripheral (PA).[52] The vast majority, approximately 92%, of ameloblastomas are SMA, with approximately 6% being UA, and 2% being PA.[53]

SMA classically present as a slow-growing, asymptomatic, painless, expansile mass. They have a striking propensity for buccolingual expansion and are seen most frequently in the posterior mandible. Radiographically, SMA are often multi-locular radiolucencies, but they may be unilocular (**Fig. 22**A). Straight edge blunting root resorption may be present. Lesions may be associated with an impacted tooth. SMA occur over a wide age range, with a mean age of presentation of approximately 35 years.[53]

Desmoplastic ameloblastomas, a subtype of SMA, have a unique presentation, with a nearly equal predilection for the mandible and maxilla versus a 5.4:1 mandibular predilection in SMA. In approximately one-half of cases, a mixed radi-opaque/radiolucent appearance is seen and tumor margins are less frequently well-defined than in SMA (**Fig. 23**A).[54] The clinical differential diagnosis for a desmoplastic ameloblastoma may include mixed density lesions, namely benign fibroosseous lesions.

UA are clinically cystic ameloblastomas that present a decade earlier than SMA. They differ from SMA in presentation, treatment, and prognosis. These present as well-defined unilocular radiolucencies often surrounding the crown of an impacted tooth.[55]

PA are extraosseous ameloblastomas, presenting most commonly on the gingiva as firm nodules that may have a roughened appearance. Radiographic features may be lacking or cupping resorption may be present.

MAPK pathway mutations are seen in ameloblastomas. *BRAF* V600E have been described in approximately 60% of mandibular ameloblastomas.[56] Other mutations in this pathway including *FGFR2* and the Ras genes (*HRAS, KRAS,* and *NRAS*) are described.[56–58] Non-MAPK mutations, including *SMO* are seen.[56] *SMO* mutations are seen most frequently in the

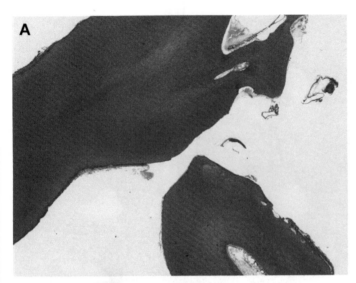

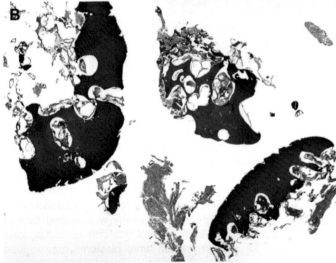

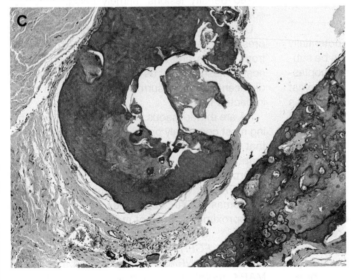

Fig. 17. (*A*) Compound odontoma showing 2 tooth forms. As seen here, much of the enamel is lost during demineralization owing to the high mineral content. (*B*) Complex odontoma, a haphazard array of dentin, with adjacent enamel and odontogenic epithelium. (*C*) Focal area of ghost cells within a complex odontoma.

Fig. 18. Cropped panoramic radiograph depicting a keratocystic odontogenic tumor (odontogenic keratocyst). Significant anterior–posterior growth is present without significant expansion of the mandible, a characteristic growth pattern of keratocystic odontogenic tumors.

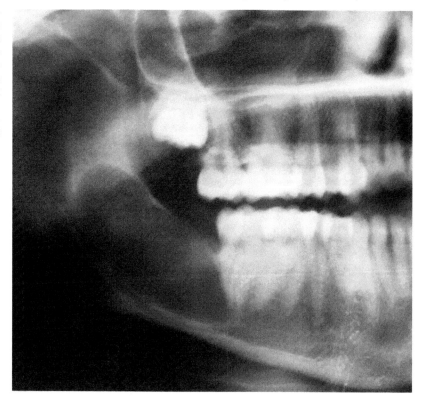

Box 1
Features of nevoid basal cell carcinoma syndrome

Rare, autosomal-dominant disorder

About 50% of cases sporadic

High penetrance, variable expression

Defects in the hedgehog signaling pathway, *PTCH* gene mutation

Multiple basal cell carcinomas developing at an early age

Multiple gnathic cysts (keratocystic odontogenic tumors)

Palmar and plantar pitting

Rib and spine abnormalities

Calcification of the falx cerebri

Frontoparietal bossing with hypertelorism with broad nasal root

Cleft lip/cleft palate

Associated with other pathologies:

Desmoplastic medulloblastoma

Meningioma

Ovarian and cardiac fibroma

Rhabdomyosarcoma

Agenesis of the corpus callosum

Data from Bresler SC, Padwa BL, Granter SR. Nevoid basal cell carcinoma syndrome (gorlin syndrome). Head Neck Pathol 2016;10(2):119–24; Johnson RL, Rothman AL, Xie J, et al. Human homolog of patched, a candidate gene for the basal cell nevus syndrome. Science 1996;272(5268):1668–71.

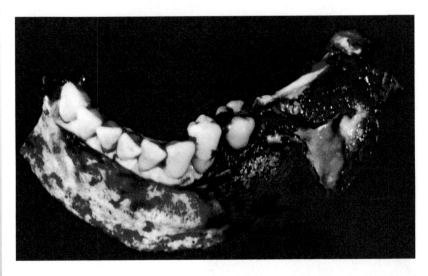

Fig. 19. Keratocystic odontogenic tumor (odontogenic keratocyst), gross appearance. Prominent anterior-posterior growth is seen. Within the lumen of the cyst, "cheesy" yellow material is seen.

maxilla and tend to be mutually exclusive with *BRAF* V600E mutations.[56,58]

GROSS FEATURES

SMA are expansile gray–white tumors that cut easily, lacking calcified material (**Fig. 22**B). SMA may be solid or often have cystic areas, with wide variation in the cystic component (**Fig. 22**C). Grossly, UA has a single smooth cystic lining, resembling other gnathic cysts. Nodules of growth are present in the lumen. Of note, SMA may resemble UA grossly.[59]

MICROSCOPIC FEATURES

The histopathologic features of ameloblastoma include hyperchromatism of basal cell nuclei, palisading and polarization of the basal cell nuclei of luminal epithelium away from the basement membrane, and subnuclear vacuolization of the luminal basal cells.[60] The center of the epithelial nests

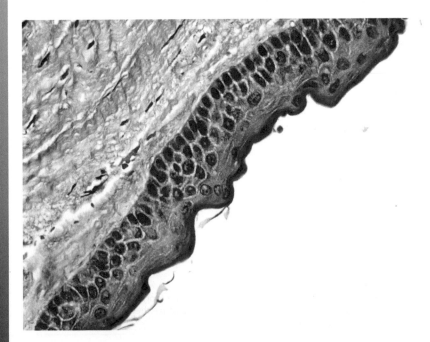

Fig. 20. Keratocystic odontogenic tumor (odontogenic keratocyst) exhibiting classic histologic features (uniform epithelial thickness with a flat connective tissue interface, prominent palisaded hyperchromatic basal cell layer, surfaced by wavy parakeratin).

Fig. 21. Orthokeratinized odontogenic cyst. Prominent orthokeratinization is present within the cyst lumen. A prominent, palisaded basal layer is lacking.

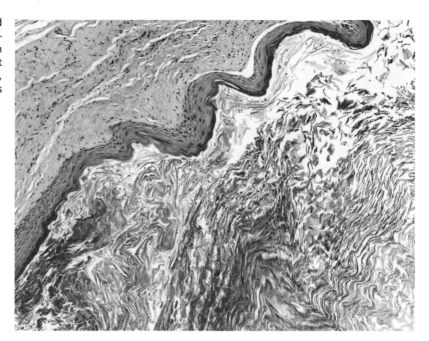

may have a loose pattern compared with the stellate reticulum of the dental organ. The overall architecture may be variable. Mitotic figures are rare. Cytokeratin 14 and 19 as well as CD56 expression may be seen in the peripheral cells, with calretinin staining seen in the stellate reticulum areas.[43,61]

Common patterns include the follicular and plexiform pattern, but tumors may also have an acanthomatous, granular, desmoplastic, basal, or clear cell pattern. Mixed patterns are seen frequently.[53] In the follicular pattern, tumors are composed of discrete, rounded epithelial islands. Tumor cells at the periphery of islands may be tall and columnar, exhibiting reverse polarity away from the basement membrane (**Fig. 24**A). Cystic degeneration may be present. In the plexiform pattern, the tumor is composed of connecting cords of epithelium (**Fig. 24**B). Subepithelial hyalinization may be seen surrounding tumor nests. In the acanthomatous pattern, tumors exhibits prominent squamous metaplasia, including keratin formation (**Fig. 24**C). The keratin pearls may calcify. In the granular cell pattern, a follicular pattern in seen most commonly with granular cells replacing the central stellate reticulum (**Fig. 24**D). No clinical significance is associated with these patterns. Infiltration into the bony trabeculae is frequently seen (**Fig. 24**E).

Desmoplastic ameloblastomas occur in a distinctive stroma with dense collagenization of the fibrous stroma or desmoplasia. The epithelium consists of strands or cords in irregular shapes surrounded by a myxoid rim (**Fig. 23**B). The classic peripheral palisading at the periphery of the epithelium is often lacking or focally present, making these more challenging to diagnose.[54]

As previously noted, UA are radiographically, grossly, and microscopically unilocular. UA are cystic lesions with 3 different patterns of growth having been described.[59] Luminal UA exhibit a lining with reverse polarity and looser areas of stellate reticulum, and are surrounded by a fibrous capsule (**Fig. 25**). Intraluminal UA exhibit nodules of ameloblastoma projecting into the lumen, but no infiltration into the wall is seen. Mural UA has areas in which the ameloblastic lining infiltrates the surrounding wall. The diagnosis of UA should be reserved for when the entire tumor is available for examination.

PA have ameloblastic epithelium exhibiting reverse polarity, which may fuse with the overlying epithelium (**Fig. 26**). The loose stellate reticulum is not a prominent feature. Tumors may exhibit clear cell change or have a prominent acanthomatous appearance.[62]

DIFFERENTIAL DIAGNOSIS

Ameloblastic fibroma (AF) and AFO must be distinguished from ameloblastoma. The characteristic stroma AF and AFO aid in this distinction. Other

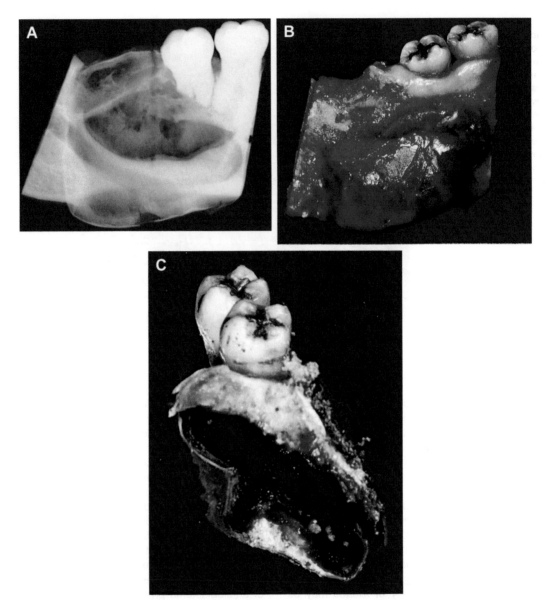

Fig. 22. Ameloblastoma, gross features. (*A*) Radiographically, the specimen is multilocular and expansile with well-defined borders and straight edge tooth root resorption. (*B*) The propensity for buccal–lingual expansion is grossly evident with rounded margins present and cortical perforation. (*C*) Cut section of a solid multicystic ameloblastoma may reveal large cystic spaces.

odontogenic lesions, such as adenomatoid odontogenic tumor (AOT) and CCOT, may exhibit "ameloblastic" epithelium. However, the other coinciding histologic features not seen in ameloblastoma should aid in this distinction (whirled epithelium/rosettes or ghost cells/calcifications, respectively). Hyperplastic follicles and dentigerous cysts may contain islands of odontogenic epithelium that exhibits reverse polarity, especially in younger patients. Clinicopathologic correlation distinguishes these tumors quickly.

Ameloblastomas, particularly at peripheral sites, may also mimic basaloid salivary gland tumors. However, salivary gland tumors do not demonstrate a stellate reticulum, and will demonstrate a structured distribution of myoepithelial and true ductal cells. Acanthomatous ameloblastomas may be mistaken for squamous cell carcinoma if the reverse polarity, and peripheral palisading of tumor nests, are not recognized. Additionally, the level of atypia in squamous cell carcinoma is beyond that expected in ameloblastoma.

Fig.   23. Desmoplastic ameloblastoma. (*A*) On computed tomography in the axial plane, an ill-defined, mixed density expansile lesion is evident. (*B*) Histology reveals compressed epithelial islands in a dense collagenous stroma. A myxoid appearance surrounds the islands.

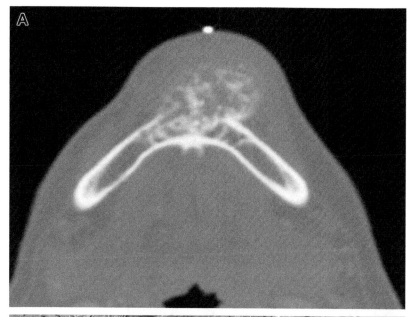

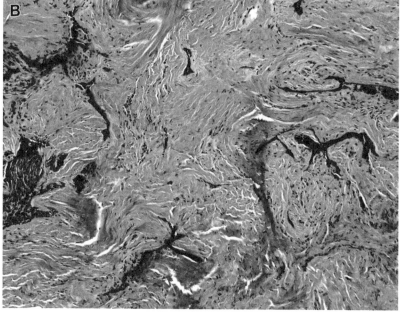

UA are cystic lesions that may surround an impacted tooth in a young patient, similar to a dentigerous cyst. These entities should not be confused, because UA have reverse polarity of the cystic lining, nuclear hyperchromatism, and stellate reticulum.

PROGNOSIS

Treatment is of SMA is resection with 1.5-cm margins.[63] Treatment with enucleation or curettage results in a high rate of recurrence reported at around 50%.[63,64]

UA are clinically less aggressive and are often treated with curettage alone with are recurrence rate of 15%.[56,59] When a prominent mural component is present, more aggressive treatment is often recommended.

It must be emphasized that the biologic behavior of PA is different than of SMA and conservative treatment is warranted.[62]

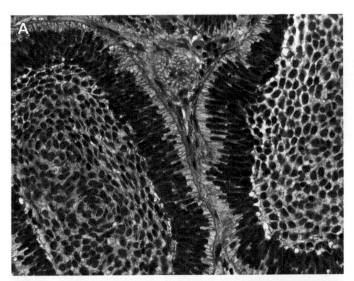

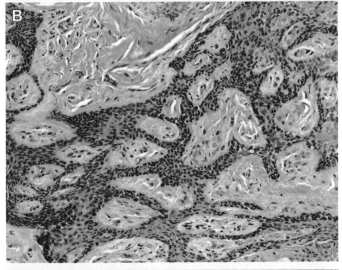

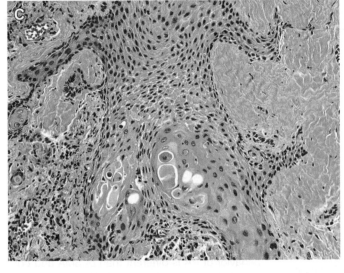

Fig. 24. Ameloblastoma. (*A*) Follicular ameloblastoma exhibiting rounded epithelial islands in a mature collagenous stroma with columnar peripheral cells exhibiting prominent reverse polarity. (*B*) Thin strands of epithelium intersect in this plexiform ameloblastoma and squamous metaplasia is present in the areas normally composed of a stellate reticulum-like appearance. (*C*) High-power view of keratin pearl formation in an acanthomatous ameloblastoma.

Fig. 24. (*continued*). (*D*) In this granular cell pattern ameloblastoma, the center of the tumor nests are replaced with cells exhibiting an eosinophilic granular cytoplasm. (*E*) Low-power view of a solid multicystic ameloblastoma that is infiltrating the bone. Tumor islands are centered with loose stellate reticulum with cystic degeneration.

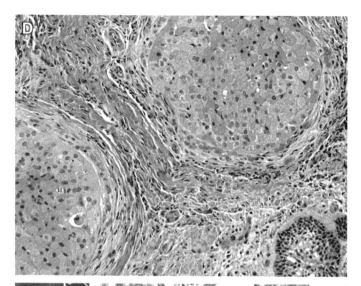

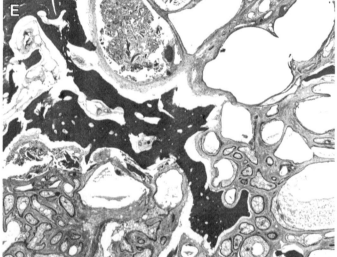

Malignant (metastasizing) ameloblastomas are diagnosed retrospectively when a morphologically "benign" ameloblastoma results in a morphologically similar metastases.[65] Typically, these neoplasms occur after multiple recurrences with an average 18-year time course from initial diagnosis of the primary tumor to diagnosis of malignant ameloblastoma.[66] Malignant ameloblastomas metastasize most frequently the lung or the regional lymph nodes.[67]

Pitfalls
AMELOBLASTOMA

! Desmoplastic ameloblastoma may lack prominent reverse polarity; focally, it will be present.

! Unlike solid/multicystic ameloblastoma, desmoplastic ameloblastomas have a predilection for the anterior jaws.

! Desmoplastic ameloblastomas can be unilocular or multilocular and may have a mixed density, confounding the surgical and radiographic impression.

Key Points
AMELOBLASTOMA

Benign, aggressive, persistent tumor

Unilocular or multilocular "soap bubble" radiolucent appearance, never show calcification

Posterior mandible, molar/ramus area affected, cortical expansion is common

En bloc resection recommended for solid/multicystic ameloblastoma owing to recurrence potential

Histologic Vickers-Gorlin criteria[60]

1. Hyperchromatism of basal cell nuclei of epithelial-lined cysts

2. Palisading and polarization of the basal cell nuclei of luminal epithelium

3. Cytoplasmic vacuolization (subnuclear vacuolization) of the luminal basal cells

Hyalinization or inductive effect on subjacent connective tissue

Epithelial spongiosis above the basal layer (resembling stellate reticulum of tooth development)

AMELOBLASTIC FIBROMA AND AMELOBLASTIC FIBROODONTOMA

AF and AFO are benign tumors presenting most frequently in the first 2 decades of life (72% of cases) with a slight male predilection (1.26:1), but uncommonly can be seen in older patients. Tumors are seen most frequently in the posterior mandible presenting with swelling. Radiographically, AF present as radiolucencies, whereas AFO may have a mixed density appearance, often associated with an impacted tooth (Fig. 27). They may be asymptomatic lesions, detected incidentally, or patients may present with pain.[68] Limited data are available, but *BRAF* V600E mutations have been found in AF and AFO.[56]

MICROSCOPIC FEATURES

AF and AFO usually show nests or thin, elongated cords of ameloblastic odontogenic epithelium set in a primitive myxoid mesenchymal stroma (Fig. 28A). AFO are distinguished from AF by the presence of hard tissue formation (dentin or enamel; Fig. 28B).[56]

DIFFERENTIAL DIAGNOSIS

Failure to appreciate the hard tissue component of an AFO may lead to difficulty in distinguishing it from an AF. Differentiating AF from an ameloblastoma is an important distinction. The epithelial tumor islands are larger and more prominent in an ameloblastoma, whereas the islands in AF are more attenuated cords and strands. Furthermore, ameloblastoma lacks the primitive myxoid to mesenchymal stroma that is characteristic in AF and AFO. Distinguishing an AFO from a developing odontoma is a potential diagnostic pitfall.

PROGNOSIS

Treatment strategy varies, most commonly using conservative therapy (enucleation and curettage)

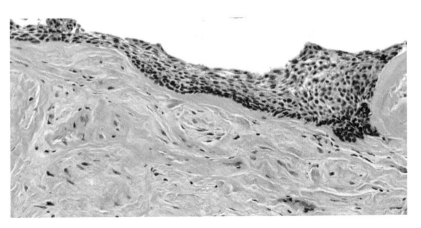

Fig. 25. Unicystic ameloblastoma. Ameloblastic epithelium lines the cystic cavity adjacent to dense connective tissue.

Fig. 26. Peripheral amelo-blastoma. Infiltrative ame-loblastic island coalescence with overlying stratified squamous epithelium.

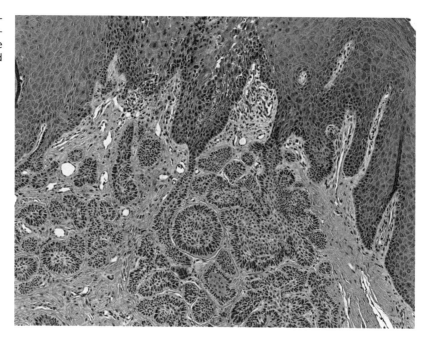

Fig. 27. Ameloblastic fi-broodontoma.   Large mixed density mass is present over an impacted mandibular left third molar.

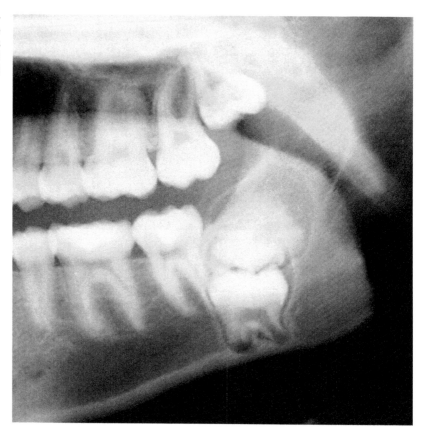

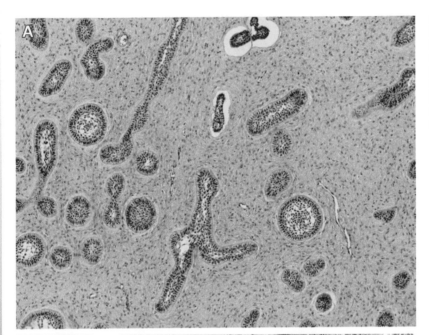

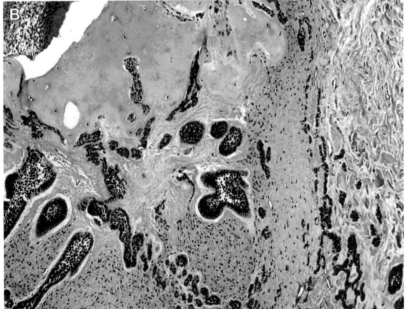

Fig. 28. (*A*) Ameloblastic fibroma exhibiting ameloblastic islands and cords of epithelium in a primitive myxoid mesenchymal stroma. (*B*) Ameloblastic fibroodontoma exhibiting eosinophilic dentinoid formation.

or less commonly more aggressive modalities (wide local excision or resection). Recurrence is reported in 18% of tumors.[69] Malignant transformation to ameloblastic fibrosarcoma (AFS), seen in the mesenchymal component, is reported in 11% of cases, most commonly after recurrence.[68] Some authors recommend wide local excision with long-term follow-up, given the risk or recurrence or malignant transformation.[70]

ADENOMATOID ODONTOGENIC TUMOR

AOTs are uncommon, benign, slow-growing lesions. Three variants exist: (1) follicular or pericoronal, (2) extrafollicular or extracoronal, and (3) peripheral variant.[71] They are sometimes referred to as the "two-thirds tumor," because roughly "two-thirds" of AOTs present before the second decade of life, roughly "two-thirds" of

AOTs present in the maxilla (most commonly the anterior), roughly "two-thirds" of AOTs present in females, roughly "two-thirds" of AOTs surround an impacted tooth (the follicular variant), and roughly "two-thirds" of the time that impacted tooth is a canine.[72] Radiographically, a unique characteristic of AOTs is in the follicular variant, the radiolucency surrounding the impacted tooth extends beyond the cemento–enamel junction, enveloping the crown and part of the root (**Fig. 29**). Also, fine radiopaque foci that represents calcifications is seen in "two-thirds" of cases.[73]

GROSS FEATURES

Grossly, AOTs are well-defined with a thick capsule. They may be solid or cystic, often with a tooth embedded in the tumor mass.[74]

MICROSCOPIC FEATURES

AOTs are solid and cystic epithelial tumors with ductlike structures surrounded by a well-defined capsule. The epithelium has been described exhibiting an inductive effect on the adjacent mesenchymal tissue. The tumor is characterized by rounded nests or rosettelike areas (**Fig. 30A, B**). Amyloid material and calcifications are present. Apple green birefringence is present under polarized light. CEOT-like areas in an otherwise classic AOT should be considered a normal variant, because this is part of the accepted spectrum of AOT.

DIFFERENTIAL DIAGNOSIS

AOTs may be confused with other mixed-density lesions that have calcifications. CCOTs have calcifications and ameloblastic epithelium; however, they also contain ghost cells.

PROGNOSIS

Treatment is enucleation or curettage, which is curative.

CALCIFYING CYSTIC ODONTOGENIC TUMOR (CALCIFYING ODONTOGENIC CYST, GORLIN CYST)

CCOTs present over a wide range of ages, and most commonly anterior to the molar region. Most commonly these are central radiolucencies, but focal radiopacities contributing to a mixed density appearance may be radiographically present. Calcifications are present more frequently in late stage lesions and this variability leads to a wide radiographic differential diagnosis. Peripheral lesions are less common. A solid variant, lacking cystic areas, is termed an odontogenic ghost cell tumor. CCOTs often coexist with other odontogenic lesions, most frequently odontomas.[75]

GROSS FEATURES

The gross features of CCOT correlate with the subtype of the odontogenic ghost cell lesion. The simple cystic variant is cystic with variability in the proliferation of the epithelial lining (**Fig. 31A**).

MICROSCOPIC FEATURES

Anucleate ghost cells are present and frequently calcify (similar to the cutaneous pilomatrixoma). These are lined by "ameloblastic" epithelium, which can exhibit peripheral palisading (**Fig. 31B**). Usually, these are cystic lesions. Beta-catenin and LEF-1 positivity are frequently seen in CCOTs, 82% and 64%, respectively.[76]

DIFFERENTIAL DIAGNOSIS

Correctly differentiating CCOT from ameloblastoma is important, because both have

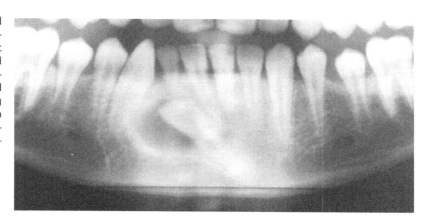

Fig. 29. Adenomatoid odontogenic tumor, radiographic features. Classic follicular adenomatoid odontogenic tumor presenting a well-defined radiolucency enveloping an impacted tooth, with the radiolucency extending beyond the cemento–enamel junction.

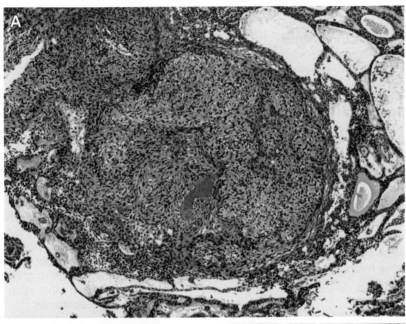

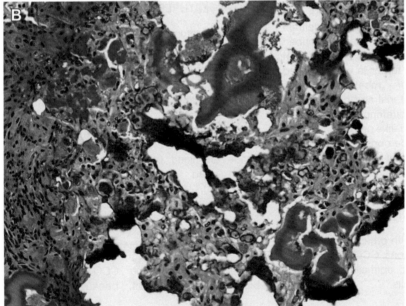

Fig. 30. Adenomatoid odontogenic tumor. (*A*) At a low power, the lesion has a mixed cystic/solid appearance containing epithelial whorls and ductlike structures. (*B*) A higher power view illustrates amyloid and irregular calcifications.

ameloblastic epithelium. The presence of numerous ghost cells and calcification should aid in this discrimination. Very rarely are ghost cells seen in ameloblastoma and hard tissue formation is not tolerated. Beta-catenin mutation is useful in discriminating CCOT from ameloblastoma.[77]

Craniopharyngiomas may mimic CCOTs. However, CCOTs are restricted to the gnathic region.

PROGNOSIS

Treatment is enucleation with a variable recurrence rate.

CALCIFYING EPITHELIAL ODONTOGENIC TUMOR (PINDBORG TUMOR)

Calcifying epithelial odontogenic tumor (CEOTs) are uncommon odontogenic tumors that present

Fig. 31. Calcifying cystic odontogenic tumor. (*A*) A thin cystic lesion is seen with focal luminal thickenings. (*B*) A basal layer of ameloblastic epithelium is seen exhibiting reverse polarity with underlying stellate reticulum. Coalescing ghost cells are seen with some undergoing mineralization.

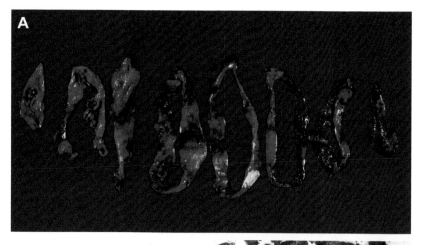

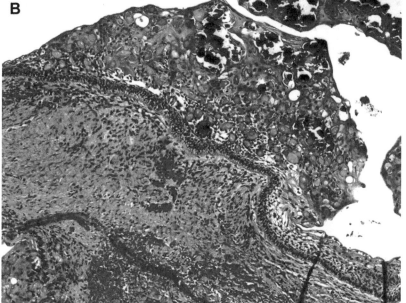

over a wide range of ages, with no strong gender predilection and a mandibular predilection (2:1). Most cases are intraosseous, but 6% of cases are peripheral.[78] Radiopacities may be seen on imaging, in approximately 50% of cases on plain films. More than one-half of these tumors are associated with an impacted tooth (**Fig. 32**A).[78]

GROSS FEATURES

Tumors are grossly solid fleshy masses (**Fig. 32**B). Sectioning may reveal calcifications.

MICROSCOPIC FEATURES

CEOTs are composed of eosinophilic polyhedral epithelial cells that exhibit prominent intercellular bridging. Significant nuclear pleomorphism may

be seen with variable nuclear size, staining, and multinucleated cells (**Fig. 33**A). An amorphous acellular amyloid is a characteristic finding in CEOTs, which is odontogenic ameloblastic associated protein (**Fig. 33**B).[79,80] This material calcifies and the resulting concentric calcifications are termed Liesegang rings (**Fig. 33**C). The amyloid may be stained for Congo red, exhibiting an apple green birefringence (**Fig. 33**D). Variable amounts of amyloid may be present and tumors may range from highly cellular to amyloid predominant.

DIFFERENTIAL DIAGNOSIS

Areas resembling CEOT, including concentric calcifications and amyloid, are frequently seen in AOTs. However, in these tumors, the AOT features

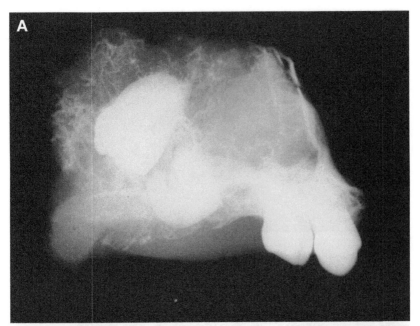

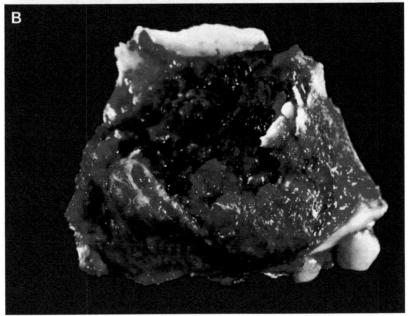

Fig. 32. Calcifying epithelial odontogenic tumor (CEOT). (*A*) Radiographically, the tumor may exhibit a mixed radiolucent radiopaque appearance and be associated with an impacted tooth. (*B*) A clinically aggressive CEOT that exhibits significant bony destruction. The tumor is a fleshy mass and calcifications are noted on sectioning.

dominate, as a whole. Clear cell change in CEOTs is a challenge, and clear cell CEOTs may be confused with clear cell odontogenic carcinoma (CCOC).[81,82] However, amyloid is not seen with CCOC. Care should be exercised on small biopsies in the diagnosis of clear cell odontogenic tumors.

PROGNOSIS

Treatment is resection with tumor-free margins. Recurrence is seen more frequently in the maxilla,

with an overall recurrence rate of approximately 20%.

CENTRAL ODONTOGENIC FIBROMA

Central odontogenic fibroma (COF) is a rare tumor of undetermined origin with possible derivation from pluripotent mesenchymal cells of the periodontal ligament, the dental follicle, or the dental papilla (primitive pulp). The tumor incidence is reported at 0.1% of all odontogenic tumors. The

Fig. 33. Calcifying epithelial odontogenic tumor. (*A*) Polygonal epithelial cells are seen with prominent intercellular bridging and pleomorphism. Scant amyloid is present. (*B*) As seen here, some tumors demonstrate a dominant amyloid component.

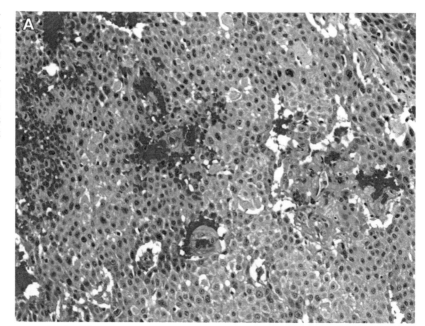

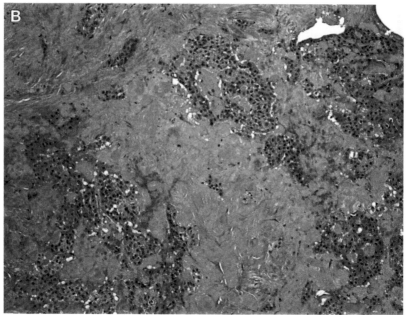

COF is a tumor of adults with a roughly equal distribution across the maxilla and mandible, although some case series show a slight predilection for the mandible. Maxillary lesions occur in the anterior areas and mandibular lesions occur in the posterior regions.[83] Radiographically, the tumor is a unilocular, well-corticated radiolucency. Larger lesions may be multilocular.[83]

MICROSCOPIC FEATURES

Microscopically, there are 2 histomorphic patterns characteristic of COF. The simple type is largely fibrous connective tissue with few or any epithelial rests or dentinoid. The fibroblasts may be stellate or fusiform, with long anastomosing tails (**Fig. 34**).

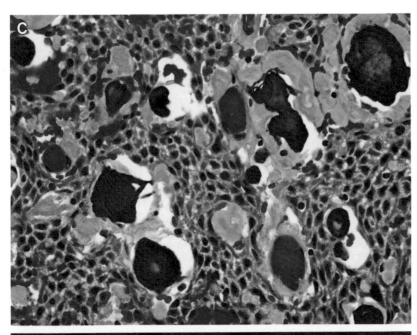

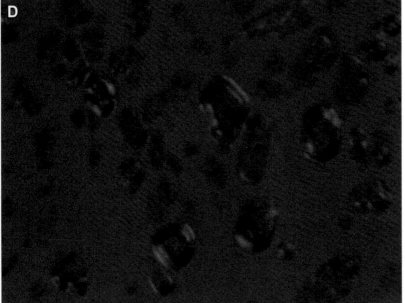

Fig. 33. (*continued*). (*C*) The amyloid calcifies leading to Liesegang ring formation. (*D*) Under polarized light, apple green birefringence highlighting immature Liesegang rings, is seen.

The complex or World Health Organization type shows mature fibrous connective tissue with numerous odontogenic epithelial rests and scattered foci of calcific material that represents either dentin or cementum.

The peripheral odontogenic fibroma is a gingival lesion with the same histopathologic appearance.

DIFFERENTIAL DIAGNOSIS

The differential diagnosis of the simple type of COF is a desmoplastic fibroma. When there is accumulation of glycosaminoglycans, the myxoid look is similar to fibromyxoma. The differential diagnosis of a complex or World Health Organization type of COF includes hyperplastic or thickened dental follicle.[83]

PROGNOSIS

Surgical excision or enucleation is the treatment of choice, because the lesions are well-demarcated. Recurrence is uncommon (approximately 4.0%)[83].

Fig. 34. Central odontogenic fibroma. Scattered attenuated odontogenic islands are seen in fibromyxoid stroma.

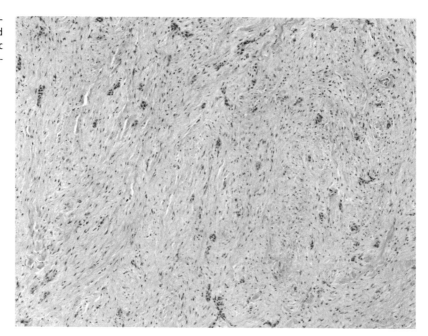

ODONTOGENIC MYXOMA

Odontogenic myxomas are slow growing but potentially large destructive odontogenic tumors that present most commonly in the posterior jaws during the second to fifth decades of life.[84] Radiographically, these are most commonly multilocular radiolucencies with fine, lacey or netlike septae present. Clinically, they most commonly present with swelling and cortical expansion, which may be accompanied by tooth displacement, root resorption, pain, or paresthesia.[84–86]

GROSS FEATURES

Grossly, the lesions are infiltrative, appearing soft, loose, glistening, white-gray, at times having a jellylike consistency (**Fig. 35**A, B). The gross density of the lesion depends on the amount of collagen, which is highly variable in odontogenic myxomas.

MICROSCOPIC FEATURES

Overall, the tumor has a bland myxoid appearance. The lesion is composed of fine delicate stellate or spindly mesenchymal cells with tapered processes in a mucoid or myxoid matrix. Uncommonly, in about 8% of cases, odontogenic epithelial islands may be noted.[86] Variable amounts of collagen may be seen, leading to the names fibromyoma or myxofibroma when collagen is abundant in the stroma. Clinically, these represent the same lesions. The stroma is positive for vimentin in all cases, actin in 46.7% of cases, and HHF35 in 22.6% of cases.[86] Extensive bony invasion may be present (**Fig. 35C**).[86]

DIFFERENTIAL DIAGNOSIS

Histopathologic diagnostic dilemmas can be resolved with adequate clinicopathologic correlation. Odontogenic myxomas resemble dental pulp (**Fig. 35** D, E), which may be displaced from a tooth at the time of extraction or gross examination. This dental papilla is no larger than 1.5 cm in size and is rimmed by odontoblasts. Dental follicles may also be mistake for myxoma, but these are more fibrous in nature with epithelial odontogenic rests common and are often rimmed by reduced enamel epithelium.[87] Another diagnostic dilemma is oral focal mucinosis, which histologically also has a loose myxoid appearance with scattered spindled to stellate cells. This lesion has been termed a soft tissue myxoma, given that it is found in the soft tissue of the jaws, commonly as a peripheral lesion.

PROGNOSIS

Treatment is resection with wide margins. Recurrence is approximately 25%, and long-term follow-up is warranted.[88,89]

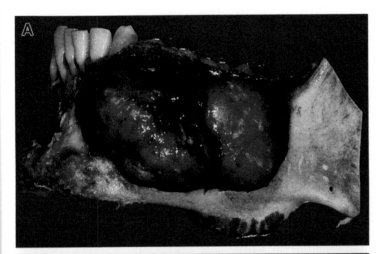

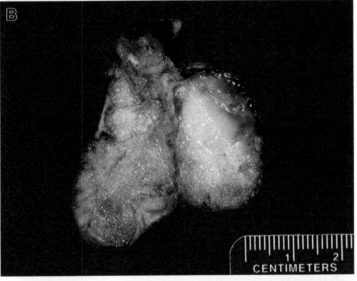

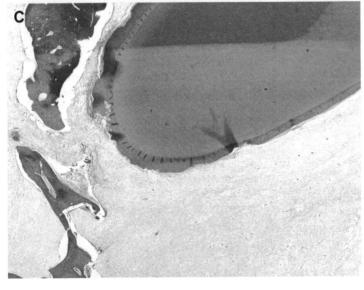

Fig. 35. Odontogenic myxoma. (*A*) Grossly, the lesion is expansile and destructive. (*B*) On cut section, the tumor exhibits a glistening grey-white appearance. (*C*) Extensive bony destruction is seen with early microscopic root resorption.

Fig. 35. (*continued*). (*D*) Delicate spindled cells of odontogenic myxoma. (*E*) Dental papilla exhibiting tapered cells in loose myxoid stroma.

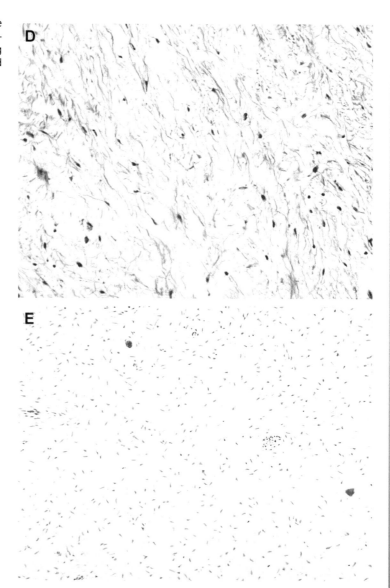

SQUAMOUS ODONTOGENIC TUMOR

Squamous odontogenic tumor (SOT) is a very rare, symptomless to occasionally tender benign tumor that can cause tooth mobility. The SOT occurs across a broad age range from children to the elderly, and affects males and females essentially equally.[90] Tumor origin is likely from residual odontogenic epithelial rests. Radiographically SOT can seem to be noncorticated, but delineated; like inflammatory lesions, it can be crestal or periradicular, and have the angular bone resorptive pattern of vertical bone loss in periodontal disease. Interestingly, the tumor can affect multiple quadrants,

another feature of periodontal disease. Tumors occur in the maxilla and mandible with equal frequency, with maxillary lesions present in anterior segments, whereas the mandibular lesions are more posterior. This is similar to the anatomic occurrence of COF. Other radiographic appearances can be semilunar, triangular, and well-corticated.

GROSS FEATURES

Grossly, circumscribed rubbery, compressible connective tissue is noted.

MICROSCOPIC FEATURES

Microscopically, bland-appearing round or irregularly shaped squamous epithelial islands with normal cytologic maturation are embedded in a stroma of mature fibrous connective tissue (**Fig. 36**). Although the variably sized epithelial islands are commonly solid, microcystic change does occur. The lesions in close proximity to the oral environment will show chronic inflammatory cells in the connective tissue stroma.

DIFFERENTIAL DIAGNOSIS

Although sometimes confused with acanthomatous ameloblastoma, SOT lacks the peripheral palisaded and polarized columnar basal cells characteristic of ameloblastomas. An SOT-like histopathologic appearance is sometimes evident in the connective tissue wall of a dentigerous cyst and also in the retromolar trigone.

PROGNOSIS

The SOT is readily "shelled out" surgically, and curettage is curative.[90]

PRIMORDIAL ODONTOGENIC TUMOR

A recently described odontogenic tumor, the primordial odontogenic tumor, albeit controversial, deserves brief mention here.[91] This rare benign tumor of children and adolescents has been described in the molar ramus region of the mandible surrounding the crown of an unerupted molar tooth, radiographically similar to a dentigerous cyst.[92,93] Radiographically, the lesion is expansile, shows cortical thinning, and is well-corticated with clear demarcation from the surrounding bone affording ease of surgical removal or "shelling out."[92,93]

GROSS FEATURES

Grossly, the primordial odontogenic tumor is described as ellipsoidal and slick to the gloved hand owing to a thin peripheral membrane of ameloblastic epithelium, and intraepithelial connective tissue mucins in exposed stellate reticulum.[92]

MICROSCOPIC FEATURES

Abundant dental papilla-like myxoid connective tissue is delimited peripherally by ameloblastic epithelium.[93] The myxoid connective tissue adjacent to the epithelium is more cellular, "cambium layer–like," whereas centrally the mesenchyme is paucicellular and more mature (**Fig. 37**). Immunohistochemically, the primordial odontogenic tumor shows low Ki 67 positivity, cytokeratin positivity for AE1/AE3, CK5, 14 and 19, and it is negative for CK 18 and 20. The mesenchyme is positive for vimentin.[93]

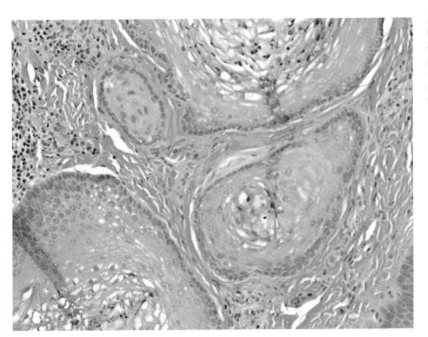

Fig. 36. Squamous odontogenic tumor. Bland epithelial islands lacking pleomorphism and peripheral palisading are noted in a fibrous stroma.

Fig. 37. Primordial odontogenic tumor. Ameloblastic epithelium is attached cellular mesenchyme without an intervening odontoblastic layer. (*Courtesy of* Dr Lee Slater, San Diego, CA.)

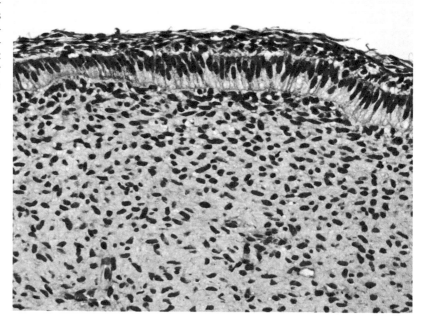

DIFFERENTIAL DIAGNOSIS

The primordial odontogenic tumor has been referred to as a soft tissue odontoma, too primitive to produce dental hard tissue, and it has been noted as a lobular mass coincident with a complex odontoma.[92] The differential diagnosis may include AF, odontogenic myxoma, or a hyperplastic dental follicle.[93]

AMELOBLASTIC CARCINOMA

Ameloblastic carcinoma are rare, aggressive, gnathic malignancies that present as swelling, at times associated with rapid growth, pain, or paresthesia, and most commonly in the mandible (**Fig. 38**A). Radiographically, poorly defined borders are seen (**Fig. 38**B). As with other ameloblastic neoplasms, *BRAF* V600E mutations have been reported.[94]

MICROSCOPIC FEATURES

In ameloblastic carcinoma, often the bulk of tumor lacks the classic features of ameloblastoma (such as palisading and reverse polarity) in the majority of the tumor, making it difficult to determine their origin.[95] Ameloblastic carcinoma may exhibit features associated with malignancy including, angiolymphatic invasion, perineural invasion, nuclear pleomorphic, and increased mitotic activity (**Fig. 38**C). A threshold of 2 mitotic figures in a high-power field in a high-grade area is proposed for the discrimination of ameloblastic carcinoma from ameloblastoma, but diagnostically borderline cases, sometimes dubbed "atypical ameloblastomas," remain challenging.[95] SOX2 has shown usefulness in discriminating ameloblastomas from ameloblastic carcinoma.[96]

PROGNOSIS

Ameloblastic carcinoma may recur locally or metastasize to locoregional lymph nodes or distant sites, most frequently the lung.[97]

AMELOBLASTIC FIBROSARCOMA

AFS are rare malignant odontogenic tumors that may arise de novo or in recurrent AFs or AFOs, with 44% arising in preexisting AF or AFO, and presenting more than decade later at 33 versus 21.9 years of age.[70] These tumors are seen over a very wide age range, with a mean of 27.5 years. A female predilection exists (1.5:1) and tumors present most frequently in the mandible (4:1).[70] Similar tumors containing enamel or dentin termed ameloblastic odontosarcoma and ameloblastic dentinosarcoma have been described. These are thought to be variants of AFS.[70,98] Clinically, patients present with pain and swelling. Radiographically, these are destructive radiolucent lesions with ill-defined borders.

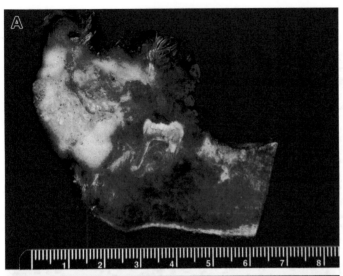

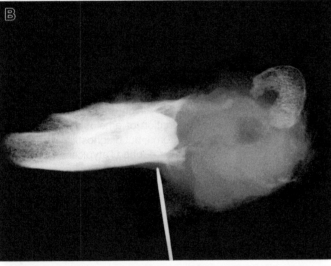

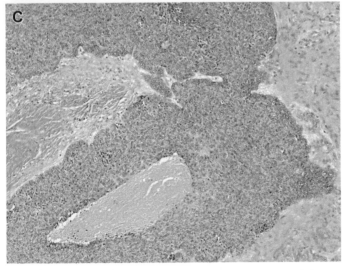

Fig. 38. Ameloblastic carcinoma. (*A*) Grossly, the tumor is infiltrative and destructive exhibiting a grey-white appearance on cut surface. (*B*) Radiographically, the tumor demonstrates irregular, poorly defined borders. (*C*) Hypercellular islands and tongues of hyperchromatic odontogenic epithelium rimmed by a mature fibrous connective tissue stroma. Peripheral palisading characteristic of ameloblastoma is not readily evident and epithelial islands show atypical mitoses and comedo necrosis.

MICROSCOPIC FEATURES

AFS are neoplasms that are similar histologically to an AF, but the mesenchymal components resemble a sarcoma.[99] Thus, increased cellularity, pleomorphism, and mitotic activity will be present in the mesenchymal stroma and the epithelium will be benign (**Fig. 39**). Thin cords or small odontogenic islands of odontogenic epithelium arranged in a follicular pattern edged with columnar cells exhibiting reverse polarity. The epithelium may be lacking, especially after multiple recurrences, and the tumor may resemble a fibrosarcoma.[70]

DIFFERENTIAL DIAGNOSIS

When considering the diagnosis of gnathic fibrosarcoma, the diagnosis of AFS lacking the epithelial component should be considered. Although the epithelium exhibits features seen in ameloblastoma or ameloblastic carcinoma, the dysplastic mesenchymal stroma is characteristic of AFS.

PROGNOSIS

Given the rarity of AFS, prognostic information is limited. However, AFS are treated aggressively with resection. Treatment with adjuvant chemo or radiotherapy has been used. Recurrence has been reported in approximately 40% of adequately treated AFS and 20% of AFS patients have died of disease.[70] Metastasis both distant or to locoregional lymph nodes has been reported, but is uncommon.[100]

CLEAR CELL ODONTOGENIC CARCINOMA

CCOCs are rare, locally aggressive, low-grade malignancies found most commonly the mandible with a slight female predilection. Radiographically, they may present as ill-defined radiolucencies, with ill-defined margins and root resorption may be present.

MICROSCOPIC FEATURES

The tumor is composed of sheets, cords, or nests of polygonal cells separated by a hyalinized to fibrous stroma. Periodic Acid-Schiff–positive and diastase-sensitive clear cells may predominate. Peripheral palisading of the tumor islands is seen in 58% of cases (**Fig. 40**).[101] High-molecular-weight keratins and P63 are positive in the tumor islands.[101]

DIFFERENTIAL DIAGNOSIS

The diagnosis of CCOC is made after ruling out clear cell metastases, clear cell odontogenic tumors, and clear cell salivary tumors. The differential diagnosis of CCOC includes metastatic renal cell carcinoma, clear cell CEOT, and (hyalinizing) clear cell carcinoma of salivary origin.[101] CCOC can be distinguished from metastatic renal cell carcinoma and clear cell CEOT by the presence

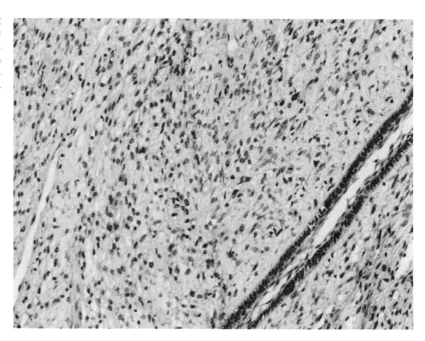

Fig. 39. Ameloblastic fibrosarcoma. Increased cellularity and mitotic activity present in the stroma surrounding ribbons of benign ameloblastic epithelium.

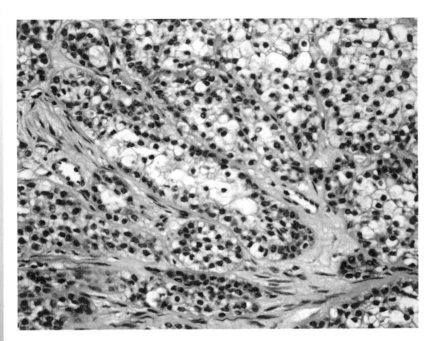

Fig. 40. Clear cell odontogenic carcinoma. Clear cells with a palisaded border comprise epithelial tumor islands.

of *EWSR1-ATF1* translocation. The vast majority (88%) of CCOC have *EWSR1* rearrangements detectable by fluorescent in situ hybridization.[82] CCOC and hyalinizing clear cell carcinoma show considerable morphologic overlap and also share the *EWSR1-ATF1* translocation. The only reliable method of distinction is location as they are likely biologic counterparts.

PROGNOSIS

Treatment is resection, because cases treated with curettage recur at a significantly higher rate (80%) when compared with resection (43%).[102] Adjuvant therapy may also be considered.[102] CCOC may recur locally (34%), in regional lymph nodes, or rarely metastasize to distant sites, most frequently the lungs.[101,103–106]

REFERENCES

1. Nanci A. Ten Cate's oral histology: development, structure, and function. 8th edition. St Louis (MO): Mosby; 2013. p. 400.
2. Avery J. Oral development and histology. 3rd edition. New York: Thieme; 2002.
3. Philipsen H, Reichart A. The development and fate of epithelial residues after completion of the human odontogenesis with special reference to the origins of epithelial odontogenic neoplasms, hamartomas and cysts. Oral Biosci Med 2004;1:171–9.
4. Johnson NR, Gannon OM, Savage NW, et al. Frequency of odontogenic cysts and tumors: a systematic review. J Investig Clin Dent 2014;5(1):9–14.
5. Carrillo C, Penarrocha M, Ortega B, et al. Correlation of radiographic size and the presence of radiopaque lamina with histological findings in 70 periapical lesions. J Oral Maxillofac Surg 2008; 66(8):1600–5.
6. Carrillo C, Penarrocha M, Bagan JV, et al. Relationship between histological diagnosis and evolution of 70 periapical lesions at 12 months, treated by periapical surgery. J Oral Maxillofac Surg 2008; 66(8):1606–9.
7. McMillan MD, Kardos TB, Edwards JL, et al. Giant cell hyalin angiopathy or pulse granuloma. Oral Surg Oral Med Oral Pathol 1981;52(2):178–86.
8. Dunlap CL, Barker BF. Giant-cell hyalin angiopathy. Oral Surg Oral Med Oral Pathol 1977;44(4):587–91.
9. Henriques AC, Pereira JS, Nonaka CF, et al. Analysis of the frequency and nature of hyaline ring granulomas in inflammatory odontogenic cysts. Int Endod J 2013;46(1):20–9.
10. Martin RW 3rd, Lumadue JA, Corio RL, et al. Cutaneous giant cell hyalin angiopathy. J Cutan Pathol 1993;20(4):356–8.
11. Chrcanovic BR, Reis BM, Freire-Maia B. Paradental (mandibular inflammatory buccal) cyst. Head Neck Pathol 2011;5(2):159–64.
12. Bsoul SA, Flint DJ, Terezhalmy GT, et al. Paradental cyst (inflammatory collateral, mandibular infected buccal cyst). Quintessence Int 2002;33(10):782–3.

13. Robinson R, Vincent S. Tumors and cysts of the jaws. In: Silverberg S, editor. 4th edition. Silver Spring (MD): ARP Press; 2012. p. 11–37.

14. Daley TD, Wysocki GP. The small dentigerous cyst. A diagnostic dilemma. Oral Surg Oral Med Oral Pathol Oral Radiol Endod 1995;79(1):77–81.

15. Wolf J, Hietanen J. The mandibular infected buccal cyst (paradental cyst). A radiographic and histological study. Br J Oral Maxillofac Surg 1990; 28(5):322–5.

16. Philipsen HP, Reichart PA, Ogawa I, et al. The inflammatory paradental cyst: a critical review of 342 cases from a literature survey, including 17 new cases from the author's files. J Oral Pathol Med 2004;33(3):147–55.

17. Takeda Y, Oikawa Y, Furuya I, et al. Mucous and ciliated cell metaplasia in epithelial linings of odontogenic inflammatory and developmental cysts. J Oral Sci 2005;47(2):77–81.

18. Fowler CB, Brannon RB, Kessler HP, et al. Glandular odontogenic cyst: analysis of 46 cases with special emphasis on microscopic criteria for diagnosis. Head Neck Pathol 2011;5(4):364–75.

19. Roofe SB, Boyd EM Jr, Houston GD, et al. Squamous cell carcinoma arising in the epithelial lining of a dentigerous cyst. South Med J 1999;92(6):611–4.

20. McMillan MD, Smillie AC. Ameloblastomas associated with dentigerous cysts. Oral Surg Oral Med Oral Pathol 1981;51(5):489–96.

21. Piattelli A, Lezzi G, Fioroni M, et al. Ki-67 expression in dentigerous cysts, unicystic ameloblastomas, and ameloblastomas arising from dental cysts. J Endod 2002;28(2):55–8.

22. Johnson LM, Sapp JP, McIntire DN. Squamous cell carcinoma arising in a dentigerous cyst. J Oral Maxillofac Surg 1994;52(9):987–90.

23. Cohen DA, Neville BW, Damm DD, et al. The lateral periodontal cyst. A report of 37 cases. J Periodontol 1984;55(4):230–4.

24. Wysocki GP, Brannon RB, Gardner DG, et al. Histogenesis of the lateral periodontal cyst and the gingival cyst of the adult. Oral Surg Oral Med Oral Pathol 1980;50(4):327–34.

25. Altini M, Shear M. The lateral periodontal cyst: an update. J Oral Pathol Med 1992;21(6):245–50.

26. Gurol M, Burkes EJ Jr, Jacoway J. Botryoid odontogenic cyst: analysis of 33 cases. J Periodontol 1995;66(12):1069–73.

27. Arora P, Bishen KA, Gupta N, et al. Botryoid odontogenic cyst developing from lateral periodontal cyst: a rare case and review on pathogenesis. Contemp Clin Dent 2012;3(3):326–9.

28. Kaplan I, Anavi Y, Hirshberg A. Glandular odontogenic cyst: a challenge in diagnosis and treatment. Oral Dis 2008;14(7):575–81.

29. Noffke C, Raubenheimer EJ. The glandular odontogenic cyst: clinical and radiological features; review of the literature and report of nine cases. Dentomaxillofac Radiol 2002;31(6):333–8.

30. Kaplan I, Anavi Y, Manor R, et al. The use of molecular markers as an aid in the diagnosis of glandular odontogenic cyst. Oral Oncol 2005; 41(9):895–902.

31. Tonon G, Modi S, Wu L, et al. t(11;19)(q21;p13) translocation in mucoepidermoid carcinoma creates a novel fusion product that disrupts a Notch signaling pathway. Nat Genet 2003; 33(2):208–13, [Erratum appears in Nat Genet 2003;33(3):430].

32. Bishop J, Yonescu R, Batista D, et al. Glandular odontogenic cysts consistently lack the MAML2 rearrangements that are frequently found in central mucoepidermoid carcinomas. Mod Pathol 2014; 27:315A–6A.

33. Kaplan I, Gal G, Anavi Y, et al. Glandular odontogenic cyst: treatment and recurrence. J Oral Maxillofac Surg 2005;63(4):435–41.

34. Philipsen HP, Reichart PA, Praetorius F. Mixed odontogenic tumours and odontomas. Considerations on interrelationship. Review of the literature and presentation of 134 new cases of odontomas. Oral Oncol 1997;33(2):86–99.

35. Titinchi F, Nortje CJ. Keratocystic odontogenic tumor: a recurrence analysis of clinical and radiographic parameters. Oral Surg Oral Med Oral Pathol Oral Radiol 2012;114(1):136–42.

36. Chirapathomsakul D, Sastravaha P, Jansisyanont P. A review of odontogenic keratocysts and the behavior of recurrences. Oral Surg Oral Med Oral Pathol Oral Radiol Endod 2006;101(1):5–9, [discussion: 10].

37. Bresler SC, Padwa BL, Granter SR. Nevoid basal cell carcinoma syndrome (gorlin syndrome). Head Neck Pathol 2016;10(2):119–24.

38. Gailani MR, Bale SJ, Leffell DJ, et al. Developmental defects in Gorlin syndrome related to a putative tumor suppressor gene on chromosome 9. Cell 1992;69(1):111–7.

39. Hahn H, Wicking C, Zaphiropoulous PG, et al. Mutations of the human homolog of Drosophila patched in the nevoid basal cell carcinoma syndrome. Cell 1996;85(6):841–51.

40. Robinson R, Vincent SD. Tumor and cysts of the jaws. In: Silverberg S, editor. Silver Spring (MD): ARP press; 2012. p. 49–86.

41. Guthrie D, Peacock ZS, Sadow P, et al. Preoperative incisional and intraoperative frozen section biopsy techniques have comparable accuracy in the diagnosis of benign intraosseous jaw pathology. J Oral Maxillofac Surg 2012;70(11):2566–72.

42. Brannon RB. The odontogenic keratocyst. A clinicopathologic study of 312 cases. Part II. Histologic features. Oral Surg Oral Med Oral Pathol 1977; 43(2):233–55.

43. Hunter KD, Speight PM. The diagnostic usefulness of immunohistochemistry for odontogenic lesions. Head Neck Pathol 2014;8(4):392–9.

44. Mendes RA, Carvalho JF, van der Waal I. A comparative immunohistochemical analysis of COX-2, p53, and Ki-67 expression in keratocystic odontogenic tumors. Oral Surg Oral Med Oral Pathol Oral Radiol Endod 2011;111(3):333–9.

45. Gadbail AR, Chaudhary M, Patil S, et al. Actual Proliferating Index and p53 protein expression as prognostic marker in odontogenic cysts. Oral Dis 2009;15(7):490–8.

46. Pogrel MA. The keratocystic odontogenic tumor. Oral Maxillofacial Surg Clin North Am 2013;25(1): 21–30, v.

47. Cottom HE, Bshena FI, Speight PM, et al. Histopathological features that predict the recurrence of odontogenic keratocysts. J Oral Pathol Med 2012;41(5):408–14.

48. Rao K, Kumar S. The use of enucleation and chemical cauterization (Carnoy's) in the management of odontogenic keratocyst of the jaws. Indian J Otolaryngol Head Neck Surg 2014;66(1):8–12.

49. Johnson NR, Batstone MD, Savage NW. Management and recurrence of keratocystic odontogenic tumor: a systematic review. Oral Surg Oral Med Oral Pathol Oral Radiol 2013;116(4):e271–6.

50. Dong Q, Pan S, Sun LS, et al. Orthokeratinized odontogenic cyst: a clinicopathologic study of 61 cases. Arch Pathol Lab Med 2010;134(2):271–5.

51. Cheng YS, Liang H, Wright J, et al. Multiple orthokeratinized odontogenic cysts: a case report. Head Neck Pathol 2015;9(1):153–7.

52. Chae MP, Smoll NR, Hunter-Smith DJ, et al. Establishing the natural history and growth rate of ameloblastoma with implications for management: systematic review and meta-analysis. PLoS One 2015;10(2):e0117241.

53. Reichart PA, Philipsen HP, Sonner S. Ameloblastoma: biological profile of 3677 cases. Eur J Cancer B Oral Oncol 1995;31B(2):86–99.

54. Philipsen HP, Reichart PA, Takata T. Desmoplastic ameloblastoma (including "hybrid" lesion of ameloblastoma). Biological profile based on 100 cases from the literature and own files. Oral Oncol 2001; 37(5):455–60.

55. Philipsen HP, Reichart PA. Unicystic ameloblastoma. A review of 193 cases from the literature. Oral Oncol 1998;34(5):317–25.

56. Brown NA, Rolland D, McHugh JB, et al. Activating FGFR2-RAS-BRAF mutations in ameloblastoma. Clin Cancer Res 2014;20(21):5517–26.

57. Kurppa KJ, Caton J, Morgan PR, et al. High frequency of BRAF V600E mutations in ameloblastoma. J Pathol 2014;232(5):492–8.

58. Sweeney RT, McClary AC, Myers BR, et al. Identification of recurrent SMO and BRAF mutations in ameloblastomas. Nat Genet 2014; 46(7):722–5.

59. Gardner DG. Some current concepts on the pathology of ameloblastomas. Oral Surg Oral Med Oral Pathol Oral Radiol Endod 1996;82(6):660–9.

60. Vickers RA, Gorlin RJ. Ameloblastoma: delineation of early histopathologic features of neoplasia. Cancer 1970;26(3):699–710.

61. Jaafari-Ashkavandi Z, Dehghani-Nazhvani A, Razmjouyi F. CD56 expression in odontogenic cysts and tumors. J Dent Res Dent Clin Dent Prospects 2014;8(4):240–5.

62. Philipsen HP, Reichart PA, Nikai H, et al. Peripheral ameloblastoma: biological profile based on 160 cases from the literature. Oral Oncol 2001;37(1): 17–27.

63. Hertog D, van der Waal I. Ameloblastoma of the jaws: a critical reappraisal based on a 40-years single institution experience. Oral Oncol 2010;46(1): 61–4.

64. Muller H, Slootweg PJ. The ameloblastoma, the controversial approach to therapy. J Maxillofac Surg 1985;13(2):79–84.

65. Woolgar JA, Triantafyllou A, Ferlito A, et al. Intraosseous carcinoma of the jaws: a clinicopathologic review. Part II: odontogenic carcinomas. Head Neck 2013;35(6):902–5.

66. Van Dam SD, Unni KK, Keller EE. Metastasizing (malignant) ameloblastoma: review of a unique histopathologic entity and report of Mayo Clinic experience. J Oral Maxillofac Surg 2010;68(12): 2962–74.

67. Kunze E, Donath K, Luhr HG, et al. Biology of metastasizing ameloblastoma. Pathol Res Pract 1985;180(5):526–35.

68. Takeda Y. Ameloblastic fibroma and related lesions: current pathologic concept. Oral Oncol 1999;35(6):535–40.

69. Zallen RD, Preskar MH, McClary SA. Ameloblastic fibroma. J Oral Maxillofac Surg 1982;40(8): 513–7.

70. Muller S, Parker DC, Kapadia SB, et al. Ameloblastic fibrosarcoma of the jaws. A clinicopathologic and DNA analysis of five cases and review of the literature with discussion of its relationship to ameloblastic fibroma. Oral Surg Oral Med Oral Pathol Oral Radiol Endod 1995;79(4):469–77.

71. Philipsen HP, Reichart PA, Zhang KH, et al. Adenomatoid odontogenic tumor: biologic profile based on 499 cases. J Oral Pathol Med 1991;20(4): 149–58.

72. Philipsen HP, Reichart PA. Adenomatoid odontogenic tumour: facts and figures. Oral Oncol 1998; 35(2):125–31.

73. Philipsen H, Reichart P, Nikai H. The adenomatoid odontogenic tumour (AOT): an update. Oral Med Pathol 1997;2:55–60.

74. Reichart PA, Philipsen H. Adenomatoid odonto-genic tumour. In: Odontogenic tumors and allied lesions. London: Quintessence; 2004. p. 105–15.

75. Hong SP, Ellis GL, Hartman KS. Calcifying odontogenic cyst. A review of ninety-two cases with reevaluation of their nature as cysts or neoplasms, the nature of ghost cells, and subclassification. Oral Surg Oral Med Oral Pathol 1991;72(1):56–64.

76. Bilodeau EA, Acquafondata M, Barnes EL, et al. A comparative analysis of LEF-1 in odontogenic and salivary tumors. Hum Pathol 2015;46(2):255–9.

77. Sekine S, Sato S, Takata T, et al. Beta-catenin mutations are frequent in calcifying odontogenic cysts, but rare in ameloblastomas. Am J Pathol 2003;163(5):1707–12.

78. Philipsen HP, Reichart PA. Calcifying epithelial odontogenic tumour: biological profile based on 181 cases from the literature. Oral Oncol 2000; 36(1):17–26.

79. Kestler DP, Foster JS, Macy SD, et al. Expression of odontogenic ameloblast-associated protein (ODAM) in dental and other epithelial neoplasms. Mol Med 2008;14(5–6):318–26.

80. Murphy CL, Kestler DP, Foster JS, et al. Odontogenic ameloblast-associated protein nature of the amyloid found in calcifying epithelial odontogenic tumors and unerupted tooth follicles. Amyloid 2008;15(2):89–95.

81. Schmidt-Westhausen A, Philipsen HP, Reichart PA. Clear cell calcifying epithelial odontogenic tumor. A case report. Int J Oral Maxillofac Surg 1992;21(1): 47–9.

82. Bilodeau EA, Weinreb I, Antonescu CR, et al. Clear cell odontogenic carcinomas show EWSR1 rearrangements: a novel finding and a biological link to salivary clear cell carcinomas. Am J Surg Pathol 2013;37(7):1001–5.

83. de Matos FR, de Moraes M, Neto AC, et al. Central odontogenic fibroma. Ann Diagn Pathol 2011; 15(6):481–4.

84. Li TJ, Sun LS, Luo HY. Odontogenic myxoma: a clinicopathologic study of 25 cases. Arch Pathol Lab Med 2006;130(12):1799–806.

85. Simon EN, Merkx MA, Vuhahula E, et al. Odontogenic myxoma: a clinicopathological study of 33 cases. Int J Oral Maxillofac Surg 2004;33(4):333–7.

86. Martinez-Mata G, Mosqueda-Taylor A, Carlos-Bregni R, et al. Odontogenic myxoma: clinicopathological, immunohistochemical and ultrastructural findings of a multicentric series. Oral Oncol 2008;44(6): 601–7.

87. Kim J, Ellis G. Dental follicular tissue: misinterpretation as odontogenic tumors. J Oral Maxillofac Surg 1993;51(7):762–7.

88. Lo Muzio L, Nocini P, Favia G, et al. Odontogenic myxoma of the jaws: a clinical, radiologic, immunohistochemical, and ultrastructural study. Oral Surg Oral Med Oral Pathol Oral Radiol Endod 1996; 82(4):426–33.

89. Kaffe I, Naor H, Buchner A. Clinical and radiological features of odontogenic myxoma of the jaws. Dentomaxillofac Radiol 1997;26(5):299–303.

90. Jones BE, Sarathy AP, Ramos MB, et al. Squamous odontogenic tumor. Head Neck Pathol 2011;5(1): 17–9.

91. Ide F, Kikuchi K, Kusama K, et al. Primordial odontogenic tumour: is it truly novel? Histopathology 2015;66(4):603–4.

92. Slater LJ, Eftimie LF, Herford AS. Primordial odontogenic tumor: report of a case. J Oral Maxillofac Surg 2016;74(3):547–51.

93. Mosqueda-Taylor A, Pires FR, Aguirre-Urizar JM, et al. Primordial odontogenic tumour: clinicopathological analysis of six cases of a previously undescribed entity. Histopathology 2014;65(5):606–12.

94. Brunner P, Bihl M, Jundt G, et al. BRAF p.V600E mutations are not unique to ameloblastoma and are shared by other odontogenic tumors with ameloblastic morphology. Oral Oncol 2015;51(10): e77–8.

95. Hall JM, Weathers DR, Unni KK. Ameloblastic carcinoma: an analysis of 14 cases. Oral Surg Oral Med Oral Pathol Oral Radiol Endod 2007;103(6): 799–807.

96. Lei Y, Jaradat JM, Owosho A, et al. Evaluation of SOX2 as a potential marker for ameloblastic carcinoma. Oral Surg Oral Med Oral Pathol Oral Radiol 2014;117(5):608–16.e1.

97. Slootweg PJ, Muller H. Malignant ameloblastoma or ameloblastic carcinoma. Oral Surg Oral Med Oral Pathol 1984;57(2):168–76.

98. Altini M, Thompson SH, Lownie JF, et al. Ameloblastic sarcoma of the mandible. J Oral Maxillofac Surg 1985;43(10):789–94.

99. Reichart PA, Philipsen H. Ameloblastic Fibrosarcoma. In: Odontogenic tumors and allied lesions. London: Quintessence; 2004. p. 255–67.

100. Chomette G, Auriol M, Guilbert F, et al. Ameloblastic fibrosarcoma of the jaws–report of three cases. Clinico-pathologic, histoenzymological and ultrastructural study. Pathol Res Pract 1983;178(1):40–7.

101. Bilodeau EA, Hoschar AP, Barnes EL, et al. Clear cell carcinoma and clear cell odontogenic carcinoma: a comparative clinicopathologic and immunohistochemical study. Head Neck Pathol 2011; 5(2):101–7.

102. Ebert CS Jr, Dubin MG, Hart CF, et al. Clear cell odontogenic carcinoma: a comprehensive analysis of treatment strategies. Head Neck 2005;27(6): 536–42.

103. Kumar M, Fasanmade A, Barrett AW, et al. Metastasising clear cell odontogenic carcinoma: a case report and review of the literature. Oral Oncol 2003;39(2):190–4.

104. Piattelli A, Sesenna E, Trisi P. Clear cell odonto-genic carcinoma. Report of a case with lymph node and pulmonary metastases. Eur J Cancer B Oral Oncol 1994;30B(4):278–80.

105. de Aguiar MC, Gomez RS, Silva EC, et al. Clear-cell ameloblastoma (clear-cell odontogenic carcinoma): report of a case. Oral Surg Oral Med Oral Pathol Oral Radiol Endod 1996;81(1):79–83.

106. Chera BS, Villaret DB, Orlando CA, et al. Clear cell odontogenic carcinoma of the maxilla: a case report and literature review. Am J Otolaryngol 2008;29(4):284–90.

Distinctive Head and Neck Bone and Soft Tissue Neoplasms

Bibianna Purgina, MD, FRCPC[a],*, Chi K. Lai, MD, FRCPC[b]

KEYWORDS

- Chondrosarcoma • Chordoma • Osteosarcoma • Biphenotypic sinonasal sarcoma • Angiofibroma
- Glomangiopericytoma • Rhabdomyosarcoma

Key Points

- Pathologic features of the recently described biphenotypic sinonasal sarcoma (BSNS).
- Association of angiofibroma (AF) and familial adenomatous polyposis (FAP).
- Differentiate between skull base chondroid chordoma and chondrosarcoma.
- Unique features of gnathic osteosarcomas.
- Rhabdomyosarcoma (RMS) of the head and neck.
- Diagnosis of glomangiopericytoma (GPC).

ABSTRACT

Benign and malignant primary bone and soft tissue lesions of the head and neck are rare. The uncommon nature of these tumors, combined with the complex anatomy of the head and neck, pose diagnostic challenges to pathologists. This article describes the pertinent clinical, radiographic, and pathologic features of selected bone and soft tissue tumors involving the head and neck region, including angiofibroma, glomangiopericytoma, rhabdomyosarcoma, biphenotypic sinonasal sarcoma, chordoma, chondrosarcoma, and osteosarcoma. Emphasis is placed on key diagnostic pitfalls, differential diagnosis, and the importance of correlating clinical and radiographic information, particularly for tumors involving bone.

ANGIOFIBROMA

OVERVIEW

AF, also known as juvenile nasopharyngeal AF, is an uncommon benign vascular neoplasm of the head and neck, making up 0.05% of head and neck tumors and occurring almost exclusively in adolescent boys (9–19 years of age).[1] AF originates from a fibrovascular nidus in the posterolateral nasal cavity near the sphenopalatine foramen or pterygoid canal.[2] The blood supply of AFs typically arises from the ipsilateral internal maxillary artery, but any branch from the internal or external carotid artery is a possible feeder vessel.[1]

Symptoms include unilateral nasal obstruction; epistaxis, which can be massive; nasal discharge; and otitis media. Although pathologically benign, larger tumors may behave aggressively, bulging into the soft palate and extending into the maxillary and sphenoid sinuses, orbit, and medial cranial fossa, causing facial deformities, headaches, and proptosis.[1] Approximately 10% to 20% of AFs extend intracranially.[3,4]

Routine radiographs and CT and MRI scans reveal a soft tissue density in the nasopharynx. Angiography allows identification of the feeder vessel, which is crucial for selecting the appropriate surgical approach and reveals characteristic irregular, tortuous vessels and the tumor blush of

[a] Division of Anatomical Pathology, Department of Pathology and Laboratory Medicine, The Ottawa Hospital, University of Ottawa, 501 Smyth Road, 4th Floor CCW, Room 4250, Ottawa, Ontario K1H 8L6, Canada;
[b] Division of Anatomical Pathology, Department of Pathology and Laboratory Medicine, The Ottawa Hospital, University of Ottawa, 501 Smyth Road, 4th Floor CCW, Room 4114, Ottawa, Ontario K1H 8L6, Canada
* Corresponding author.
E-mail address: bpurgina@ottawahospital.on.ca

Surgical Pathology 10 (2017) 223–279
http://dx.doi.org/10.1016/j.path.2016.11.003
1875-9181/17/© 2016 Elsevier Inc. All rights reserved.

surgpath.theclinics.com

AF.[5] One of the more commonly adopted preoperative staging systems to determine extent of surgery is proposed by Radkowski and colleagues[6] (**Table 1**).

The pathogenesis of AF is unknown, and developmental, hormonal, and genetic causes have been proposed. The role of testosterone in tumor development and growth is suggested by its gender predilection, incidence during puberty, and possible regression after maturation.[7] Patients with FAP, an autosomal dominant disorder characterized by a germline mutation of the *APC* gene, are 25 times more likely to develop AFs.[8,9] Approximately 20% of patients with FAP do not have a family history and the diagnosis of AF may precede the diagnosis of FAP.[10]

PATHOLOGIC FEATURES

AFs vary in size depending on the extent of disease. The mean size is approximately 4 cm.[5] They have a polypoid shape with a rounded or bosselated contour. Cut sections demonstrate porous and focally hemorrhagic tissue.

Microscopically, AFs are unencapsulated lesions covered by nasopharyngeal mucosa that may be focally ulcerated. At low power, a prominent hemangiopericytoma (HPC)-like vascular pattern is appreciated (**Fig. 1**). The blood vessels have an irregular smooth muscle layer that may be focally attenuated or absent, and the endothelial layer is typically thin and lacks atypia. The dense fibrous stroma contains scattered plump, epithelioid, or stellate fibroblasts and coarse and

fine collagen fibers (see **Fig. 1**). Up to mild nuclear atypia may be occasionally present, but mitotic activity is low. Stromal mast cells are frequently identified.

In long-standing lesions, focal myxoid areas may be seen and the center of the tumor tends to be more collagenous with diminished vascularity. Embolization material in vessels and adjacent reactive changes are identified in resected specimens after embolization. Other degenerative features include multinucleated stromal cells.

Key Pathologic Features

- Unencapsulated, hypocellular submucosal lesion involving the nasopharynx
- Prominent HPC-like vascular pattern
- Blood vessels with irregular smooth muscle coats
- Dense fibrous stroma with scattered plump epithelioid or stellate fibroblasts and coarse and fine collagen fibers
- At most mild atypia but low mitotic activity
- Stromal mast cell frequently identified
- In long-standing lesions, the center of the tumor tends to be more collagenous with diminished vasculature.
- Other degenerative changes include focal myxoid change and multinucleated stromal cells.
- Embolization material in blood vessels

IMMUNOHISTOCHEMICAL AND MOLECULAR FEATURES

The stromal cells of AFs are positive for vimentin and negative for desmin and smooth muscle actin (SMA) (**Fig. 2**).[5] SMA may highlight occasional myofibroblasts, which are likely regressive in nature.[11] CD117 may be positive in both the stromal cells and the vascular endothelial cells.[12] AFs also frequently demonstrate nuclear β-catenin staining (see **Fig. 2**).[13]

Studies of sex hormone receptors have shown inconsistent results.[14,15] In general, AF demonstrates nuclear staining for AR and infrequently for estrogen receptor (ER) (see **Fig. 2**). ER-β, however, which is found in normal mesenchymal tissues, is often positive in AF, unlike ER-α.[15] CD34, CD31, FLI-1, and factor VIII–related antigen (FVIIIRAg) are positive in the vascular component

Table 1
Radkowski classification of angiofibromas

Stage	Extent
Ia	Limited to the nose and nasopharyngeal area
Ib	Extension into 1 or more sinuses
IIa	Minimal extension into pterygopalatine fossa
IIb	Occupation of the pterygopalatine fossa without orbital erosion
IIc	Infratemporal fossa extension without cheek or pterygoid plate involvement
IIIa	Erosion of the skull base (middle cranial fossa or pterygoids)
IIIb	Erosion of the skull base with intracranial extension with or without cavernous sinus involvement

From Radkowski D, McGill T, Healy GB, et al. Angiofibroma. Changes in staging and treatment. Arch Otolaryngol Head Neck Surg 1996;122(2):122–9.

Fig. 1. AF. (*A*) Low-power view demonstrates an un-encapsulated, hypocellular lesion, covered by nasopharyngeal mucosa, with a prominent HPC-like vascular pattern. (H&E, ×40) (*B*) Many of the ectatic, irregular vessels have an irregular smooth muscle coat, that may be focally attenuated or absent. The endothelial layer is thin and lacks atypia. (H&E, ×40) (*C*) Embolization material identified within a vessel. (H&E, ×100).

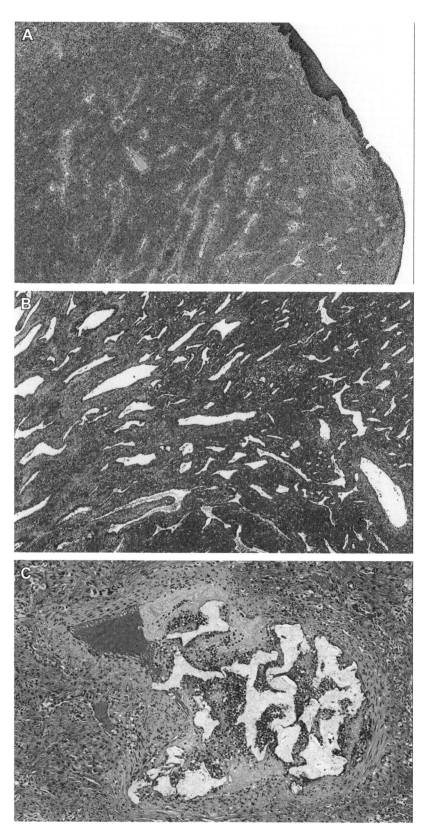

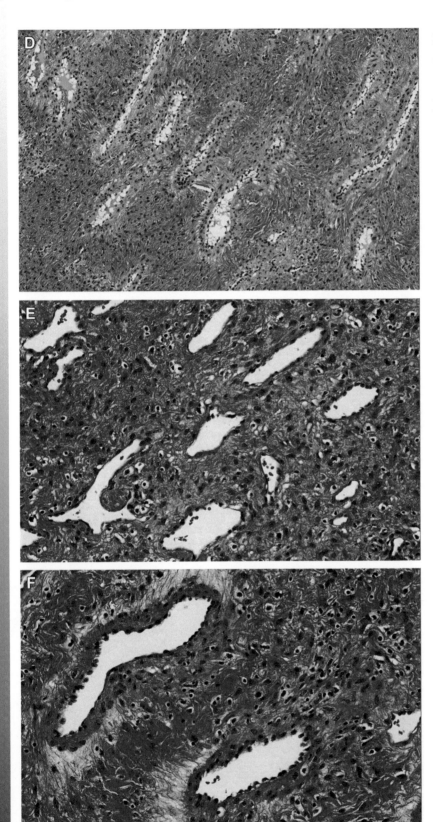

Fig. 1. (*continued*). (*D–G*) The fibrous stroma of AF contains scattered epithelioid or stellate fibroblasts, with at most mild atypia, and coarse and fine collagen fibers. (*D*) (H&E, ×100) (*E*) (H&E, ×200) (*F*) (H&E, ×200).

Fig. 1. (continued). (*G*) Stromal mast cells are identified. (H&E, ×400).

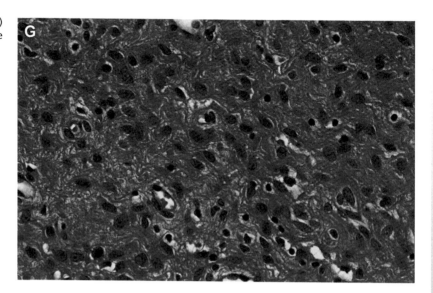

of AF. CD34 may additionally demonstrate weak stromal cell staining.[16] AFs are negative for podoplanin (D2-40) and glucose transporter 1.[16]

Most AFs are sporadic and harbor activating β-catenin gene (*CTNNB1*) mutations in up to 75% of cases.[13] Even though some patients with FAP develop AF, genetic evidence of an *APC* gene mutation is documented in only 1 case of AF in an affected FAP carrier.[9]

DIFFERENTIAL DIAGNOSIS

The differential diagnosis of AF includes fibrosed sinonasal polyp (SNP), lobular capillary hemangiomas (LCHs), fibromatosis, solitary fibrous tumor (SFT), and GPC (also known as sinonasal HPC).[5] Typical SNPs have edematous, paucicellular stroma with delicate, dilated capillaries and scattered inflammatory cells. Fibrosed SNPs, which tend to have increased fine stromal collagen with scattered stromal spindle cells, can mimic an AF. The histologic distinction between AF and SNP is summarized in **Table 2**.

An LCH (also known as pyogenic granuloma) enters the differential diagnosis if there are abundant degenerative changes. Unlike AF, resolving LCH retains its lobular proliferation of small capillaries with a central feeder vessel. This feature of LCH is best appreciated at low magnification.

Fibromatosis, which can occur in the head and neck, is a hypocellular proliferation of bland spindle cells in a collagenous stroma demonstrating frequent nuclear β-catenin staining and, thus, is included in the differential diagnosis. The spindle cells of fibromatosis have a fascicular growth pattern with elongated nuclei containing small, punctate nucleoli. Although focal ectatic vessels may be seen, the vascularity in fibromatosis is not a dominant feature distinguishing it from AF.

Due to the prominent HPC-like vascular pattern, GPC and SFT involving the sinonasal cavity are both considered in the differential diagnosis. SFT is a proliferation of fibroblast-like cells arranged in a patternless pattern with thick bands of collagen and prominent branching vessels. Cracking in the thick collagen and between tumor cells is a useful histologic feature. Clinically, SFTs occur in older patients with a median age of 50 years. Classically, SFTs are positive for CD34, B-cell lymphoma 2 (Bcl-2), and CD99. Recent studies have demonstrated that nearly all SFTs harbor an *NAB2-STAT6* gene fusion and, subsequently, STAT6 immunohistochemistry has been shown specific for SFTs.[17,18] GPCs tend to have a more cellular stroma with a perivascular myoid phenotype expressing SMA, muscle-specific actin (MSA), and factor XIIIA. Although GPCs demonstrate nuclear staining with β-catenin, the uniform ovoid cell morphology, perivascular hyalinization, and diffuse muscle marker reactivity distinguish it from AF.

△△ *Differential Diagnosis*

- Fibrosed SNP
- LCH (also known as pyogenic granuloma)
- Fibromatosis
- SFT
- GPC

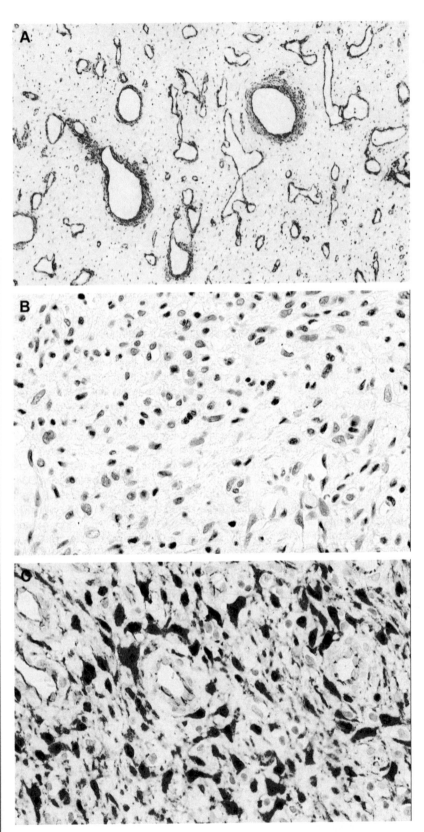

Fig. 2. AF. (*A*) SMA highlights the smooth muscle of vessel walls but is typically negative in the stromal cells of AF. (H&E, ×100) (*B*) AF with focal nuclear expression of androgen receptor. (H&E, ×400) (*C*) AFs can also demonstrate strong nuclear β-catenin staining. (H&E, ×400).

Table 2
Comparison of histologic features of angiofibromas and fibrosed sinonasal polyps

Feature	Angiofibromas	Fibrosed Sinonasal Polyps
Surface epithelium	Absent (ulcerated) or on 1 side	On 3 sides
Inflammation	Not prominent	Prominent eosinophils
Basement membrane	Normal	Hyalinized
Mucoserous glands	Absent	Present
Stromal collagen	Fine and coarse	Fine
Stromal cells	Plump-stellate	Elongated

TREATMENT AND PROGNOSIS

Due to the classic clinical and radiographic features, preoperative biopsy of AF is not recommended due to the significant risk of bleeding. Typically, patients undergo preoperative embolization to reduce intraoperative blood loss[1] followed by surgical resection, by endoscopic, open, or combined approaches depending on Radkowski stage. Radiotherapy is generally avoided due to the adjacent critical structures, the risk of malignant transformation, and the development of radiation-induced neoplasms in later decades.[1,19]

The recurrence rate of AF is approximately 25%, most commonly in those with intracranial extension, and usually occurs within the first year after surgery.[5] Death from disease is exceedingly uncommon and usually in larger tumors with intracranial involvement secondary to exsanguination or infections, such as meningitis and pneumonia.[5] Sarcomatous transformation of AF has been reported in 5 patients, 4 of which developed after radiotherapy.[19,20]

Key Points

- Preoperative biopsy of AF is not recommended due to the risk of massive bleeding.

- Low-stage AFs are resected endoscopically.

- Recurrence rate is approximately 25%, more frequently seen in tumor with intracranial extension.

- FAP should be considered in patients with newly diagnosed AF:

  ○ Approximately 20% of patients with FAP have no family history of the syndrome.

  ○ AF may precede the diagnosis of FAP.

GLOMANGIOPERICYTOMA

OVERVIEW

GPC (also known as sinonasal-type HPC) is an uncommon, indolent tumor that exhibits a perivascular myoid phenotype and occurs almost exclusively in the sinonasal tract, where it accounts for less than 0.5% of all neoplasms.[21] GPC can affect patients of all ages, ranging from in utero to 86 years, with a peak incidence in the 7th decade.[21–23] There is a slight female-to-male predominance of 1.2 to 1.5.[22,23]

The most common site of occurrence is the nasal cavity by itself (45%) followed by the nasal cavity with associated paranasal sinus involvement (25%).[23] Only a minor proportion of cases involve the paranasal sinuses alone. Furthermore, most tumors are unilateral with an equal distribution between the right and left sides.

CLINICAL FEATURES

Clinically, most patients present nonspecifically, with nasal obstruction and/or epistaxis and associated symptoms.[22–25] Symptom duration may be long, with an average of 10 months (range of 1 month to 5 years). Rarely, oncogenic (tumor-induced) osteomalacia has been reported in association with GPC.[24,26]

Endoscopically, GPC shows a red to gray-tan, obstructive, polypoid mass lesion located high in the nasal cavity that has a propensity to bleed profusely when biopsied or manipulated.[22,24] Radiographic studies commonly demonstrate a polypoid mass lesion that opacifies the nasal cavity or paranasal sinus, often associated with sinusitis, bone erosion, and sclerosis.[23] The mass lesion may be obscured by the sinusitis, thus potentially delaying diagnosis.

PATHOLOGIC FEATURES

Intact GPC specimens show polypoid tumors, which measure between 0.8 cm and 8.0 cm (mean 3.1 cm).[23] The mucosal surfaces are generally intact without evidence of ulceration. Cut surfaces are solid to spongelike, soft to rubbery, maroon red to gray-tan, and fleshy to friable, with edematous and/or hemorrhagic areas.[22,23]

Microscopically, GPC consists of a nonencapsulated, well-demarcated, submucosal, ovoid to spindle, cellular proliferation that effaces the normal submucosal constituents or surrounds the residual minor salivary glands (**Fig. 3**).[22–25] The overlying respiratory epithelium is usually intact but it may occasionally exhibit traumatic erosion/ulceration or squamous metaplasia. A tumor-free zone akin to the grenz zone of the skin is often present between the subepithelial basement membrane and the tumor. At low power, a complex, ramifying, and highly vascular network can be observed that separates the tumor cells. The vascular channels are highly variable in size ranging from small, capillary-sized vessels to large, thin-walled, and patulous vessels, with some exhibiting a staghorn configuration. Characteristically, prominent perivascular hyalinization is present in the small vessels in most cases.

The uniform, ovoid to spindled tumor cells are typically closely packed with indistinct cell borders producing a syncytial appearance.[22–24] They may be arranged in a variety of architectural patterns, including diffuse/sheetlike, short fascicular, storiform, whorled, meningothelial-like, reticular, or palisaded. A mixed pattern is commonly seen. The nuclei are round, oval to spindle-shaped with smooth nuclear contours, evenly distributed and pale chromatin, and 1 or more small inconspicuous nucleoli. The cytoplasm ranges from clear to lightly eosinophilic. Mild nuclear pleomorphism and rare mitoses may be seen, but no tumor necrosis or atypical mitoses are identified. In addition, extravasated red blood cells, mast cells, and eosinophils are virtually always present. Scattered tumor giant cells formed from aggregation of tumor cells, which likely represent a degenerative phenomenon, may be identified in occasional cases. Typically, there is little intervening stroma between the tumor cells; however, a small proportion of cases may focally exhibit fibrosis or myxoid change.

IMMUNOHISTOCHEMISTRY AND MOLECULAR FINDINGS

Most cases demonstrate immunoreactivity for vimentin and muscle markers compatible with a perivascular myoid phenotype.[23,25] In addition, factor XIIIA is frequently expressed by these tumors.[23,24] Focal and weak positivity for CD34 is identified in a small proportion of tumors. Laminin highlights pericellular basal laminar material surrounding individual cells. Other immunohistochemical markers, including S100, CD31, FVIIIRAg, CD117, Bcl-2, cytokeratin (CK), epithelial membrane antigen (EMA), desmin, glial fibrillary acidic protein (GFAP), CD68, CD99, and neuron-specific enolase (NSE), are usually negative in these tumors.[23] STAT6, a specific immunohistochemical marker of SFTs, has been reported negative in most tumors.[17,25]

Using whole-genome sequencing combined with RNA sequencing, Haller and colleagues[27] found recurrent missense mutations in exon 3 of the *CTTNB1* gene (clustering at positions 33–45) in all 6 GPC cases analyzed. These mutations resulted in amino acid substitutions in the amino-terminal region of β-catenin, which corresponds to the recognition site of the β-catenin destruction complex, preventing β-catenin phosphorylation and proteasomal degradation and leading to nuclear accumulation of β-catenin as demonstrated by diffuse and strong nuclear β-catenin immunoreactivity (see **Fig. 3**).

Key Pathologic Features

- Nonencapsulated, well-demarcated, submucosal, ovoid to spindle, cellular proliferation that effaces or surrounds normal submucosal constituents

- Overlying respiratory epithelium usually intact, but occasionally exhibits traumatic erosion/ulceration or squamous metaplasia

- Prominent HPC-like vascular pattern with perivascular hyalinization of smaller vessels present in most cases

- Uniform, tightly packed, ovoid to spindle cells with clear to lightly eosinophilic cytoplasm and indistinct cell borders arranged in diffuse/sheetlike, short fascicular, storiform, whorled, meningothelial-like, reticular, or palisaded patterns

- Mild nuclear pleomorphism and rare mitoses may be seen

- Little intervening stroma between tumor cells

- Extravasated red blood cells, mast cells, and eosinophils almost always present

- Multinucleated tumor cells occasionally present

Fig. 3. GPC. (*A*) Low-power magnification demonstrates nonencapsulated, well-demarcated, submucosal, cellular tumor with prominent HPC-like vascular pattern and an intact overlying epithelium exhibiting squamous metaplasia. Note the presence of a tumor-free zone between the subepithelial basement membrane and the tumor. (H&E, ×40) (*B*) A complex, ramifying, and highly vascular network separates syncytial clusters of tightly packed, ovoid to spindle tumor cells with indistinct cell borders and little intervening stroma. (H&E, ×100) (*C*) Prominent perivascular hyalinization of small vessels is identified in most cases. Note presence of focal myxoid change of the stroma. (H&E, ×200).

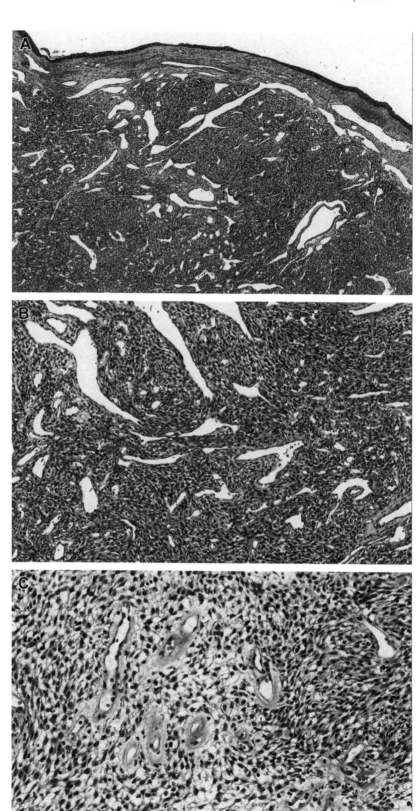

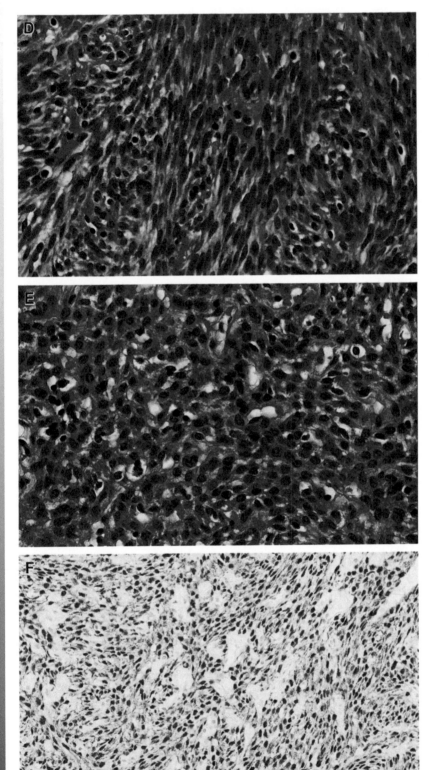

Fig. 3. (continued). (D) Short fascicular arrangement of ovoid to spindle tumor cells with lightly eosinophilic cytoplasm and bland nuclei exhibiting smooth nuclear contours, evenly distributed and pale chromatin, and 1 or more, small, inconspicuous nucleoli. (H&E, ×400) (E) Occasional tumors exhibit focal areas with a more round cell appearance resembling a glomus tumor. (H&E, ×400) (F) Nuclear immunoreactivity for β-catenin in tumors cells. Note the lack of nuclear staining in endothelial cells of adjacent blood vessels. (beta-catenin, ×200).

DIFFERENTIAL DIAGNOSIS

The differential diagnosis for GPC includes LCH, AF, SFT, leiomyoma, monophasic spindle cell synovial sarcoma, schwannoma, and meningioma. For the most part, these differential diagnostic considerations can be distinguished from GPC with selective use of a small panel of immunohistochemical stains in conjunction with the histologic and clinical findings. Although the HPC-like vascular pattern is characteristic of GPC, it is not a specific feature because it can be seen in a wide variety of other benign and malignant tumors.

LCH (also known as pyogenic granuloma) is more frequently seen in the sinonasal tract than GPC. Unlike the latter, it consists of a lobular proliferation of small, slitlike vascular channels often with identifiable larger central feeder vessels embedded within a myxohyaline stroma containing scattered inflammatory cells. Surface erosion is often present. The small vessels are lined by plump endothelial cells, which stain for vascular markers (CD31, CD34, FVIIIRAg, ERG, and FLI-1), and are surrounded by SMA-positive pericytic cells. Perivascular hyalinization is not seen. Unlike GPC, mitotic figures are frequently seen, but none is atypical.

AF arises in the posterolateral nasal wall with extension into the nasopharynx of mostly adolescent boys. The differential diagnosis is discussed previously.

SFT uncommonly involves the sinonasal tract and consists of a patternless pattern of variably cellular, bland, haphazard, spindle cell proliferation with associated ropey keloidal collagen bundles and HPC-like vasculature. The vessels of this tumor typically do not exhibit perivascular hyalinization. In contrast to GPC, SFT typically expresses CD34, STAT6, Bcl-2, and CD99 with inconsistent immunoreactivity for SMA (often negative).

Leiomyoma and leiomyosarcoma are rare tumors in the sinonasal tract consisting of a bland cellular spindle proliferation with a fascicular growth pattern characterized by long sweeping fascicles. In comparison to GPC, the neoplastic cells have more elongated, blunt-ended, and cigar-shaped nuclei with perinuclear vacuoles and a coarser chromatin pattern. They also possess more abundant fibrillary eosinophilic cytoplasm. Immunohistochemically, the tumor cells are positive for desmin and h-caldesmon in addition to actins (SMA and MSA).

Monophasic spindle cell synovial sarcoma is characterized by fairly uniform, small spindle cells having scant cytoplasm and bland, ovoid, hyperchromatic nuclei with inconspicuous nucleoli. The tumor cells are arranged in tightly packed sheets or vague fascicles and often exhibit alternating areas of hypercellularity and hypocellularity. An HPC-like vascular pattern is often present at least focally. A variable amount of wiry collagen and stromal calcification can be seen. Mitoses and necrosis are not frequently identified in tumors that are not poorly differentiated. Immunophenotypically, these tumors focally express EMA and CKs (more commonly CKs 7, 8, 18, and 19) as well as TLE-1, CD99, CD56, and Bcl-2. Other markers inconsistently expressed include calretinin, nuclear β-catenin, S100, and FLI-1. Tumor cells are usually not immunoreactive with CD34, SMA, and MSA.

Schwannomas show more elongated wavy nuclei in keeping with nerve sheath origin and may show microcystic change more frequently and demonstrate Verocay bodies. They are diffusely positive for S100 and SOX10 and negative for actins.

Sinonasal tract meningioma may overlap with whorled pattern predominant GPC. These are usually positive for EMA and vimentin, however, but negative for CKs, S100, SMA, CD34, STAT6, and nuclear β-catenin. Progesterone receptor (PR) and ER may be expressed. Additionally, they demonstrate psammoma bodies more frequently and do not show the perivascular hyalinization typical of GPC.

Pitfalls

! Although the HPC-like vascular pattern is characteristic of GPC, it is a nonspecific histologic feature and can be seen in many other benign and malignant tumors.

! GPCs may exhibit only focal and weak immunoreactivity for SMA.

! Focal and weak CD34 staining can be seen in GPCs, potentially causing diagnostic confusion with SFTs.

! In addition to GPCs, other sinonasal tract tumors may exhibit nuclear β-catenin, including AFs, SFTs, and synovial sarcomas.

TREATMENT AND PROGNOSIS

The mainstay of therapy for GPC is wide surgical excision with adequate surgical margins to achieve local control and prevent future recurrences.[22–24] Due to the vascular nature of this tumor, preoperative angiographic embolization is often performed to diminish intraoperative blood loss. Radiotherapy may be used for incompletely resected or unresectable tumors.

The clinical behavior of GPC is typically indolent, with a more than 90% 5-year survival rate after complete surgical resection.[21] The recurrence rate has been reported to be as high as 40%.[23,24,28] Most local recurrences are due to incomplete removal. Aggressive-behaving (malignant) GPCs, including those with metastases, have rarely been reported.[21] Such tumors may exhibit a large size (>5 cm) bone invasion, profound nuclear pleomorphism, increased mitotic activity (>4/10 high-power fields [HPFs]),

necrosis, and a Ki-67 proliferation index of greater than 10%.

RHABDOMYOSARCOMA

OVERVIEW

RMS is a malignant mesenchymal neoplasm that exhibits a skeletal muscle phenotype. It accounts for 3.9% of all soft tissue sarcomas.[29] Although it represents the most common type of soft tissue sarcoma seen in children and adolescents comprising 40.2% of all pediatric soft tissue sarcomas, it is an uncommon type in adults, comprising only 1.7% of all adult soft tissue sarcomas. There is a slight male predominance and a predilection for white patients.[30] In pediatric RMS, the head and neck region represents the most common primary site, comprising 34.9% of cases. The most frequent sites are the orbit, nasopharynx, nasal cavity, and maxillary sinus (Table 3).[31]

There are 4 histologic subtypes of malignant skeletal muscle tumors: embryonal (including botryoid and anaplastic variants) RMS (ERMS), alveolar (including solid variant) RMS (ARMS), pleomorphic RMS (PRMS), and spindle cell/sclerosing RMS (SCSRMS).[32–35] Most head and neck RMS cases seem sporadic in origin; however, a small subset of cases have been associated with various genetic syndromes caused by germline mutations.[36] Most are of the embryonal subtype; however, those with an alveolar morphology have been reported to a lesser extent, typically without the *PAX-FOXO1* translocations.

The embryonal and alveolar subtypes comprise 54.7% and 24.0% of head and neck RMSs,

Table 3
Distribution of 558 head and neck rhabdomyosarcomas by primary site

Primary Site	Number	Percentage
Orbit	143	25.6
Nasopharynx	84	15.1
Nasal cavity	59	10.6
Maxillary sinus	59	10.6
Other sinuses	48	8.6
Ethmoid sinus	35	6.3
Middle ear	22	3.9
Tongue[a]	21	3.8
Palate[a]	17	3.0
Parotid gland[a]	17	3.0

[a] Nonorbital/nonparameningeal sites.

From Turner JH, Richmon JD. Head and neck rhabdomyosarcoma: a critical analysis of population-based incidence and survival data. Otolaryngol Head Neck Surg 2011;145(6):967–73.

respectively.[31] The botryoid variant of ERMS involves the head and neck region in 15% of cases,[37] typically of mucosal sites, such as the nasal cavity, nasopharynx, auditory canal, and conjunctiva. ARMS in the head and neck region preferentially involves the nose and paranasal sinuses. In adults, the spindle cell subtype most commonly involves the deep soft tissues of the head and neck, accounting for greater than 50% of cases.[33,38–41] PRMS typically involves the extremities and is not frequently seen in the head and neck region.[42,43]

Clinical manifestations of head and neck RMSs depend on the site of occurrence and tumor-related mass effect, obstruction, and destructive growth at the involved site.[44] Orbital RMSs most commonly present with unilateral proptosis, eyelid swelling, and blepharoptosis. For nasal tumors, patients can present with nasal obstruction, pain, facial swelling, proptosis, numbness, and serous otitis. For paranasal sinus tumors, sinusitis, headache, toothache, and visual problems are more frequently encountered. The botryoid variant of ERMS may mimic a nasal polyp or an aural polyp if involving ear canal.

PATHOLOGIC FEATURES

Macroscopically, ERMSs are poorly circumscribed with infiltrative margins and fleshy, tan to white, hemorrhagic, or necrotic masses. The botryoid variant typically forms an exophytic mass with a bunch of grapes–like or polypoid appearance. The cut surface has a gelatinous appearance. ARMSs exhibit infiltrative, fleshy, tan-grey, hemorrhagic, or necrotic masses with a variable amount of fibrous tissue. SCSRMSs form firm, fibrous, grey-white masses with a whorled cut surface. Necrosis or hemorrhage may be seen. PRMSs develop masses that appear seemingly well circumscribed, large, white to tan, and fleshy with often extensively necrotic and variably hemorrhagic areas. The recently described epithelioid RMSs have nodular, fleshy, and necrotic cut surfaces with poorly circumscribed and infiltrative margins.

Histologically, the conventional variant of ERMS exhibits primitive mesenchymal cells that recapitulate various stages of embryonic myogenesis (**Fig. 4**). Effectively the morphology ranges from small ovoid to spindled undifferentiated cells to mature fetal-type rhabdomyoblasts with cross-striations (two-thirds of cases) and eosinophilic cytoplasm. Multinucleated giant wreath cells are rarely seen. Stroma is myxoid rather than sclerotic. The botryoid variant of ERMS (see **Fig. 4**) characteristically grows in a polypoid fashion at mucosal surfaces to produce a grapelike appearance, although this is not a requisite.[45] Only the presence of a cambium layer is required to diagnose this variant, which consists of a variably thick, linear condensation of primitive undifferentiated tumor cells immediately subjacent to the surface epithelium separated by a zone of loose stroma. The anaplastic variant exhibits markedly atypical tumor cells with large, lobated, hyperchromatic nuclei that are at least 3 times the size of neighboring nuclei.[46] Bizarre, multipolar atypical mitotic figures are commonly present. Anaplasia can be quantified as focal (anaplastic cells loosely scattered among nonanaplastic cells) or diffuse (anaplastic cells aggregating in clusters or forming continuous sheets).

Both the classic and solid variants of ARMS (**Fig. 5**) consist predominantly of small-to-medium, primitive round tumor cells with round-to-oval nuclei and sparse cytoplasm. The nuclei are hyperchromatic and uniform with inconspicuous nucleoli. As the name suggests, cell dyshesion within tumor nests is characteristic, but solid ARMS may not show this. Variable rhabdomyoblastic differentiation is noted, but strap cells with cross-striations are rare. Multinucleated giant wreath cells with peripherally oriented nuclei and eosinophilic cytoplasm are also characteristic of ARMS. Clear cell change is common in the head and neck, although rare overall, as is anaplasia.

Most PRMSs histologically resemble an undifferentiated pleomorphic sarcoma. The tumor cells have diverse morphologic appearances that range from markedly atypical spindled to large polygonal to undifferentiated round cells with severely pleomorphic, vesicular to hyperchromatic nuclei and abundant, deeply eosinophilic cytoplasm (**Fig. 6**).

Spindle cell RMS exhibits a predominant population (>50%) of elongated, thin, spindled tumor cells embedded within a variable collagenous matrix (**Fig. 7**). The tumor cells have centrally located, cigar-shaped, vesicular nuclei, with variably prominent nucleoli and amphophilic to eosinophilic, fibrillar cytoplasm with prominent cell borders. Few scattered spindled to polygonal rhabdomyoblasts with occasional cross-striations may be observed. Mitotic figures, including atypical forms, are usually apparent. Round cell or pleomorphic areas are not typically present. Sclerosing RMS overlaps with spindle cell RMS but the tumor cells are separated into lobules and cords embedded in a densely hyalinizing stroma reminiscent of osteoid (see **Fig. 7**). Tumor cells are typically dyshesive, imparting a pseudovascular pattern. Mixed SCSRMSs are described.[33,38]

Key Pathologic Features

Rhabdomyo-sarcoma Subtype	Gross	Microscopic	Immunohistochemistry	Genetics/Molecular
ERMS	Poorly circumscribed, fleshy, tan-white	Undifferentiated round, stellate, and spindle cells forming loose fascicles and nondescript sheets with variable cellularity and myxoid stroma; variable number of rhabdomyoblasts in different stages of differentiation	Positive for desmin; variable expression for MYOD1 and myogenin (usually less diffuse and intense than ARMS)	Complex structural and numeric chromosomal abnormalities; trisomy 8 common; loss of heterozygosity at 11p15.5; genomic amplification infrequent except anaplastic variant; somatic mutations in key signaling pathways
Botryoid variant	Bunch of grapes–like, polypoid appearance	Linear condensation of undifferentiated cells immediately subjacent to surface epithelium separated by a zone of loose stroma (cambium layer) overlying conventional ERMS	—	—
Anaplastic variant	—	Multifocal/diffuse, markedly atypical cells with large, lobated, hyperchromatic nuclei, often with bizarre atypical mitoses	—	—
ARMS	Fleshy, tan-grey, hemorrhagic/necrotic with variable fibrous tissue	Small-to-medium, primitive round cells; variable rhabdomyoblastic differentiation (strap cells rarely seen); scattered wreath cells; fibrovascular septa separate variably sized nests, which exhibit central discohesion forming pseudoalveolar spaces	Positive for desmin; diffuse and strong myogenin expression (often much stronger than MYOD1); PAX5 positivity seen only in ARMS (not ERMS)	t(2;13) (q35;q14) (PAX3-FOXO1) in 54%–76% and t(1;13) (p36;q14) (PAX7-FOXO1) in 8%–24% of cases; genomic amplification common in fusion-positive cases, whereas somatic mutations infrequent
Solid variant	—	Sheets of tightly packed cells without fibrovascular septa or central discohesion	—	More likely to be fusion-negative
PRMS	Deceptively well-circumscribed, large, extensively necrotic and hemorrhagic	Spindle, large polygonal, or undifferentiated round cells with markedly pleomorphic nuclei and abundant eosinophilic cytoplasm arranged in haphazard, fascicular, or storiform patterns; cross-striations rarely seen; no alveolar or embryonal histology	Positive for desmin and/or MYOD1/myogenin	No characteristic cytogenetic abnormality; highly complex karyotype with numerous numeric and unbalanced structural chromosomal abnormalities
SCSRMS	Firm, fibrous, gray-white with whorled cut surface	Spindle cell morphology: elongated, thin, spindle cells within variable collagenous matrix with centrally located, cigar-shaped nuclei arranged in fascicular pattern; few scattered rhabdomyoblasts; round cell or pleomorphic areas not present Sclerosing morphology: primitive, round to spindle cells separated into lobules, small nests, microalveoli, cords, trabeculae, and linear arrays by eosinophilic-to-basophilic, hyalinizing fibrous stroma that mimics osteoid or chondroid matrix; rare, scattered rhabdomyoblasts	Strong positivity for MYOD1 with absent to focal myogenin expression; desmin positivity often focal (may exhibit dotlike pattern)	Aneuploidy with numeric abnormalities and nonrecurrent structural rearrangements; PAX3-FOXO1 and PAX7-FOXO1 gene fusions not identified; NCOA2 or VGLL2 gene rearrangements in congenital/infantile SCSRMS; MYOD1 p.L122R mutations, some with coexisting PIK3CA mutations

Fig. 4. ERMS. (*A*) Primitive undifferentiated cellular component arranged in nondescript sheet within a myxoid stroma containing little collagen. (H&E, ×200) (*B*) An area with denser cellularity and less myxoid stroma. (H&E, ×200) (*C*) Round, spindle, and stellate primitive undifferentiated tumor cells with central, ovoid to spindle, mildly pleomorphic, hyperchromatic nuclei and scant amphophilic cytoplasm. The nuclei contain smooth, dense chromatin with small and inconspicuous nucleoli. (H&E, ×400).

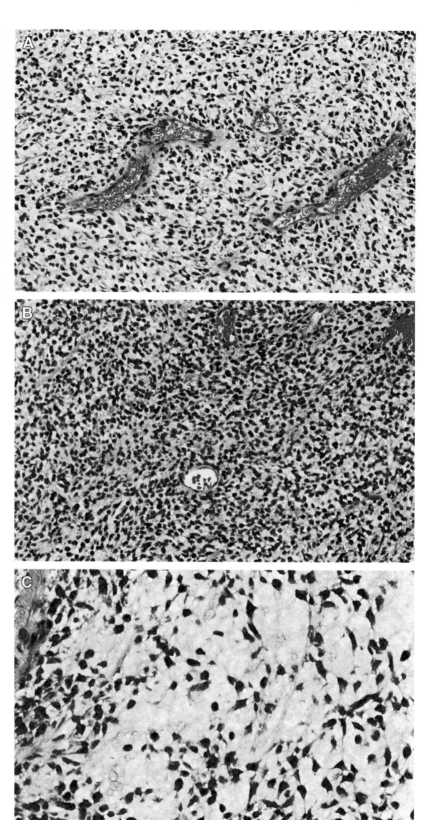

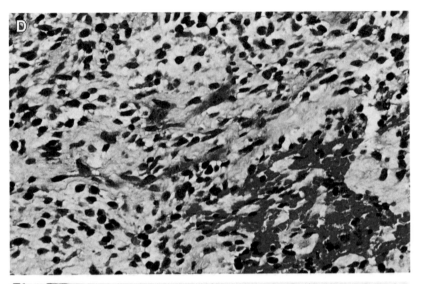

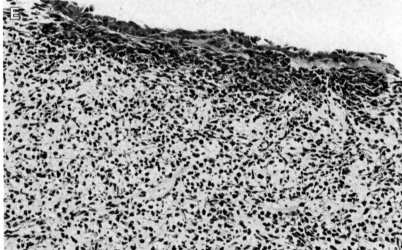

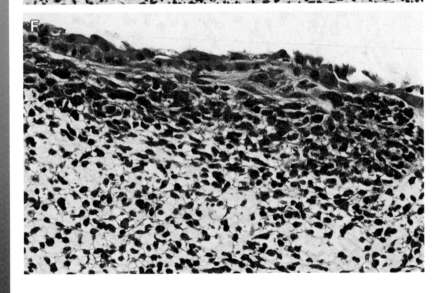

Fig. 4. (continued). (D) Terminally differentiated rhabdomyoblasts exhibiting intensely cytoplasmic eosinophilia with cross-striations and peripherally located nuclei. (H&E, ×400) (E, F) The botryoid variant of ERMS with characteristic cambium layer, which consists of a variably thick, linear condensation of primitive undifferentiated tumor cells immediately subjacent to the surface epithelium separated by a zone of loose stroma. The rest of the tumor below the cambium layer appears histologic identical to the conventional variant of ERMS. (E) (H&E, ×200) (F) (H&E, ×400).

Fig. 5. ARMS. (*A*) The classic variant consisting of variably sized nests of tumor cells separated by highly vascularized fibrous septa. There is central discohesion and peripherally situated tumor cells lining the fibrovascular septa imparting a pseudoalveolar pattern. (H&E, ×100) (*B*) Classic variant comprised of predominantly small-to-medium, primitive round tumor cells with round-to-oval nuclei and sparse cytoplasm. The nuclei are hyperchromatic and relatively uniform with inconspicuous nucleoli. (H&E, ×400) (*C*) The discohesive tumor cells within the central portions of the nests are free-floating and appear degenerated. The peripherally lining tumor cells attached to the fibrovascular septa appear better preserved. Note the round to oval rhabdomyoblasts with more abundant eosinophilic fibrillary cytoplasm with eccentrically placed nuclei. (H&E, ×400).

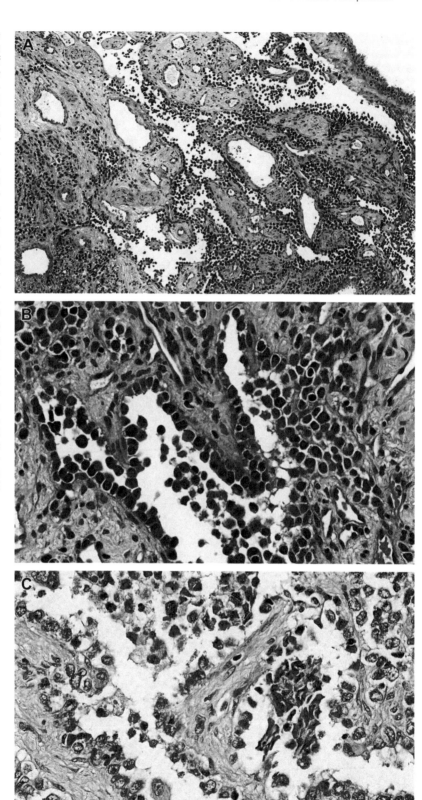

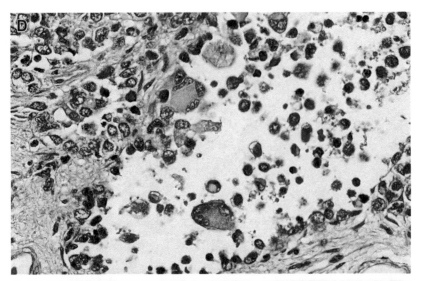

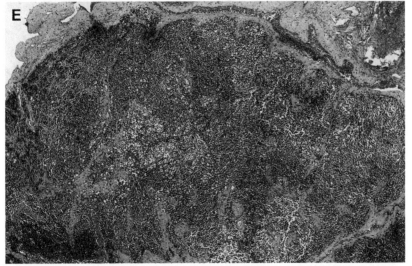

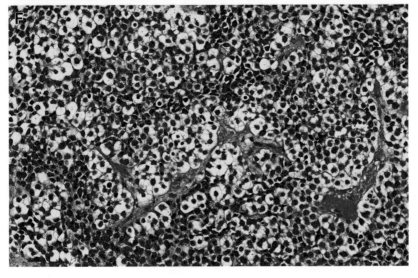

Fig. 5. (continued). (*D*) Scattered multinucleated giant wreath cells with peripherally oriented nuclei and eosinophilic cytoplasm are characteristic of the ARMS. (H&E, ×400) (*E*) Solid variant forms tightly packed sheets of tumor cells without fibrovascular septa and central discohesion. Focally, fibrovascular septa and incipient central discohesion is observed. The cellular morphology is similar to the classic variant of ARMS. (H&E, ×40) (*F*) Occasionally, clear tumor cells exhibiting abundant glycogen-rich cytoplasmic contents. (H&E, ×200).

Fig. 6. PRMS. (*A*) Markedly atypical, spindle, cellular proliferation arranged in intersecting fascicles. (H&E, ×100) (*B*) Focal areas of large polygonal to undifferentiated round cells are present in a more haphazard pattern. (H&E, ×100).

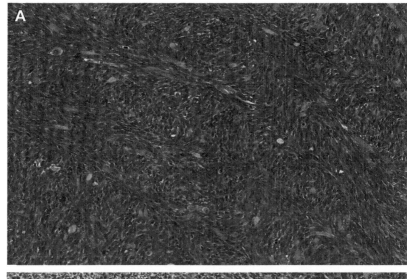

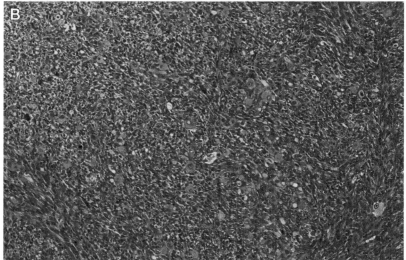

IMMUNOHISTOCHEMICAL AND MOLECULAR FEATURES

RMS can express a variety of skeletal muscle antigens, such as desmin, MSA, myoglobin, myogenin, and MyoD1. Myogenin and MyoD1 are myogenic transcriptional regulatory proteins whose expression determines commitment and differentiation of primitive mesenchymal cells into skeletal muscle and are expressed early on in skeletal muscle differentiation. Desmin, MSA, and myoglobin are typically expressed later in more differentiated rhabdomyoblasts.[43,47–49] ERMS typically exhibits variable expression for MyoD1 and myogenin in contrast to the diffuse and strong nuclear staining of ARMS, which can help

distinguish between these 2 RMS types.[47] Sclerosing RMS frequently exhibits strong positivity for MyoD1 with absent to focal myogenin expression. Desmin immunoreactivity is often focal and may exhibit a dotlike pattern.[33,38]

ERMS demonstrate numerous copy number alterations,[50] although gain of chromosome 8 seems particularly common, occurring in up to 74% of cases.[51]

Most ARMSs exhibit a characteristic t(2;13) (q35;q14) (*PAX3-FOXO1*) and t(1;13) (p36;q14) (*PAX7-FOXO1*), in 55% and 22% of cases, respectively.[52] The remaining cases lack either of these gene fusions and are considered to be fusion-negative. Only few cytogenetic studies of PRMSs exist in the literature, which reveal that such

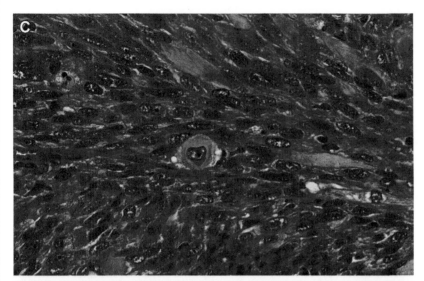

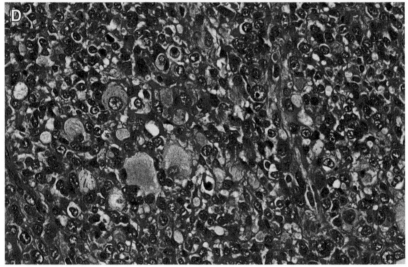

Fig. 6. (*continued*). (*C, D*) At higher magnification, the tumors cells have severely pleomorphic, vesicular to hyperchromatic nuclei with prominent nucleoli and abundant, deeply eosinophilic cytoplasm. Large, pleomorphic rhabdomyoblasts with various shapes are seen. No cross-striations are identified. (H&E, ×400).

tumors exhibit highly complex karyotypes with numerous numeric and unbalanced structural abnormalities.[32,53] SCSRMS shows novel findings. A subset of pediatric spindle cell RMS shows *NCOA2* gene rearrangements.[54] A significant proportion of spindled and sclerosis RMS, however, demonstrate homozygous c.365 T>G, p.L122R mutations in the *MYOD1* gene, in both adults and children.[55] Sclerosing RMS may demonstrate *PIK3CA* mutations.

DIFFERENTIAL DIAGNOSIS

The differential diagnosis of RMS depends primarily on the histologic subtype. Cellular ERMS and ARMS may overlap with small round blue cell tumors, including sinonasal undifferentiated carcinoma, small cell undifferentiated neuroendocrine carcinoma, undifferentiated type of non-keratinizing nasopharyngeal carcinoma, NUT midline carcinoma, Ewing sarcoma/primitive neuroectodermal tumor, olfactory neuroblastoma, ectopic pituitary adenoma, malignant melanoma, melanotic neuroectodermal tumor of infancy, granulocytic sarcoma, non-Hodgkin lymphoma (NHL), poorly differentiated synovial sarcoma, small cell osteosarcoma, mesenchymal chondrosarcoma, and extrarenal rhabdoid tumor. For the most part, positive staining for desmin, myogenin, and MyoD1 can distinguish ERMSs and ARMSs from other small round blue cell tumors. RMS may show aberrant CK expression and CD56, which may be diagnostic pitfalls.

Fig. 7. SCSRMS. (*A*) Spindle cell component consisting of a spindle cell proliferation arranged in a fascicular pattern with little intervening collagenous stroma. (H&E, ×200) (*B*) The tumor cells have centrally located, cigar-shaped, vesicular nuclei with variably prominent nucleoli and amphophilic to eosinophilic, fibrillar cytoplasm with prominent cell borders. (H&E, ×400) (*C*) Sclerosing component consisting of tumor cells separated by eosinophilic, hyalinizing fibrous stroma mimicking the appearance of lacelike osteoid matrix of osteosarcoma. Note, however, the lack of matrix calcification. (H&E, ×200).

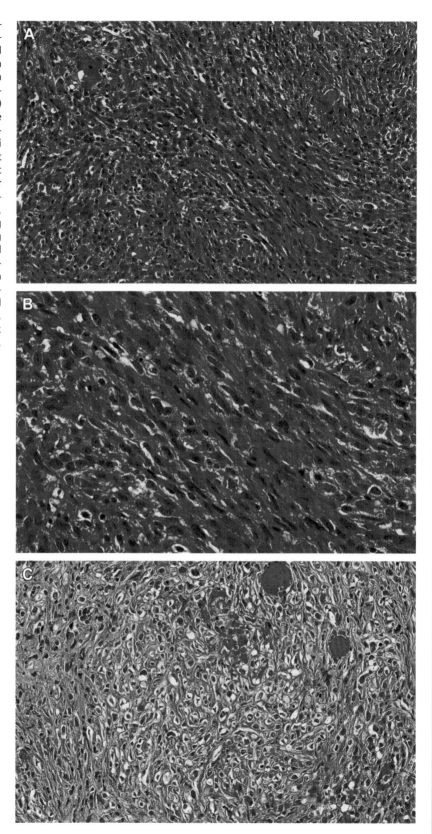

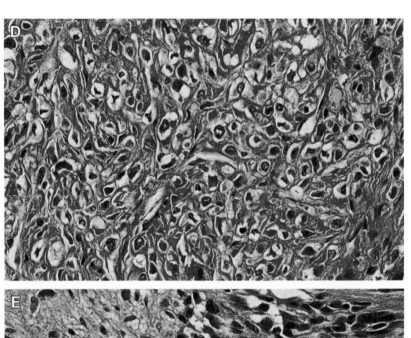

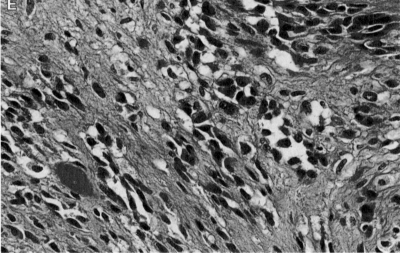

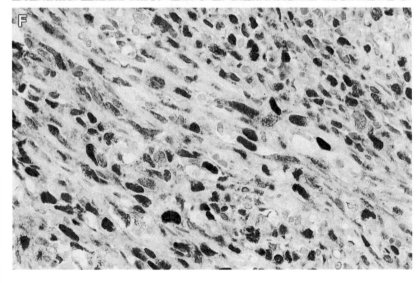

Fig. 7. (*continued*). (*D*) The tumor cells are round to spindle shaped with scant eosinophilic cytoplasm and hyperchromatic nuclei exhibiting irregular nuclear contours with coarse chromatin and inconspicuous nucleoli. (H&E, ×400) (*E*) Focal areas exhibit microalveolar or pseudovascular structures. (H&E, ×400) (*F*) Diffuse and strong MyoD1 immunoreactivity in tumor cells with (original magnification, ×400) (*G*) occasional, scattered, weak-to-moderate staining for myogenin. (original magnification, ×400).

Fig. 7. (continued).

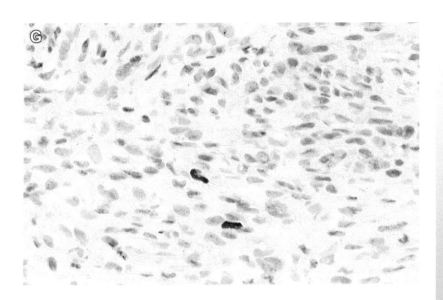

The main differential diagnostic consideration for well-differentiated ERMS and spindle cell RMS is fetal rhabdomyoma. Unlike well-differentiated ERMS and spindle cell RMS, fetal rhabdomyoma is a well circumscribed but nonencapsulated tumor without significant nuclear atypia, necrosis, or hyperchromasia. Mitoses are typically absent or few in number. In ERMS, a subepithelial cambium layer in mucosal sites and reversed zonation, in which more primitive cells are seen peripherally and more mature cells are seen centrally, may be observed. Other spindle cell proliferations enter the differential diagnosis of spindle cell RMS, including cellular schwannoma, nodular fasciitis, desmoid fibromatosis, SFT, inflammatory myofibroblastic tumor, dermatofibrosarcoma protuberans, infantile fibrosarcoma, monophasic spindle cell synovial sarcoma, leiomyosarcoma, malignant peripheral nerve sheath tumor (MPNST) with rhabdomyoblastic differentiation (malignant Triton tumor), spindle cell melanoma, and spindle cell (sarcomatoid) carcinoma. Most of these differential diagnostic considerations can be resolved by demonstration of myogenic markers (desmin, myogenin, and MyoD1) in RMS.

The morphologic differential diagnosis of sclerosing RMS includes extraskeletal osteosarcoma, mesenchymal and extraskeletal myxoid chondrosarcomas, sclerosing epithelioid fibrosarcoma, angiosarcoma, primary or metastatic carcinomas, and sclerosing NHL. Again, inclusion of myogenic markers in the panel of immunohistochemical work-up distinguishes sclerosing RMS from these considerations. Similarly, PRMS may overlap with various pleomorphic carcinomas, lymphomas, and melanoma, although they should not generally express myogenic markers.

 Differential Diagnosis

- ERMS
  - Fetal rhabdomyoma
  - Sinonasal undifferentiated carcinoma
  - Small cell undifferentiated neuroendocrine carcinoma
  - Undifferentiated type of nonkeratinizing nasopharyngeal carcinoma
  - NUT midline carcinoma
  - Ewing sarcoma/primitive neuroectodermal tumor

- Olfactory neuroblastoma
- Ectopic pituitary adenoma
- Malignant melanoma
- Melanotic neuroectodermal tumor of infancy
- Granulocytic sarcoma
- NHL
- Poorly differentiated synovial sarcoma
- Small cell osteosarcoma
- Mesenchymal chondrosarcoma
- Extrarenal rhabdoid tumor
- ARMS
  - Same differential diagnosis as ERMS with the exception of fetal rhabdomyoma
- Spindle cell RMS
  - Fetal rhabdomyoma
  - Cellular schwannoma
  - Nodular fasciitis
  - Desmoid fibromatosis
  - SFT
  - Inflammatory myofibroblastic tumor
  - Dermatofibrosarcoma protuberans
  - Infantile fibrosarcoma
  - Leiomyosarcoma
  - MPNST with rhabdomyoblastic differentiation (malignant Triton tumor)
  - Spindle cell melanoma
  - Spindle cell (sarcomatoid) carcinoma
- Sclerosing RMS
  - Extraskeletal osteosarcoma
  - Mesenchymal osteosarcoma
  - Extraskeletal myxoid chondrosarcoma
  - Sclerosing epithelioid fibrosarcoma
  - Angiosarcoma
  - Primary or metastatic carcinoma
  - Sclerosing NHL
- PRMS
  - Pleomorphic carcinoma
  - Anaplastic lymphoma
  - Malignant melanoma
  - Pleomorphic undifferentiated sarcoma
  - Pleomorphic leiomyosarcoma
  - Pleomorphic liposarcoma

Pitfalls

! The dense pattern of ERMS can mimic ARMS.

! Not all ARMSs have *PAX-FOXO1* gene fusions.

! Desmin and MSA may not stain tumors comprised of the most primitive undifferentiated tumor cells.

! Several malignant tumors may exhibit heterologous   rhabdomyosarcomatous differentiation.

! RMSs can aberrantly express a variety of immunohistochemical markers, including CK, EMA, SMA, S100, NF, CD99, TLE-1, WT1, chromogranin, synaptophysin, and CD56.

! Entrapped atrophic and regenerating skeletal muscle fibers stain for myogenic immunomarkers.

TREATMENT AND PROGNOSIS

The Intergroup Rhabdomyosarcoma Study (IRS) Group, which is currently the Soft-Tissue Sarcoma Committee of the Children's Oncology Group, conducted several cooperative clinical trials that dramatically improved the long-term survival of pediatric RMS patients from 25% to 71% in the IRS-IV.[56,57] These studies recognized important prognostic patient groups and established the efficacy of risk-based multimodality treatment, that is, multiagent chemotherapy, surgery, and/or radiotherapy. The key prognostic factors include clinical group, pretreatment TNM stage, tumor location, age, and histologic subtype. Retrospective analysis of this TNM staging system in a subset of 505 patients in the IRS-II study showed estimated 5-year survival rates of 91%, 73%, 52%, and 23% for stages I, II, III, and IV, respectively.[58] Currently, the combination of the clinical grouping and pretreatment TNM staging systems along with the tumor histologic subtype are used to risk-stratify patients into low-risk, intermediate-risk, and high-risk groups to determine the type of protocol-based therapy.[57] Site is also relevant prognostically with nonparameningeal head and neck considered favorable and parameningeal head and neck considered intermediate prognostically.[59,60] Regarding histologic subtype in children,[45] botryoid and spindle cell RMSs had a superior prognosis (5-year survival rates of 95% and 88% respectively), conventional ERMS had an intermediate prognosis (5-year survival rate of 66%), and ARMS had a poor prognosis (5-year survival rate of 54%). Anaplastic ERMS has

worse survival than conventional ERMS, however (45%–68%).[46]

Adult RMS in contrast continues to be poor, with reported 5-year survival rates ranging from 35% to 52.6%.[32,42,61] Moreover, multivariate analysis showed that the purported prognosticators, including age less than 20 years at diagnosis, absence of regional or distant spread, primary tumor size less than or equal to 5 cm, and negative surgical margin were all retained in adults, with the exception of alveolar histology and unfavorable primary tumor site. Essentially absent in children, PRMS increases in relative frequency with advancing age. This subtype is indeed aggressive with a 5-year disease-free survival rate of 27%[43] and a poor and short-lived response to standard chemotherapy. In comparison to their pediatric counterparts, adult SCSRMSs have a significantly worse prognosis. Of the approximately 95 reported adult cases of SCSRMS with follow-up information, 49.5% had local recurrence and/or metastasis and 24.2% died of disease within a median of 24 months.[33,38–41,55,62–64] The subset of pediatric SCSRMSs with *MYOD1* mutations seems to follow an aggressive behavior with high mortality.[55,65] in contrast to the favorable prognosis seen infantile cases with NCOA2 rearrangements.[65] In ARMS, fusion-positive tumors are more aggressive than those that are negative, but there are conflicting data as to whether gene fusion subtype has prognostic significance. *PAX7-FOXO1* fusion-positive patients are younger and their disease tends to be in the extremities, both of which are already prognosticators.[51,66]

BIPHENOTYPIC SINONASAL SARCOMA

OVERVIEW

BSNS, first reported as low-grade sinonasal sarcoma with neural and myogenic differentiation, is a low-grade sarcoma arising exclusively in the sinonasal tract, most commonly in the superior aspects of the nasal cavity and ethmoid sinuses and rarely extending into the orbit, cribriform plate, or cranial vault.[67] Of the 37 reported cases, it occurs more frequently in women ranging in age from 24 to 85 years (mean 51.1 years).[67–70] Presenting symptoms include difficulty breathing, facial pain and pressure, and nasal congestion.

PATHOLOGIC FEATURES

BSNSs are poorly circumscribed, infiltrative, hypercellular lesions composed of uniform spindle cells arranged in medium-to-long fascicles (**Fig. 8**). Classic herringbone areas are seen in most cases.

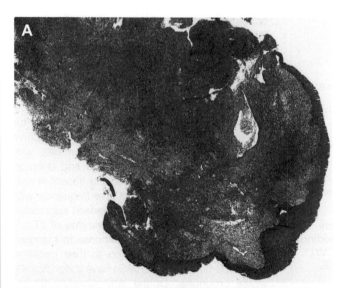

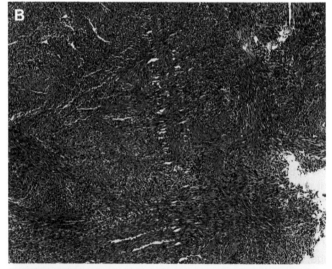

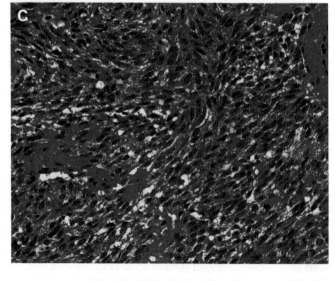

Fig. 8. BSNS. (*A*) A submucosal hypercellular, spindle cell proliferation with a focal HPC-like vascular pattern. (H&E, ×20) (*B*) BSNS consists of uniform spindle cells arranged in medium-to-long fascicles. (H&E, ×100) (*C*) The spindle cells have minimal atypia and rare mitoses. (H&E, ×200).

Fig. 8. (continued). (D) In some areas, the nuclei appear wavy or buckled, imparting a neural appearance. (H&E, ×200) *(E)* BSNS is locally aggressive with invasion and infiltration into bone. (H&E, ×100) *(F)* Non-neoplastic hyperplastic respiratory epithelium invaginates down into the tumor forming small glands or cysts and is a helpful diagnostic clue. (H&E, ×100).

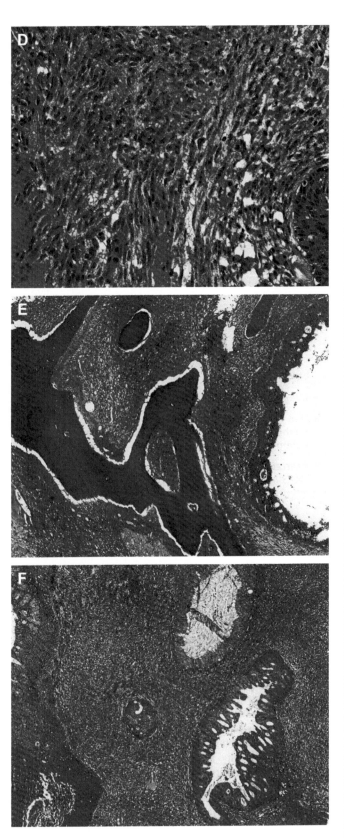

The spindle cells have elongated nuclei that are focally wavy or buckled. Delicate strands of collagen are frequently found between the tumor cells. As with other translocation sarcomas, the nuclear atypia is uniform without significant nuclear pleomorphism. Mitoses are rare and necrosis is absent. An HPC-like vascular pattern is frequently identified (see Fig. 8). A helpful diagnostic clue is the entrapment of non-neoplastic hyperplastic respiratory epithelium that invaginates down into the tumor, forming small glands or cysts (see Fig. 8). Focal rhabdomyoblastic differentiation is seen in some cases.[69,71]

Key Pathologic Features

- Infiltrative
- Hypercellular, uniform spindle cells with minimal atypia
- Focal herringbone pattern and HPC-like vascular pattern
- Coexpress S100 and actins
- Non-neoplastic hyperplastic respiratory epithelium forming small glands or cysts within tumor
- Rearrangements of *PAX3*, most commonly *PAX3-MAML3* fusion

---

IMMUNOHISTOCHEMISTRY AND MOLECULAR FINDINGS

By immunohistochemistry, BSNSs typically coexpress actins (SMA and MSA) and S100 (Fig. 9). Staining for S100 and actins is most often diffuse but may be patchy or show only isolated tumor cell positivity (see Fig. 9).[67] SOX10 has been consistently negative.[69] Other immunohistochemical markers that may be focally positive include CD34, desmin, CK AE1/3, and EMA (weakly). Diffuse h-caldesmon staining was reported in 1 case.[70] Nuclear β-catenin staining has also been reported.[70] In cases of focal rhabdomyoblastic differentiation, myogenin and/or MyoD1 nuclear expression has been demonstrated.[69,71] Thus far, no immunoreactivity for ER and PR has been demonstrated.[70] Nearly all of the reported cases demonstrate rearrangements of *PAX3*, most commonly *PAX3-MAML3* fusion, which at present is specific for this entity.[67,70] A subset of BSNS demonstrates 2 fusions previously described in ARMS, *PAX3-NCOA1*, and *PAX3-FOXO1*. These cases also had focal rhabdomyoblastic differentiation with nuclear myogenin immunoreactivity.[69,71]

DIFFERENTIAL DIAGNOSIS

The differential diagnosis of BSNS includes a variety of both benign and malignant spindle cell neoplasms, including adult-type (low-grade) fibrosarcoma, cellular schwannoma, MPNST, malignant melanoma, monophasic spindle cell synovial sarcoma, SFT, and GPC. The presence of classic herringbone areas makes adult-type fibrosarcoma a strong diagnostic consideration. The immunoprofile of BSNS, however, with coexpression of S100 and actins eliminates fibrosarcoma from the differential diagnosis.

Cellular schwannomas of the sinonasal tract are commonly unencapsulated and may be infiltrative,[72] with strong and diffuse positivity for S100, but they lack staining with muscle markers. MPNST may be a consideration, particularly on biopsy, due to the infiltrative nature of BSNS and at least focal neural appearance. Also both MPNST and BSNS may demonstrate focal rhabdomyoblastic differentiation. MPNSTs typically demonstrate significant nuclear pleomorphism and necrosis, however. BSNS can be distinguished from other nerve sheath tumors and from malignant melanoma by its lack of SOX10 immunoreactivity.

An HPC-like vascular pattern raises the possibilities of SFT and GPC. BSNS, however, lacks variable cellularity, ropey collagen, and cracking of collagen, which are characteristic of SFT. In addition, SFTs are strongly and diffusely CD34-positive and demonstrate nuclear immunoreactivity for STAT6 and negative staining for S100.[17,18] The lesional cells of GPC are more epithelioid and S100 negative, unlike BSNS.

As a result of immunoreactivity for actins and possibly desmin and h-caldesmon, a low-grade leiomyosarcoma may enter the differential diagnosis, particularly on a biopsy. Leiomyosarcoma is negative for S100, however, and the tumor cells have cigar-shaped/blunt-ended nuclei with ample eosinophilic fibrillary cytoplasm with perinuclear vacuoles. In addition, low-grade leiomyosarcomas are diffusely positive for actin, desmin, and h-caldesmon, a pattern of staining not seen in BSNS.

Monophasic spindle cell synovial sarcoma is a strong diagnostic consideration with its uniform nuclear atypia and focal S100, CK, and EMA staining, a pattern of staining that may be seen in BSNS. BSNS lacks the synovial sarcoma fusion transcripts, however, and demonstrates *PAX3* rearrangements.[67,68]

TREATMENT AND PROGNOSIS

Most patients are treated with surgical resection with or without adjuvant radiotherapy. Local recurrence has been reported in approximately 40% of cases. Thus far, there have been no reported cases of metastasis or tumor-related death.[67,68]

CHORDOMA

OVERVIEW

Chordoma is a rare notochordal tumor (0.08 per 100,000 people).[73,74] The skull base accounts for approximately 32% of cases and the cervical spine approximately 5% of cases.[73,74] At these sites, there is an equal gender predilection, and presentation is 1 decade earlier than that of other sites. Symptoms are related to mass effect, including headache, neck pain, diplopia, or cranial nerve palsy.[75] Rarely, chordoma has been reported in extra-axial locations,[76,77] including head and neck sites, such as the nasopharynx, paranasal sinuses, oropharynx, and the soft tissue of the neck.[78–81] Rarely, in children, there seems an association with tuberous sclerosis complex.[82]

PATHOLOGIC FEATURES

Grossly, chordoma is a lobulated mass, typically extending beyond the cortex, with a gelatinous or chondroid cut surface. Histologically, conventional chordoma consists of cords of tumor cells embedded within a myxoid matrix and arranged in lobules separated by fibrous septa (Fig. 10). The tumor cells have abundant eosinophilic cytoplasm, some with intracytoplasmic vacuoles, referred to as physaliferous cells (see Fig. 10). Atypia in chordoma ranges from mild to severe. Necrosis is frequent and may be extensive.

Chondroid chordoma is a distinct histologic subtype, comprising 7% to 63% of skull base chordomas,[75,83] in which the matrix resembles neoplastic hyaline cartilage (Fig. 11).[84,85] Cellular chordoma describes a chordoma composed of sheets of tumor cells with conventional cytologic features, including physaliferous cells, without an extracellular myxoid matrix.[86] Poorly differentiated chordomas lack physaliferous cells and consist of tightly packed small epithelioid cells with increased nuclear-to-cytoplasmic ratios and irregular nuclei.[86] The tumor cells are arranged in irregular nests and sheets set in a more fibrous background. Dedifferentiated chordoma describes a conventional chordoma juxtaposed to an undifferentiated pleomorphic sarcoma or osteosarcoma.[84] Chordomas with rhabdoid morphology have been described.[83,86]

IMMUNOHISTOCHEMISTRY AND MOLECULAR FINDINGS

Chordomas, including the chondroid type, express CKs and are usually immunoreactive for EMA and S100 (Fig. 12). Nuclear expression for brachyury, a marker of notochord differentiation, is a marker highly specific for chordomas (see Fig. 12).[87,88] Poorly differentiated chordoma and dedifferentiated areas may demonstrate loss of brachyury immunoreactivity.[83,87,88] Importantly, immunoreactivity for brachyury may be lost after decalcification. On occasion, chondroid chordoma may demonstrate only focal CK expression.[83] In addition, some studies have reported a loss of INI-1 staining in poorly differentiated chordomas.[89,90]

A majority of chordomas are sporadic; however, a subset seems inherited. Duplication of brachyury, a transcription factor encoded by *T* gene, has been described in familial chordomas,[91] whereas sporadic chordomas may demonstrate *T*-gene amplification and single nucleotide polymorphism in the coding region of the *T* gene.[92,93] Recurrent clival chordomas have demonstrated MGMT promoter methylation.[94] *IDH1* and *IDH2* mutations, which are frequently seen in

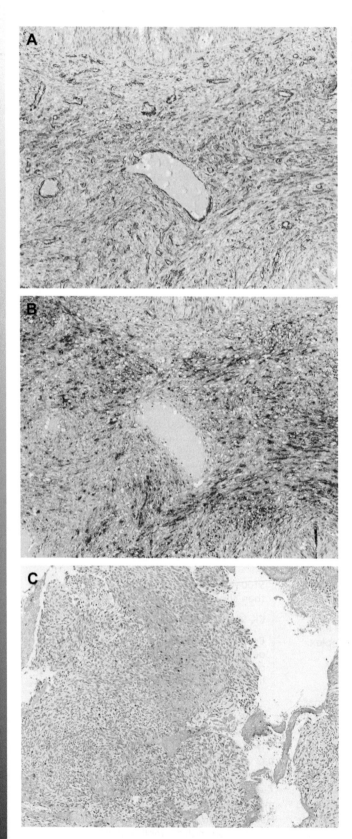

Fig. 9. BSNS typically coexpresses (*A*) actins (×100) and (*B*) S100 (×100), and staining is most often diffuse. (*C*) On occasion, staining for S100 (×100) (depicted here) and actins may be patchy or show only isolated tumor cell positivity.

Fig.   10. Conventional chordoma. (*A*) Conventional chordoma consists of cords of tumor cells within a myxoid matrix and arranged in lobules separated by fibrous septa. (H&E, ×40) (*B*) The tumor has cells with abundant eosinophilic and prominent cytoplasmic borders and vacuolated physaliferous cells. (H&E, ×400).

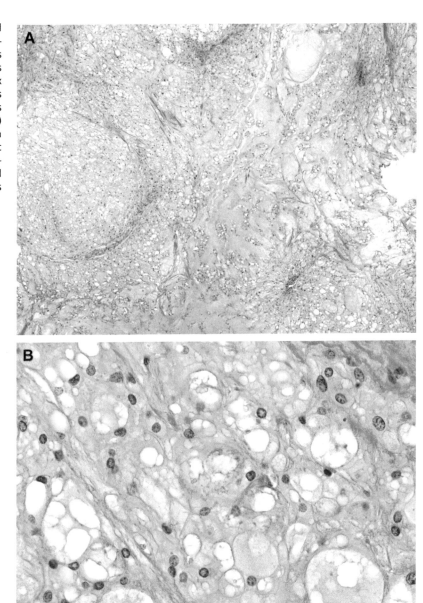

conventional chondrosarcomas, are not detected in chordomas.[95,96]

DIFFERENTIAL DIAGNOSIS

With adequate sampling, the morphology and limited panel, discussed previously, is adequate for distinction from other entities. But the histologic similarities between chondroid chordoma and chondrosarcoma may pose a diagnostic challenge on limited and crushed biopsy material typical of skull base lesions.[83] Additional markers may be needed, although they have caveats. EMA is a sensitive marker for chordoma; however, it is not entirely specific because chondrosarcomas may demonstrate immunoreactivity.[83,97] Podoplanin (D2-40) is similarly sensitive but not specific because chondroid chordomas may express this marker.[83]

The rationale for including CK, S100, and brachyury in the chordoma work-up is to ensure that considerations other than chondrosarcoma are

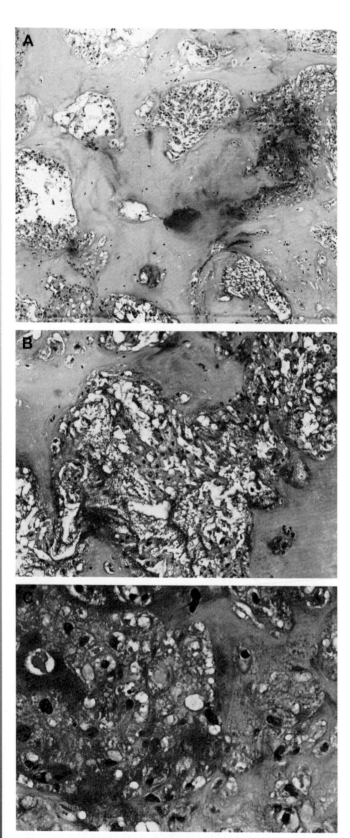

Fig. 11. Chondroid chordoma. (*A*) Chondroid chordoma consists of cords of tumor cells arranged in lobules, within a neoplastic hyaline cartilage matrix, mimicking a chondrosarcoma. (H&E, ×40) (*B*, *C*) The tumor cells are identical to conventional chordoma. (H&E, original magnification [*B*] ×200 and [*C*] ×400).

Fig. 12. Conventional chordoma demonstrating diffuse staining with (*A*) cytokeratin AE1/3 (×200), (*B*) S100 (×200), and (*C*) brachyury (×200).

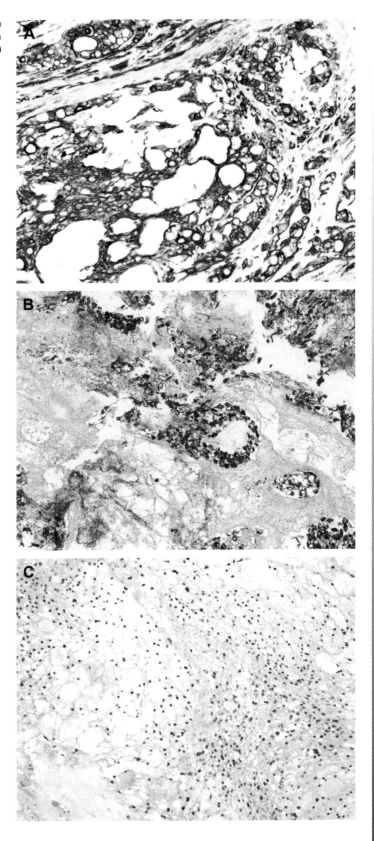

addressed. CK alone is not helpful in distinguishing chordoma from metastatic mucinous or clear cell carcinomas and even CK plus S100 is not useful in distinguishing chordoma from myoepithelial cell-rich tumors.[76,77,88] Distinguishing chordoma from myoepithelial tumors requires immunohistochemical evidence of brachyury expression, in addition to CKs and S100.[76,77]

Other morphologic mimics include extraskeletal myxoid chondrosarcoma, chordoid meningioma,

and chordoid glioma, but these are readily resolved by the panel (discussed previously). In addition, extraskeletal myxoid chondrosarcoma demonstrate rearrangements involving *NR4A3*, most commonly *NR4A3-EWSR1* fusion. Chordoid glioma is strongly positive for GFAP, although chordoma may also express this focally.[83]

Pitfalls

! Cellular and poorly differentiated chordoma may be mistaken for metastatic carcinoma, particularly on biopsy, due to the presence of epithelioid tumor cells, lack of matrix, and CK positivity.

! Chondroid chordoma may be misdiagnosed as chondrosarcoma, particularly on small crushed biopsy material from the skull base.

! Extra-axial chordomas may be mistaken for myoepithelial tumors of salivary gland or soft tissue origin.

Chordoma	Chondrosarcoma
Lobular arrangement of cells with fibrous septa	No fibrous septations
Tumor cells within lobule arranged in cords	Tumor cells are not arranged in cords
Tumor cells with abundant eosinophilic cytoplasm and vacuolated physaliferous cells	Tumor cells with less abundant to scant cytoplasm
Tumor cells immunoreactive for CKs, S100, brachyury, and EMA	Tumor cells immunoreactive for S100 but negative for brachyury and CKs. EMA staining may be seen in chondrosarcoma.

Differential Diagnosis

Chondrosarcoma

• Negative for CK and brachyury (EMA may be positive, variable S100)

Chordoid meningioma

• Negative for brachyury (EMA positive, variable S100, CK)

Chordoid glioma

• Negative for brachyury (S100 positive, variable CK and EMA; also GFAP positive)

Mixed tumor/myoepithelioma/parachordoma and myoepithelial carcinoma

• Negative for brachyury (positive for S100, CKs, and EMA)

Extraskeletal myxoid chondrosarcoma

• Negative for CK and brachyury (S100 positive)

Metastatic mucinous adenocarcinoma, clear cell renal cell carcinoma

• Negative for brachyury and S100 (CK positive); may be positive for site-specific markers

TREATMENT AND PROGNOSIS

Treatment of skull base chordomas typically consists of piecemeal surgical resection, which precludes histologic evaluation of margin status, followed by adjuvant radiotherapy. Due to the locally aggressive nature of chordoma, complete gross total resection is difficult to achieve, successful in 29% of cases,[75] and high-dose adjuvant radiotherapy near the brainstem poses difficulties in providing an effective dose. Proton beam therapy has increasingly become a strategy to circumvent this issue.[98] Although skull base chordomas and chondrosarcomas are treated similarly, distinction between the 2 is important because chondrosarcomas carries a better prognosis (Table 4).[75,99–101]

Chordomas most commonly metastasize to the lung, followed by the lymph nodes, bone, liver, and subcutaneous tissues.[84] Skull base chordomas are less likely to metastasize than their sacral counterparts.[84] Chondroid chordoma were initially thought more favorable prognostically[85,102,103] but are now considered equivalent to conventional chordoma in terms of outcome.[87,97,99,104] Skull base chordomas in children under the age of 5 years are associated with an aggressive clinical course, reflecting the frequency of poorly

Table 4
Comparison of clinical features and outcomes in skull base chordoma and chondrosarcoma

	Chordoma	Chondrosarcoma
Age (y)	Median: 45 Mean: 38 Range: 1–87	Median: 52 Mean: 46 Range: 10–79
Race	84% white	81% white
Gender (male:female)	Approximately 1:1	Approximately 1:1
Tumor size	Approximately half of the cases are between 2.0 cm and 3.9 cm	More than half of cases >6.0 cm
Complete surgical resection (%)	29	37
Adjuvant radiotherapy (%)	42	41
Local recurrence rate (%)	68	1.5 (up to 53% without adjuvant radiotherapy)
5-y overall survival (%)	63–78.4	82–88.5
10-y overall survival (%)	16–32	50
5-y tumor-specific survival (%)	73	88
10-y tumor-specific survival (%)	42	62–71

Data from Refs.[75,99–101]

differentiated chordomas (or chordomas with atypical histology) seen in this age group.[86,104] But when corrected for histology, patients seem to have similar or better survival.[86,104,105] Other adverse prognosticators include older age (≥50 years) and larger tumor size at presentation (≥4.0 cm).[75]

CHONDROSARCOMA

OVERVIEW

The head and neck region is a primary site for chondrosarcoma in approximately 1% to 12% of cases.[106] Approximately half of the chondrosarcomas of the head and neck occur in the jaw and craniofacial bones, approximately a quarter occur in the ossified cartilages of the larynx, and the remainder occur in other head and neck sites.[106] Gnathic chondrosarcomas tends to arise in the maxilla, followed by the mandible, specifically the mandibular symphysis, coronoid process, and condyle and are rare in the body.

Conventional chondrosarcomas may be classified as primary (de novo) or secondary (syndromic [ie, Ollier disease or Maffucci disease] or in a precursor [ie, synovial chondromatosis, approximately 2% at head and neck subsites]).[107] Less common histologic subtypes include mesenchymal chondrosarcoma, clear cell chondrosarcoma, and dedifferentiated chondrosarcoma. Chondrosarcomas arising in the head and neck demonstrate site specific differences in patient demographics and histologic features (**Table 5**).[75,97,108–111]

With the exception of laryngeal chondrosarcomas, which tend to arise in patients over age 50, craniofacial chondrosarcomas tends to occur in young patients, with approximately one-third of cases occurring in patients under age 40.[106,108] Mesenchymal chondrosarcoma, a rare subtype, also occurs in younger patients, with peak incidence between the second and third decades; 61.8% of patients are younger than 30 years, and there is nearly equal incidence among men and women.[106,112,113]

Plain films or CT scans demonstrate a radiolucent mass lesion with stippled or coarse popcorn calcifications. Any cartilaginous/chondroid tumor of the head and neck greater than 1.0 cm in size should be assumed to be a chondrosarcoma until proved otherwise. Invasion of adjacent structures, including soft tissue, is a helpful feature highly suggestive of malignancy.

PATHOLOGIC FEATURES

Grossly, conventional chondrosarcoma is a greyish-white lobulated mass, resembling hyaline cartilage, which expands and extends through the marrow space (**Fig. 13**). It may erode through the cortex and infiltrate the adjacent soft tissues. Scattered flecks of yellow-white calcifications impart a gritty texture. Areas of myxoid and cystic degeneration may be seen.

Table 5
Chondrosarcomas of head and neck sites

Site	Subsite	Age (y)	Gender (male:female)	Size (cm)	Histologic Features	Prognosis

Larynx	77.3% cricoid cartilage 19.2% thyroid cartilage 2.8% arytenoid cartilage Rest of other cartilages	Mean: 64.4 Range: 25–91	3.2:1	Mean: approximately 3.5 Range: 0.1–12.0	Nearly all conventional chondrosarcoma: (predominantly hyaline, approximately 5% myxoid)
					• Grade 1: 78.4%
					• Grade 2: 12.6%
					• Grade 3: 6.3%
					• Dedifferentiated: 2.7%; clear cell: <1%
						• Local recurrence rate: 18%–40%
						• Metastatic rate: 1.9%–10%
						• Disease-specific survival
						  ○ 5-y = 78.9%–88.6%
						  ○ 10-y = 47.8%–84.8%

Jaw and paranasal sinuses Approximately 2% seen in setting of Ollier disease	Maxilla/maxillary sinus: 44.6% Ethmoid, sphenoid sinuses, nasal septum: 41.1% Mandible: 7.7%–10.7%	Mean: 41.6 Range: 1.5–88	Approximately 1:1	Mean: 4.0 Range: 1.0–12.0	Majority conventional chondrosarcoma
					• Grade 1: 65%
					• Grade 2: 30%
					• Grade 3: 5%
					Variants
					• Clear cell: 1%–2%
					• Dedifferentiated: <1%
					• Mesenchymal: approximately 8%
						• Local recurrence rate: 33.3%
						• Metastatic rate: approximately 5%
						• Overall survival:
						  ○ 5-y = 80.7%
						  ○ 10-y = 65.3%
						• Mesenchymal: 5-y survival 59.1%–82%; 10-y survival 55%; local recurrence 34.8%

Skull base	Temporo-occipital junction: 66% Clivus: 28% Sphenoethmoid complex: 6%	Mean: 39 Range: 10–79	Approximately 1:1	>50% >6.0 cm	Majority conventional chondrosarcoma: (7.5% hyaline, 29.5% myxoid, 63% mixed hyaline and myxoid)
					• Grade 1: 51%
					• Grade 2: 49%
					• No grade 3; dedifferentiated: <1%
					Variants
					• Mesenchymal: 7.8%
						• Local recurrence rate: up to 1.5%
						• Overall survival:
						  ○ 5-y survival: 82%–99%
						  ○ 10-y survival: 50%
						• Mesenchymal: 5-y survival 62%; 10-y survival 22%

Data from Refs.[75,97,108–111]

Fig. 13. Conventional chondrosarcoma. (*A, B*) A conventional chondrosarcoma involving the right ala of the thyroid cartilage and invading adjacent soft tissues. (*A*) A lobulated, grey-white mass resembling hyaline cartilage with cystic degeneration. Typically, a larynx is opened longitudinally along the posterior aspect. When handling tumors of the laryngeal cartilages, it may be advantageous to serially section the larynx through its transverse or axial plane, which allows for assessment of the tumor relationship to adjacent structures and for correlation with imaging findings. (*B*) Low-power view demonstrating a low-grade conventional chondrosarcoma infiltrating adjacent soft tissue. (*C*) Grade 1 conventional chondrosarcoma with infiltrative destructive growth pattern, mildly increased cellularity, hyaline matrix, and atypical chondrocytes with small dark nuclei, some with open chromatin. (*Courtesy of* [*A, B*] Dr Raja R. Seethala, UPMC, Pittsburgh, PA.)

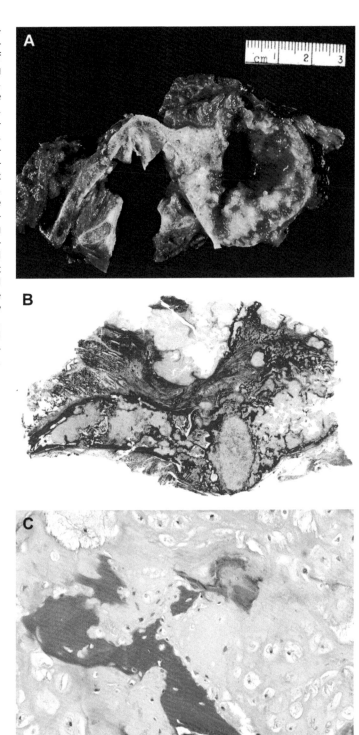

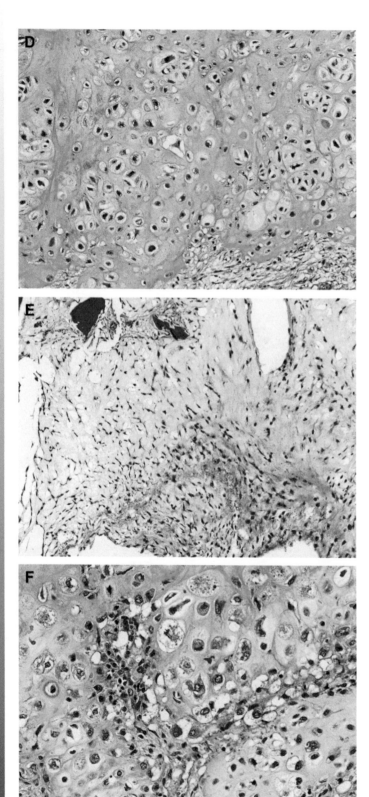

Fig. 13. (continued).   (D) Grade 2 conventional chondrosarcoma with greater cellularity, increased cytologic detail including abundant cytoplasm and nuclei with open chromatin, and scattered binucleate chondrocytes. (E) Grade 2 myxoid chondrosarcoma with stellate chondrocytes and myxoid matrix. (F) Grade 3 chondrosarcoma with greater cellularity and atypical chondrocytes with pleomorphic nuclei.

Fig. 13. (continued). (G, H) Dedifferentiated chondrosarcoma demonstrating an abrupt transition (G) from low-grade chondrosarcoma to an undifferentiated pleomorphic sarcoma (H) with pleomorphic spindled cells and numerous mitoses. (H&E, original magnification [C] ×200, [D] ×200, [E] ×200, [F] ×200, [G] ×100, and [H] ×200).

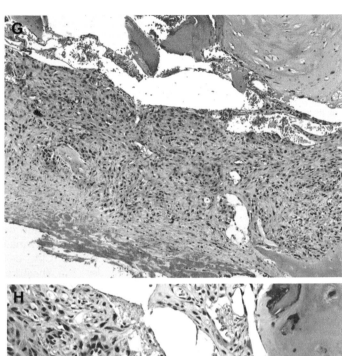

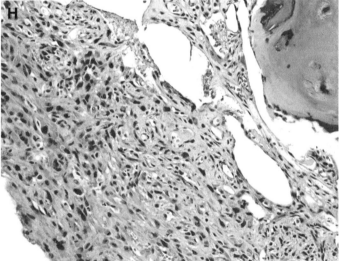

Conventional chondrosarcoma can be hyaline type with atypical chondrocytes residing in lacunae and surrounded by hyaline matrix, or myxoid type with stellate atypical chondrocytes floating within a frothy mucinous matrix (see Fig. 13). Criteria for malignancy in cartilaginous tumors are outlined in Box 1 and are best applied to central chondroid tumors. These criteria can become problematic when applied to cartilaginous tumors on the surface of bone, in soft tissue, and in the small bones of the hand and feet, because benign cartilaginous tumors in these locations may demonstrate increased cellularity, enhanced cytologic detail, and binucleate chondrocytes. An infiltrative growth pattern is the most reliable feature in these locations. Grading of conventional chondrosarcomas is summarized in Table 6.[114]

OTHER HISTOLOGIC SUBTYPES

Dedifferentiated Chondrosarcoma

Dedifferentiated chondrosarcoma is a highly malignant variant of chondrosarcoma that develops in 10% to 15% of central conventional chondrosarcomas.[115] It is characterized by sharply demarcated areas of a low-grade chondrosarcoma and noncartilaginous high-grade sarcoma, most commonly an undifferentiated pleomorphic sarcoma or osteosarcoma (see Fig. 13).

Mesenchymal Chondrosarcoma

Although mesenchymal chondrosarcoma is rare, accounting for less than 3% of chondrosarcomas, it accounts for 8.8% of head and neck chondrosarcomas and has a predilection for the jaw.[106,109,112] Approximately one-third are in

---

Box 1
General criteria for malignancy in chondroid neoplasms

- Architecture
  - Permeation of bone or extension beyond periosteum
  - Disorganized arrangement of malignant cartilage lobules
- Increased cellularity
- Enhanced cytologic detail
  - Cytoplasm becomes readily apparent
  - Nuclear membranes, chromatin distribution, and nucleoli become visible
- *More than occasional* binucleate chondrocytes

---

extraosseous locations with frequent involvement of the meninges.[112]

Mesenchymal chondrosarcoma is a high-grade, biphasic tumor composed of lobules of low-grade, conventional chondrosarcoma (hyaline type) and an undifferentiated component composed of small, round to oval tumor cells with hyperchromatic nuclei, inconspicuous nucleoli, and minimal cytoplasm associated with an HPC-like vascular pattern (**Fig. 14**). Typically, the transition between these 2 elements is usually abrupt but may be gradual. In untreated tumors, necrosis is typically absent and mitotic rate is low.

Key Points

- Accounts for 8.8% of head and neck chondrosarcomas (jaw, sinuses, and skull base)
- One-third may be extraosseous in location.
- High-grade (grade 3) biphasic tumor:
  - Low-grade (hyaline type) conventional chondrosarcoma
  - Undifferentiated, small round blue cell component with HPC-like vascular pattern
- Recurrent *HEY1-NCOA2* fusion
- Undifferentiated component positive for CD99 and SOX-9; may be focally positive for desmin, MyoD1, and SMA and typically negative for myogenin, CD45, and CKs
- Tends to be more aggressive with worse overall survival and recurrence rate than conventional chondrosarcoma

---

Clear Cell Chondrosarcoma

Clear cell chondrosarcoma is another uncommon histologic subtype, accounting for approximately 2% of chondrosarcomas. Approximately 5% of

reported cases involve the head and neck, and approximately half involve the larynx.[116]

Clear cell chondrosarcoma is characterized by a sheetlike proliferation of malignant chondrocytes, with ample, clear to eosinophilic cytoplasm; well-defined cytoplasmic borders; and small centrally located nuclei, with minimal atypia and rare mitoses (**Fig. 15**). Clear cell chondrosarcomas lack a chondroid matrix unless associated with a conventional low-grade chondrosarcoma (hyaline type) that may be focally ossified or calcified. Irregularly shaped trabeculae of immature woven bone are frequently seen scattered within the lesion (see **Fig. 15**). Cystic degeneration in the form of secondary aneurysmal bone cyst is common. Periodic acid–Schiff stain with and without diastase predigestion confirms the presence of glycogen within the cytoplasm of the clear cells.

IMMUNOHISTOCHEMICAL AND MOLECULAR FEATURES

Immunohistochemistry is of little benefit in the diagnosis of chondrosarcoma, except in certain scenarios. These include distinguishing chondrosarcoma from chondroid chordoma (discussed previously), sarcomatoid carcinoma with chondrosarcomatous differentiation, and in the work-up of mesenchymal chondrosarcoma. S100 is of limited use because it is positive in both benign and malignant cartilaginous tumors; however, it may be useful in clear cell chondrosarcoma to confirm chondroid origin, particularly in biopsy material. *IDH1* and *IDH2* mutations are noted in peripheral and central chondrosarcomas and represent early events seen even in benign chondroid neoplasms.[95]

Immunohistochemistry is often performed on biopsies of mesenchymal chondrosarcomas, particularly if the biopsy material consists of the undifferentiated component. S100 is

Table 6
Histologic grading of chondrosarcoma

Low grade	Grade 1	Atypical chondrocytes with small dark nuclei; multiple nuclei per lacuna; mild to moderate cellularity; no mitosis; mostly hyaline matrix
Includes clear cell chondrosarcoma (grade 1)	Grade 2	Atypical, moderate-sized chondrocytes with more vesicular nuclei; <2 mitoses/10 HPFs; greater cellularity; matrix more myxoid
High grade	Grade 3	Greater cellularity; atypical chondrocytes with pleomorphic nuclei; ≥2 mitoses/10 HPFs; myxoid or spindled matrix (peripheral spindling)
Includes mesenchymal chondrosarcoma (grade 3)	Dedifferentiated chondrosarcoma	

Fig. 14. (*A*, *B*) Mesenchymal chondrosarcoma with abrupt transition from the low-grade conventional chondrosarcoma and the undifferentiated component composed of small round to oval tumor cells. (*A*) (H&E, ×20) (*B*) (H&E, ×100).

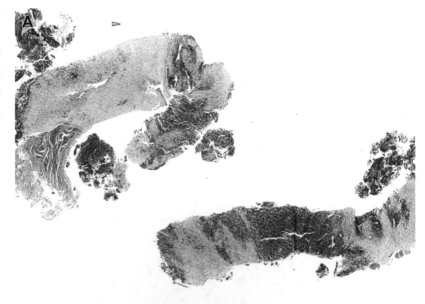

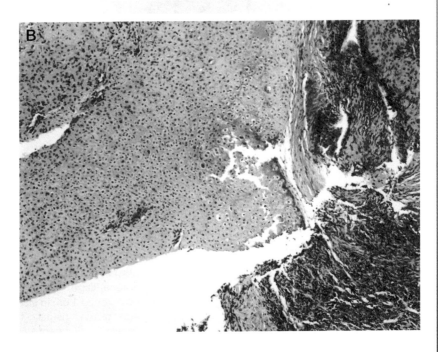

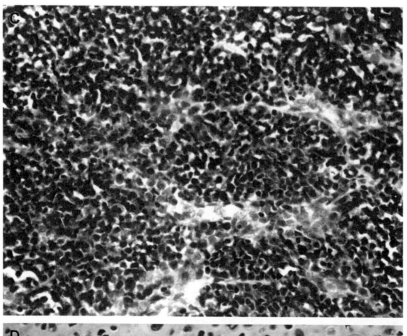

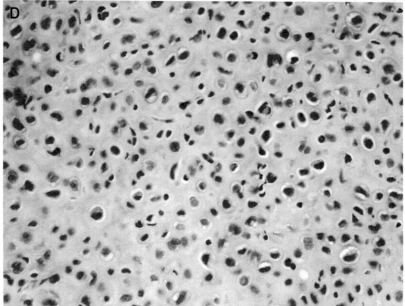

Fig. 14. (*continued*). (*C*) The undifferentiated component consists of atypical small round tumor cells with minimal cytoplasm and inconspicuous nucleoli. (H&E, ×400) (*D*) Higher-power view of the malignant hyaline-type cartilage with increased cellularity, increased cytologic details and scattered binucleate chondrocytes. (*Courtesy of* Dr Brendan Dickson, Mount Sinai Hospital, Toronto, Ontario, Canada.) (H&E, ×400).

positive in the low-grade cartilaginous component, whereas the undifferentiated component is usually positive for CD99. Both components of mesenchymal chondrosarcoma are immunoreactive for S0X-9, making it a particularly useful marker in distinguishing mesenchymal chondrosarcoma from other small round blue cell tumors.[117]

A recurrent *HEY1-NCOA2* fusion on the long arm of chromosome 8 is characteristic of mesenchymal chondrosarcoma.[118]

DIFFERENTIAL DIAGNOSIS

It is crucial to correlate imaging findings with histology when dealing with primary lesions of the bone. In the larynx, the differential for chondrosarcoma includes chondrometaplasia. Chondrometaplasia describes a small nodule of bland fibrocartilage, typically less than 0.5 cm (must not exceed 1 cm in size), found in the submucosal soft tissue, usually the vocalis ligament and Broyles ligament. In contrast, laryngeal

Fig. 15. (*A*) Low-power (H&E, ×100) and (*B*) higher-power views of a clear cell chondrosarcoma with abundant clear cytoplasm and centrally placed small dark nuclei and irregular trabeculae of immature bone that are partly mineralized. (H&E, ×400).

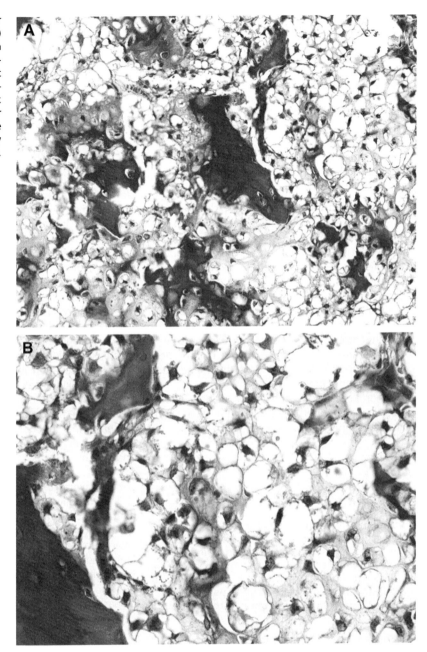

chondrosarcomas are typically located within the ossified laryngeal cartilage, consist of hyaline-type cartilage, and are larger than benign lesions.

High-grade cartilaginous neoplasms of the head and neck are sarcomatoid carcinomas (cutaneous, mucosal, or salivary) or chondroblastic osteosarcoma until proved otherwise. Review of the clinical history for prior head and neck carcinomas, adequate specimen sampling to identify a well differentiated or an in situ component, and immunohistochemical evaluation for immunoreactivity with CKs and/or p40 are helpful to identify sarcomatoid carcinomas.

In contrast to dedifferentiated chondrosarcoma, where there is a sharp demarcation between the dedifferentiated component and the low-grade chondrosarcoma component, the malignant cartilage of chondroblastic osteosarcoma is high grade and blends with the osteosarcoma (discussed later; Fig. 16). Identification of definitive malignant osteoid associated with atypical epithelioid or

Key Points

- Low-grade cartilaginous neoplasms of the head and neck greater than 1.0 cm in size are chondrosarcomas until proved otherwise.

- High-grade cartilaginous neoplasms of the head and neck are sarcomatoid carcinomas (cutaneous, mucosal, or salivary gland) or chondroblastic osteosarcoma until proved otherwise.

- Chondroid chordoma must be excluded in chondroid tumors involving the skull base.

spindle cells is a key feature to distinguish chondroblastic osteosarcoma from a high-grade or dedifferentiated chondrosarcoma.

When dealing with malignant chondroid neoplasms of the mandible, chondroblastic osteosarcoma is far more common than chondrosarcoma and a chondroblastic osteosarcoma must be carefully considered before diagnosing a high-grade conventional chondrosarcoma of the mandible, especially in the body.

Chondroid chordoma must be excluded when assessing a chondroid neoplasm of the skull base (discussed previously). A core biopsy from a

Pitfalls

! The undifferentiated component of mesenchymal chondrosarcoma mimics other small round blue cell tumors, including Ewing sarcoma/primitive neuroectodermal tumor, RMS, malignant melanoma, and poorly differentiated synovial sarcoma, particularly with overlapping immunohistochemical findings.

! Be wary of diagnosing high-grade chondrosarcomas of the mandible, particularly in the body. Grade 3 histology on a biopsy equates to chondroblastic osteosarcoma until proved otherwise.

! Benign and malignant bone tumors, including chondroid neoplasms, should only diagnosed in conjunction with radiologic findings.

! A diagnosis of low-grade chondroid neoplasm is recommended for any low-grade chondroid mass of the head and neck with equivocal radiologic findings and borderline size.

mesenchymal chondrosarcoma can be misleading if only the low-grade cartilaginous or undifferentiated components are sampled. The differential diagnosis for the undifferentiated component of mesenchymal chondrosarcoma includes other round cell tumors (discussed previously). Immunoreactivity for SOX-9 and confirmation of a *HEY1-NCOA2* fusion are useful in this context.

TREATMENT AND PROGNOSIS

Surgical resection without neck dissection is the standard initial therapy for head and neck chondrosarcomas. Complete surgical resection significantly improves prognosis, because local recurrence with extension into vital structures is the main cause of death.[108] Local recurrence of head and neck chondrosarcomas is seen in up to 40% of cases (see **Table 5**). Regional and distant spread in head and neck chondrosarcomas are rare.[106] A conservative surgical approach with the goal of organ preservation is often chosen for head and neck chondrosarcomas, except for those of skull base for which complete resection is achieved in only 37% of cases.[75] Skull base chondrosarcomas are treated similarly to chordoma. Chondrosarcomas are not chemosensitive with the exception of mesenchymal chondrosarcoma where chemotherapy has reduced risk of local recurrence and death.[113]

Overall, head and neck chondrosarcomas have a more favorable prognosis than other sites. This is likely a reflection of earlier symptoms due to anatomic constraints, leading to diagnosis at a lower stage. In the head and neck, the 5-year survival for low-grade chondrosarcomas is 93.2%, for high-grade chondrosarcomas 67.3%, and for those with regional/distant spread 71%.[106] Among tumors arising in the head and neck, the 5-year disease-specific survival for conventional chondrosarcoma (91.4%) is higher than mesenchymal chondrosarcomas (53.2%).[106] **Table 5** summarizes the prognostic difference among different head and neck sites.[75,97,108–111]

OSTEOSARCOMA

OVERVIEW

Osteosarcoma is the most common primary, non-hematopoietic malignant neoplasm of bone. Fewer than 10% of cases involve the head and neck,[119] with the jaw comprising approximately two-thirds of cases, typically the body of the mandible and the alveolar ridge or antral area of the maxilla.[110] Surface variants are rare.[120–122]

Fig. 16. (*A*) Gross image of a conventional osteoblastic osteosarcoma involving the mandible, displacing teeth and expanding the bone. (*B, C*) Gnathic conventional osteoblastic osteosarcoma in a 78-year-old man, infiltrating soft tissue. (*B*) The tumor is composed of irregular, thin trabeculae of osteoid that is partially mineralized, imparting a basophilic quality. (*Courtesy of* [*A*] Dr Raja R. Seethala, UPMC, Pittsburgh, PA.) (H&E, ×100).

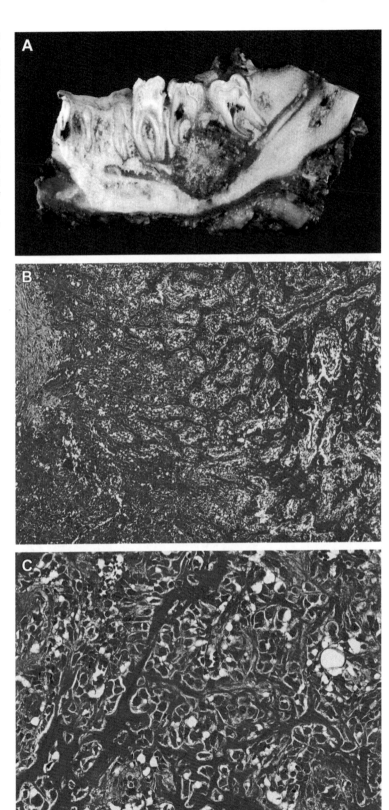

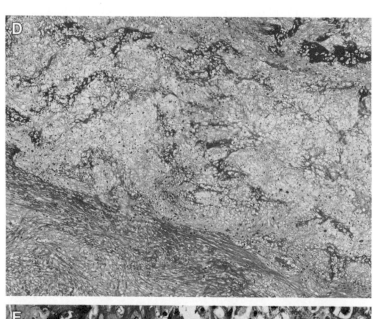

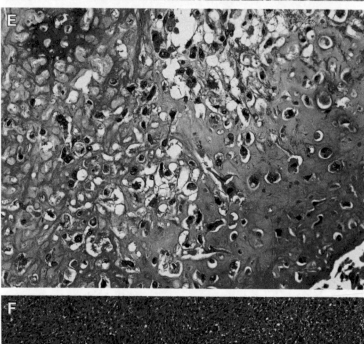

Fig. 16. (continued). (*C*) The osteoid arises from highly atypical epithelioid tumor cells. (H&E, ×400) (*D, E*) Conventional chondroblastic osteosarcoma with high-grade hyaline-type malignant cartilage blending into conventional osteoblastic osteosarcoma with filligree osteoid irregular trabeculae of woven bone. (*D*) (H&E, ×100) (*E*) (H&E, ×400).

Fig. 16. (*continued*). (*F, G*) Conventional fibroblastic osteosarcoma with pleomorphic spindle cells arranged in fascicles and focal herringbone pattern. Focal osteoid is seen associated with pleomorphic tumor cells ([*G*] *upper left*). An atypical mitotic figure is also seen. (*F*) (H&E, ×100) (*G*) (H&E, ×400).

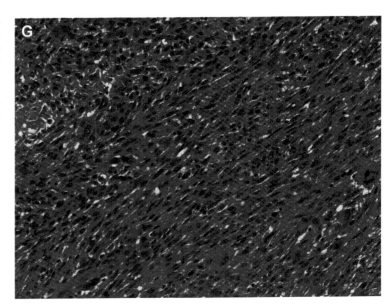

Primary osteosarcoma of the larynx also is rarely reported.[123]

There are several ways to classify osteosarcomas:

1. Primary or secondary
2. Anatomic variants: craniofacial/gnathic versus appendicular/axial
3. Compartmental variants: intramedullary (low-grade central or conventional [high-grade]), surface of bones (parosteal [low-grade] and periosteal [intermediate-grade] and high-grade surface), and extraosseous (low-grade to high-grade)
4. Histologic variants: conventional (osteoblastic, chondroblastic, fibroblastic, and so forth) and other less common variants (high grade), including telangiectatic and small cell.

Osteosarcomas may develop in association with several genetic syndromes, including Li-Fraumeni syndrome, hereditary retinoblastoma, Rothmund-Thomson syndrome, and Werner syndrome.[124] Osteosarcomas are usually primary, arising de novo. Secondary osteosarcomas may develop in the settings of Paget disease of bone, postradiation, fibrous dysplasia, and bone infarction.[125–127] Secondary osteosarcomas are typically high grade and are more aggressive than primary osteosarcomas. They are more common in older patients and are more likely to develop in craniofacial/gnathic sites.[126,128] Osteosarcomas of the jaw/craniofacial skeleton are distinct from those arising in

other locations, and the differences are summarized in **Table 7**.

Radiologic identification of gnathic osteosarcomas can be difficult and may mimic benign odontogenic lesions or reactive processes. Evidence of infiltration may be challenging to document. Displacement of teeth, aggressive pattern of tooth root resorption, widening of the space surrounding periodontal ligament and mandibular canal alterations are useful features.[129]

PATHOLOGIC FEATURES

Grossly, osteosarcomas are gritty, expansile lesions that destroy the underlying bone and may demonstrate extension into adjacent soft tissue (see **Fig. 16**).

Regardless of histologic subtype, the diagnosis of osteosarcoma relies on the identification of neoplastic immature woven bone (osteoid).[124] The neoplastic osteoid is intimately associated with the tumor cells and there is no osteoblastic rimming to distinguish it from reactive new bone formation that can be seen in a fracture, adjacent to osteonecrosis, or osteomyelitis. The organization of the osteoid is variable and may be composed of delicate strands (filigree) or coarse, lacelike patterns or thickened, irregular trabeculae. The osteoid may be mineralized imparting a basophilic appearance. A majority of gnathic osteosarcomas are high grade.[128,130]

Key Pathologic Features

- Diagnosis of osteosarcoma relies on the identification of neoplastic immature woven bone.

- The most common forms of conventional osteosarcomas are classified based on the predominant type of matrix: osteoblastic, chondroblastic, or fibroblastic.

- Neoplastic cartilage in chondroblastic osteosarcoma is almost always high grade.

- Low-grade central and parosteal osteosarcomas demonstrate amplification of *MDM2* and *CDK4* with corresponding immunohistochemical expression.

Conventional Osteosarcoma

The 3 main types of conventional osteosarcoma include osteoblastic, chondroblastic, and fibroblastic, based on the predominant matrix and account for 70%. All 3 types may be identified in the same tumor. Other less common types of conventional osteosarcoma include giant cell rich, osteoblastoma-like, chondroblastoma-like, epithelioid, and clear cell.[124]

In osteoblastic osteosarcoma, neoplastic bone and osteoid is the predominant matrix (see **Fig. 16**). The osteoid/bone matrix can vary from thin and lacelike to sclerotic.[124] If the predominant matrix is cartilage, it is a chondroblastic osteosarcoma (see **Fig. 16**). The neoplastic cartilage is usually high grade and hyaline-type but may be myxoid-type, especially in those arising in the jaw.[124] If the dominant matrix is scarce or absent with atypical spindled tumor cells associated with extracellular collagen, the diagnosis is fibroblastic osteasarcoma (see **Fig. 16**).

Surface Variants

Surface variants of osteosarcoma are rare. Parosteal osteosarcoma is a low-grade osteosarcoma that consists of spindle cells with minimal atypia forming bone trabeculae arranged in parallel long seams. Periosteal osteosarcoma is an intermediate-grade osteosarcoma with malignant bone and cartilage. High-grade surface osteosarcomas either occur de novo or represent dedifferentiation of parosteal osteosarcoma.[120–122]

Secondary Osteosarcomas

In the head and neck, the most common secondary osteosarcomas are Paget osteosarcoma and radiation-induced osteosarcoma. Paget osteosarcoma is high grade and most often a conventional osteoblastic osteosarcoma. Radiation osteitis may be seen in radiation-induced osteosarcoma.[124]

Table 7
Comparison of head and neck osteosarcomas to other sites

	Appendicular Osteosarcoma	Jaw/Craniofacial Osteosarcoma
Age	Bimodal: second decade (appendicular); sixth decade (axial)	Bimodal: third–fourth decade; sixth decade
Gender (male:female)	Approximately 1.35:1	Approximately 1:1
Secondary Causes (%)	5 cases (older patients, axial locations)	Approximately 20 of cases (older patients)
Most common sign/symptom	Pain	Mass
Size (cm)	>5–10	Approximately 5.5 (range: 1.2–15.0)
Metastasic rate (%)	80–95 (presumed disseminated at time of diagnosis)	<21 (late in clinical course)
Reponse to chemotherapy	Excellent	Unclear
Overall survival (%)	Approximately 70 to >80	Approximately 65
Main predictor of outcome	Response to chemotherapy	Margin status; death due to local recurrence

Data from Refs.[124,126,128,130,141,142,144]

Low-Grade Central Osteosarcoma

Low-grade central osteosarcoma (well-differentiated osteosarcoma) is uncommon (6%–17.9%) in the head and neck.[128,131] It is characterized by a low-to-intermediate cellular proliferation of spindle cells with minimal atypia and varying amounts of osteoid; the mitotic rate is low. The pattern of immature bone production is variable and may consist of irregular branching bone trabeculae, curvilinear bone trabeculae, or long seams of lamellar-like bone. The key diagnostic finding is an infiltrative growth pattern.

Other Less Common Variants

Telangiectatic osteosarcoma is rare variant (approximately 5%) composed of loculated, blood-filled, or empty spaces lined by pleomorphic cells. Atypical mitoses are frequent and osteoid formation is often focal (**Fig. 17**).

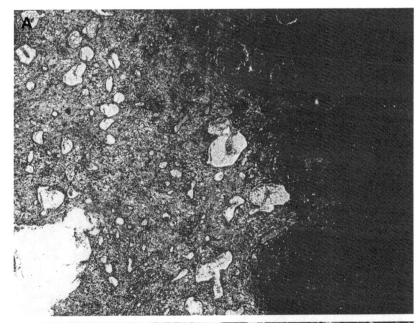

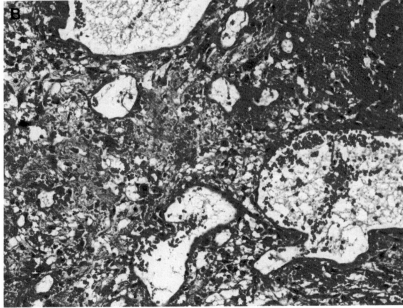

Fig. 17. (*A*) Telangiectatic osteosarcoma, with loculated-blood filled spaces, arising in the sphenoid sinus in a teenage boy with a history of bilateral retinoblastomas. Even at low power, enlarged, hyperchromatic, pleomorphic tumor cells can be seen within the walls of cysts. (H&E, ×40) (*B*) At higher magnification, there are numerous pleomorphic tumor cells in the variably thickened cyst walls. Osteoid may be focal and in the setting of abundant hemorrhage, may be difficult to distinguish from fibrin. (H&E, ×400).

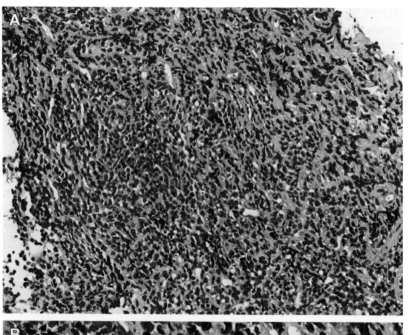

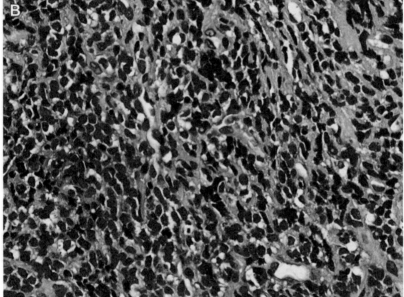

Fig. 18. (*A*) Small cell osteosarcoma is composed of cords of small round cells and neoplastic osteoid between tumor cells. A focal hemangipericytoma-like vascular pattern is present. (H&E, ×200) (*B*) Higher-power views demonstrated the small round cells with minimal cytoplasm and lacelike osteoid between the tumor cells. Molecular testing confirmed an absence of *HEY1-NCOA2* fusion or *EWSR1* rearrangements, excluding mesenchymal chondrosarcoma and Ewing sarcoma, respectively. (H&E, ×400).

Small cell osteosarcoma is composed of small cells with round-to-oval nuclei and little cytoplasm associated with osteoid, usually lacelike. A focal HPC-like vascular pattern may be present (Fig. 18).

IMMUNOHISTOCHEMISTRY AND MOLECULAR FINDINGS

Immunohistochemistry is of limited use in the setting of osteosarcoma. Osteosarcomas have been shown, however, on occasion to express CKs, a potential diagnostic pitfall.[132] Low-grade central and parosteal osteosarcomas demonstrate nuclear immunohistochemical expression of MDM2 and CDK4, which has been reported to be retained in examples of dedifferentiation.[133,134]

Low-grade central and parosteal osteosarcoma exhibit supernumerary ring chromosomes with *MDM2* and *CDK4* amplification in the region 12q13-15.[133,135] Conventional osteosarcomas demonstrate complex unstable karyotypes. Two well-known tumor suppressor genes have been implicated in conventional osteosarcoma, *TP53* and *RB1*, with either somatic or hereditary gene mutations with loss of heterozygosity.[136,137] *RB1* has an important role in regulating another cell cycle gene, *CDKN2A*, which has been shown to be mutated in osteosarcomas lacking *RB1* mutations.[138]

DIFFERENTIAL DIAGNOSIS

The greatest challenge in diagnosing a gnathic osteosarcoma is an insufficient biopsy lacking osteoid, particularly when clinically, an osteosarcoma is not considered. Often symptoms associated with gnathic osteosarcomas may be misinterpreted as odontogenic in nature, leading to a delay in obtaining the correct diagnosis. Because gnathic osteosarcomas expand the bone, they may cause mucosal ulcerations. In this situation, superficial biopsy is not representative and may be misdiagnosed as a reactive process, such as granulation tissue or pyogenic granuloma.

Low-grade central (well-differentiated) and parosteal osteosarcomas, which have been reported rarely in the head and neck, are slow-growing lesions with minimal atypia. The lack of significant cytologic atypia leads to difficulty distinguishing them from benign fibro-osseous lesions, including ossifying fibromas, fibrous dysplasia, and osteoblastoma or reactive bone lesions. Thus documentation of infiltration histologically or radiologically is the most reliable method of distinction from benign fibro-osseous lesions. MDM2/CDK4 assessment is not considered reliable to for differential diagnosis.[139]

In contrast to appendicular osteosarcomas, a greater proportion (approximately 40%) of gnathic osteosarcomas are chondroblastic and the distinction from chondroid lesions is discussed previously.[128,140,141] Telangiectatic osteosarcoma may simulate aneurysmal bone cyst, particularly radiologically and by low-power microscopic examination, but is distinguished by pleomorphic cells within the cyst walls at higher magnification and in many cases periosteal reaction on imaging. Small cell osteosarcoma overlaps with other round blue cell neoplasms, necessitating exclusionary work-up as discussed previously. Ultimately demonstration of osteoid is the most useful defining feature for this variant.

TREATMENT AND PROGNOSIS

Head and neck osteosarcomas are treated primarily with surgery, in contrast to osteosarcomas of the appendicular skeleton, which are considered a disseminated malignancy at diagnosis and treated with neoadjuvant chemotherapy followed by surgical resection. Adjuvant postoperative radiotherapy is indicated in patients with close or positive margins.[128] The role of chemotherapy in gnathic/craniofacial osteosarcomas is still unclear.[128,131]

Overall, for gnathic/craniofacial osteosarcomas, the reported 5-year disease-free and overall survival rates are approximately 50% and 65%, respectively.[128,130,131,141,142] Gnathic osteosarcomas may have a better prognosis than osteosarcomas in extragnathic craniofacial locations.[143] Secondary osteosarcomas are rapidly fatal. Complete surgical resection with clear margins is the strongest prognostic factor in craniofacial/gnathic osteosarcomas.[128,130,131,141,142] Death is due to local failure and uncontrolled disease in

---

Pitfalls

! Inadequate/limited biopsies may lack osteoid, leading to an incorrect diagnosis.

! Superficial biopsies may be misinterpretated as reactive processes or peripheral ossifying fibromas. It is crucial to review the corresponding imaging.

! Biopsies of well-differentiated osteosarcoma mimic benign fibro-osseous lesions. It is crucial to review imaging to assess for an infiltrative/invasive growth pattern, prior to classifying a fibro-osseous lesion.

! Osteosarcomas of the jaw are more common than chondrosarcomas, particularly in the body of the mandible. Chondroblastic osteosarcoma is the most common subtype at this location.

! On biopsy, a high-grade cartilaginous tumor of the jaw is assumed to be chondroblastic osteosarcoma until proved otherwise.

! Neoplastic immature woven bone is arising directly from tumor cells warrants the diagnosis of osteosarcoma.

Key Clinical Features
CRANIOFACIAL/GNATHIC OSTEOSARCOMAS

- A greater proportion of gnathic conventional osteosarcomas are chondroblastic.

- Chondroblastic osteosarcomas of the jaw may have a better prognosis than other conventional types.

- Secondary osteosarcomas are high grade and rapidly fatal.

- Complete surgical resection with clear margins is the strongest prognostic factor.

- Death is due to local failure and uncontrolled local disease.

- Adjuvant postoperative radiotherapy is indicated in patients with close or positive margins.

- The role of chemotherapy is unclear.

- Unlike appendicular osteosarcomas, metastases are late complications of craniofacial/gnathic osteosarcomas.

craniofacial/gnathic osteosarcomas. Metastases are far less common than seen in appendicular osteosarcomas.

REFERENCES

1. Lund VJ, Stammberger H, Nicolai P, et al. European position paper on endoscopic management of tumours of the nose, paranasal sinuses and skull base. Rhinol Suppl 2010;(22):1–143.
2. Liu ZF, Wang DH, Sun XC, et al. The site of origin and expansive routes of juvenile nasopharyngeal angiofibroma (JNA). Int J Pediatr Otorhinolaryngol 2011;75(9):1088–92.
3. Bremer JW, Neel HB 3rd, DeSanto LW, et al. Angiofibroma: treatment trends in 150 patients during 40 years. Laryngoscope 1986;96(12):1321–9.
4. Herman P, Lot G, Chapot R, et al. Long-term follow-up of juvenile nasopharyngeal angiofibromas: analysis of recurrences. Laryngoscope 1999;109(1):140–7.
5. Thompson LDR, Fanburg-Smith JC. Tumours of the Nasopharynx: nasopharyngeal angiofibroma. In: Barnes L, Eveson JW, Reichart P, et al, editors. Pathology and genetics of head and neck tumours. Lyon (France): IARC Press; 2005. p. 102–3.
6. Radkowski D, McGill T, Healy GB, et al. Changes in staging and treatment. Arch Otolaryngol Head Neck Surg 1996;122(2):122–9.
7. Martin H, Ehrlich HE, Abels JC. Juvenile nasopharyngeal angiofibroma. Ann Surg 1948;127(3):513–36.
8. Giardiello FM, Hamilton SR, Krush AJ, et al. Nasopharyngeal angiofibroma in patients with familial adenomatous polyposis. Gastroenterology 1993;105(5):1550–2.
9. Valanzano R, Curia MC, Aceto G, et al. Genetic evidence that juvenile nasopharyngeal angiofibroma is an integral FAP tumour. Gut 2005;54(7):1046–7.
10. Hes FJ, Nielsen M, Bik EC, et al. Somatic APC mosaicism: an underestimated cause of polyposis coli. Gut 2008;57(1):71–6.
11. Beham A, Kainz J, Stammberger H, et al. Immunohistochemical and electron microscopical characterization of stromal cells in nasopharyngeal angiofibromas. Eur Arch Otorhinolaryngol 1997;254(4):196–9.
12. Zhang PJ, Weber R, Liang HH, et al. Growth factors and receptors in juvenile nasopharyngeal angiofibroma and nasal polyps: an immunohistochemical study. Arch Pathol Lab Med 2003;127(11):1480–4.
13. Abraham SC, Montgomery EA, Giardiello FM, et al. Frequent beta-catenin mutations in juvenile nasopharyngeal angiofibromas. Am J Pathol 2001;158(3):1073–8.
14. Liu Z, Wang J, Wang H, et al. Hormonal receptors and vascular endothelial growth factor in juvenile nasopharyngeal angiofibroma: immunohistochemical and tissue microarray analysis. Acta Otolaryngol 2015;135(1):51–7.
15. Montag AG, Tretiakova M, Richardson M. Steroid hormone receptor expression in nasopharyngeal angiofibromas. Consistent expression of estrogen receptor beta. Am J Clin Pathol 2006;125(6):832–7.
16. Nonogaki S, Campos HG, Butugan O, et al. Markers of vascular differentiation, proliferation and tissue remodeling in juvenile nasopharyngeal angiofibromas. Exp Ther Med 2010;1(6):921–6.
17. Demicco EG, Harms PW, Patel RM, et al. Extensive survey of STAT6 expression in a large series of mesenchymal tumors. Am J Clin Pathol 2015;143(5):672–82.
18. Chmielecki J, Crago AM, Rosenberg M, et al. Whole-exome sequencing identifies a recurrent NAB2-STAT6 fusion in solitary fibrous tumors. Nat Genet 2013;45(2):131–2.
19. Makek MS, Andrews JC, Fisch U. Malignant transformation of a nasopharyngeal angiofibroma. Laryngoscope 1989;99(10 Pt 1):1088–92.
20. Allensworth JJ, Troob SH, Lanciault C, et al. High-grade malignant transformation of a radiation-naive nasopharyngeal angiofibroma. Head Neck 2016;38(Suppl 1):E2425–7.
21. Thompson LDR, Fanburg-Smith JC, Wenig BM. Tumours of the nasal cavity and paranasal sinuses: borderline and low malignant potential tumours of soft tissues. In: Barnes L, Eveson JW, Reichart P, et al, editors. Pathology and genetics of head

and neck tumours. Lyon (France): IARC Press; 2005. p. 43–5.

22. Compagno J, Hyams VJ. Hemangiopericytoma-like intranasal tumors. A clinicopathologic study of 23 cases. Am J Clin Pathol 1976;66(4):672–83.

23. Thompson LD, Miettinen M, Wenig BM. Sinonasal-type hemangiopericytoma: a clinicopathologic and immunophenotypic analysis of 104 cases showing perivascular myoid differentiation. Am J Surg Pathol 2003;27(6):737–49.

24. Catalano PJ, Brandwein M, Shah DK, et al. Sino-nasal hemangiopericytomas: a clinicopathologic and immunohistochemical study of seven cases. Head Neck 1996;18(1):42–53.

25. Agaimy A, Barthelmess S, Geddert H, et al. Pheno-typical and molecular distinctness of sinonasal haemangiopericytoma compared to solitary fibrous tumour of the sinonasal tract. Histopathology 2014; 65(5):667–73.

26. Lee GG, Dhong HJ, Park YS, et al. Sinonasal glo-mangiopericytoma causing oncogenic osteoma-lacia. Clin Exp Otorhinolaryngol 2014;7(2):145–8.

27. Haller F, Bieg M, Moskalev EA, et al. Recurrent mu-tations within the amino-terminal region of beta-catenin are probable key molecular driver events in sinonasal hemangiopericytoma. Am J Pathol 2015;185(2):563–71.

28. Billings KR, Fu YS, Calcaterra TC, et al. Hemangio-pericytoma of the head and neck. Am J Otolaryngol 2000;21(4):238–43.

29. Ferrari A, Sultan I, Huang TT, et al. Soft tissue sar-coma across the age spectrum: a population-based study from the surveillance epidemiology and end results database. Pediatr Blood Cancer 2011;57(6):943–9.

30. Sultan I, Qaddoumi I, Yaser S, et al. Comparing adult and pediatric rhabdomyosarcoma in the sur-veillance, epidemiology and end results program, 1973 to 2005: an analysis of 2,600 patients. J Clin Oncol 2009;27(20):3391–7.

31. Turner JH, Richmon JD. Head and neck rhabdo-myosarcoma: a critical analysis of population-based incidence and survival data. Otolaryngol Head Neck Surg 2011;145(6):967–73.

32. Montgomery EA, Barr FG. Skeletal-muscle tumours: pleomorphic rhabdomyosarcoma. In: Fletcher CDM, Bridge JA, Hogendoorn PCW, et al, editors. WHO classification of tumours of soft tissue and bone. 4th edition. Lyon (France): IARC; 2013. p. 132–3.

33. Nascimento AF, Barr FG. Skeletal-muscle tumours: spindle cell/sclerosing rhabdomyosarcoma. In: Fletcher CDM, Bridge JA, Hogendoorn PCW, et al, editors. WHO classification of tumours of soft tissue and bone. 4th edition. Lyon (France): IARC; 2013. p. 134–5.

34. Parham DM, Barr FG. Skeletal-muscle tumours: embryonal rhabdomyosarcoma. In: Fletcher CDM,

Bridge JA, Hogendoorn PCW, et al, editors. WHO classification of tumours of soft tissue and bone. 4th edition. Lyon (France): IARC; 2013. p. 127–9.

35. Parham DM, Barr FG. Skeletal-muscle tumours: alveolar rhabdomyosarcoma. In: Fletcher CDM, Bridge JA, Hogendoorn PCW, et al, editors. WHO classification of tumours of soft tissue and bone. 4th edition. Lyon (France): IARC; 2013. p. 130–2.

36. Coffin CM, Davis JL, Borinstein SC. Syndrome-associated soft tissue tumours. Histopathology 2014;64(1):68–87.

37. Newton WA Jr, Soule EH, Hamoudi AB, et al. Histo-pathology of childhood sarcomas, intergroup rhab-domyosarcoma studies I and II: clinicopathologic correlation. J Clin Oncol 1988;6(1):67–75.

38. Rekhi B, Singhvi T. Histopathological, immunohisto-chemical and molecular cytogenetic analysis of 21 spindle cell/sclerosing rhabdomyosarcomas. AP-MIS 2014;122(11):1144–52.

39. Yasui N, Yoshida A, Kawamoto H, et al. Clinicopath-ologic analysis of spindle cell/sclerosing rhabdo-myosarcoma. Pediatr Blood Cancer 2015;62(6): 1011–6.

40. Robinson JC, Richardson MS, Neville BW, et al. Sclerosing rhabdomyosarcoma: report of a case arising in the head and neck of an adult and review of the literature. Head Neck Pathol 2013;7(2): 193–202.

41. Zhao Z, Yin Y, Zhang J, et al. Spindle cell/scle-rosing rhabdomyosarcoma: case series from a sin-gle institution emphasizing morphology, immunohistochemistry and follow-up. Int J Clin Exp Pathol 2015;8(11):13814–20.

42. Ferrari A, Dileo P, Casanova M, et al. Rhabdomyo-sarcoma in adults. A retrospective analysis of 171 patients treated at a single institution. Cancer 2003;98(3):571–80.

43. Furlong MA, Mentzel T, Fanburg-Smith JC. Pleo-morphic rhabdomyosarcoma in adults: a clinico-pathologic study of 38 cases with emphasis on morphologic variants and recent skeletal muscle-specific markers. Mod Pathol 2001;14(6):595–603.

44. Fanburg-Smith JC, Lasota J, Auerbach A, et al. Tu-mors and tumor-like lesions of the soft tissues. In: Barnes L, editor. Surgical pathology of the head and neck, vol. 2. New York: Informa Healthcare USA, Inc; 2009. p. 773–949.

45. Newton WA Jr, Gehan EA, Webber BL, et al. Clas-sification of rhabdomyosarcomas and related sar-comas. Pathologic aspects and proposal for a new classification–an Intergroup Rhabdomyosar-coma Study. Cancer 1995;76(6):1073–85.

46. Qualman S, Lynch J, Bridge J, et al. Prevalence and clinical impact of anaplasia in childhood rhab-domyosarcoma: a report from the Soft Tissue Sar-coma Committee of the Children's Oncology Group. Cancer 2008;113(11):3242–7.

47. Dias P, Chen B, Dilday B, et al. Strong immuno-staining for myogenin in rhabdomyosarcoma is significantly associated with tumors of the alveolar subclass. Am J Pathol 2000;156(2):399–408.

48. Morotti RA, Nicol KK, Parham DM, et al. An immunohistochemical algorithm to facilitate diagnosis and subtyping of rhabdomyosarcoma: the Children's Oncology Group experience. Am J Surg Pathol 2006;30(8):962–8.

49. Parham DM, Webber B, Holt H, et al. Immunohistochemical study of childhood rhabdomyosarcomas and related neoplasms. Results of an Intergroup Rhabdomyosarcoma study project. Cancer 1991; 67(12):3072–80.

50. Paulson V, Chandler G, Rakheja D, et al. High-resolution array CGH identifies common mechanisms that drive embryonal rhabdomyosarcoma pathogenesis. Genes Chromosomes Cancer 2011; 50(6):397–408.

51. Williamson D, Missiaglia E, de Reynies A, et al. Fusion gene-negative alveolar rhabdomyosarcoma is clinically and molecularly indistinguishable from embryonal rhabdomyosarcoma. J Clin Oncol 2010;28(13):2151–8.

52. Sorensen PH, Lynch JC, Qualman SJ, et al. PAX3-FKHR and PAX7-FKHR gene fusions are prognostic indicators in alveolar rhabdomyosarcoma: a report from the children's oncology group. J Clin Oncol 2002;20(11):2672–9.

53. Mertens F, Fletcher CD, Dal Cin P, et al. Cytogenetic analysis of 46 pleomorphic soft tissue sarcomas and correlation with morphologic and clinical features: a report of the CHAMP Study Group. Chromosomes and MorPhology. Genes Chromosomes Cancer 1998;22(1):16–25.

54. Mosquera JM, Sboner A, Zhang L, et al. Recurrent NCOA2 gene rearrangements in congenital/infantile spindle cell rhabdomyosarcoma. Genes Chromosomes Cancer 2013;52(6):538–50.

55. Agaram NP, Chen CL, Zhang L, et al. Recurrent MYOD1 mutations in pediatric and adult sclerosing and spindle cell rhabdomyosarcomas: evidence for a common pathogenesis. Genes Chromosomes Cancer 2014;53(9):779–87.

56. Meza JL, Anderson J, Pappo AS, et al. Analysis of prognostic factors in patients with nonmetastatic rhabdomyosarcoma treated on intergroup rhabdomyosarcoma studies III and IV: the Children's Oncology Group. J Clin Oncol 2006;24(24):3844–51.

57. Raney RB, Anderson JR, Barr FG, et al. Rhabdomyosarcoma and undifferentiated sarcoma in the first two decades of life: a selective review of intergroup rhabdomyosarcoma study group experience and rationale for Intergroup Rhabdomyosarcoma Study V. J Pediatr Hematol Oncol 2001;23(4):215–20.

58. Lawrence W Jr, Anderson JR, Gehan EA, et al. Pretreatment TNM staging of childhood rhabdomyosarcoma: a report of the Intergroup Rhabdomyosarcoma Study Group. Children's Cancer Study Group. Pediatric Oncology Group. Cancer 1997;80(6):1165–70.

59. Maurer HM, Beltangady M, Gehan EA, et al. The intergroup rhabdomyosarcoma study-I. A final report. Cancer 1988;61(2):209–20.

60. Maurer HM, Gehan EA, Beltangady M, et al. The Intergroup Rhabdomyosarcoma Study-II. Cancer 1993;71(5):1904–22.

61. Hawkins WG, Hoos A, Antonescu CR, et al. Clinicopathologic analysis of patients with adult rhabdomyosarcoma. Cancer 2001;91(4):794–803.

62. Chen Q, Lu W, Li B. Primary sclerosing rhabdomyosarcoma of the scalp and skull: report of a case and review of literature. Int J Clin Exp Pathol 2015;8(2):2205–7.

63. Hartmann S, Lessner G, Mentzel T, et al. An adult spindle cell rhabdomyosarcoma in the head and neck region with long-term survival: a case report. J Med Case Rep 2014;8:208.

64. Warner BM, Griffith CC, Taylor WD, et al. Sclerosing rhabdomyosarcoma: presentation of a rare sarcoma mimicking myoepithelial carcinoma of the parotid gland and review of the literature. Head Neck Pathol 2015;9(1):147–52.

65. Alaggio R, Zhang L, Sung YS, et al. A molecular study of pediatric spindle and sclerosing rhabdomyosarcoma: identification of novel and recurrent VGLL2-related fusions in infantile cases. Am J Surg Pathol 2016;40(2):224–35.

66. Skapek SX, Anderson J, Barr FG, et al. PAX-FOXO1 fusion status drives unfavorable outcome for children with rhabdomyosarcoma: a children's oncology group report. Pediatr Blood Cancer 2013;60(9):1411–7.

67. Lewis JT, Oliveira AM, Nascimento AG, et al. Low-grade sinonasal sarcoma with neural and myogenic features: a clinicopathologic analysis of 28 cases. Am J Surg Pathol 2012;36(4):517–25.

68. Wang X, Bledsoe KL, Graham RP, et al. Recurrent PAX3-MAML3 fusion in biphenotypic sinonasal sarcoma. Nat Genet 2014;46(7):666–8.

69. Huang SC, Ghossein RA, Bishop JA, et al. Novel PAX3-NCOA1 fusions in biphenotypic sinonasal sarcoma with focal rhabdomyoblastic differentiation. Am J Surg Pathol 2016;40(1):51–9.

70. Powers KA, Han LM, Chiu AG, et al. Low-grade sinonasal sarcoma with neural and myogenic features–diagnostic challenge and pathogenic insight. Oral Surg Oral Med Oral Pathol Oral Radiol 2015;119(5):e265–9.

71. Wong WJ, Lauria A, Hornick JL, et al. Alternate PAX3-FOXO1 oncogenic fusion in biphenotypic sinonasal sarcoma. Genes Chromosomes Cancer 2016;55(1):25–9.

72. Hasegawa SL, Mentzel T, Fletcher CD. Schwannomas of the sinonasal tract and nasopharynx. Mod Pathol 1997;10(8):777–84.

73. McMaster ML, Goldstein AM, Bromley CM, et al. Chordoma: incidence and survival patterns in the United States, 1973-1995. Cancer Causes Control 2001;12(1):1–11.

74. Smoll NR, Gautschi OP, Radovanovic I, et al. Incidence and relative survival of chordomas: the standardized mortality ratio and the impact of chordomas on a population. Cancer 2013; 119(11):2029–37.

75. Bohman LE, Koch M, Bailey RL, et al. Skull base chordoma and chondrosarcoma: influence of clinical and demographic factors on prognosis: a SEER analysis. World Neurosurg 2014;82(5): 806–14.

76. Tirabosco R, Mangham DC, Rosenberg AE, et al. Brachyury expression in extra-axial skeletal and soft tissue chordomas: a marker that distinguishes chordoma from mixed tumor/myoepithelioma/parachordoma in soft tissue. Am J Surg Pathol 2008; 32(4):572–80.

77. Lauer SR, Edgar MA, Gardner JM, et al. Soft tissue chordomas: a clinicopathologic analysis of 11 cases. Am J Surg Pathol 2013;37(5):719–26.

78. Khurram SA, Biswas D, Fernando M. A parapharyngeal soft tissue chordoma presenting with synchronous cervical lymph node metastasis: an unusual presentation. Head Neck Pathol 2016;10(3):400–4.

79. Kataria SP, Batra A, Singh G, et al. Chordoma of skull base presenting as nasopharyngeal mass. J Neurosci Rural Pract 2013;4(Suppl 1):S95–7.

80. Tao ZZ, Chen SM, Liu JF, et al. Paranasal sinuses chordoma in pediatric patient: a case report and literature review. Int J Pediatr Otorhinolaryngol 2005;69(10):1415–8.

81. Gladstone HB, Bailet JW, Rowland JP. Chordoma of the oropharynx: an unusual presentation and review of the literature. Otolaryngol Head Neck Surg 1998;118(1):104–7.

82. Lee-Jones L, Aligianis I, Davies PA, et al. Sacrococcygeal chordomas in patients with tuberous sclerosis complex show somatic loss of TSC1 or TSC2. Genes Chromosomes Cancer 2004;41(1): 80–5.

83. Oakley GJ, Fuhrer K, Seethala RR. Brachyury, SOX-9, and podoplanin, new markers in the skull base chordoma vs chondrosarcoma differential: a tissue microarray-based comparative analysis. Mod Pathol 2008;21(12):1461–9.

84. Flanagan AM, Yamaguchi T. Notocordal tumours: chordoma. In: Fletcher CDM, Bridge JA, Hogendoorn PCW, et al, editors. WHO classification of tumours of soft tissue and bone. 4th edition. Lyon (France): IARC; 2013. p. 323–30.

85. Heffelfinger MJ, Dahlin DC, MacCarty CS, et al. Chordomas and cartilaginous tumors at the skull base. Cancer 1973;32(2):410–20.

86. Hoch BL, Nielsen GP, Liebsch NJ, et al. Base of skull chordomas in children and adolescents: a clinicopathologic study of 73 cases. Am J Surg Pathol 2006;30(7):811–8.

87. Vujovic S, Henderson S, Presneau N, et al. Brachyury, a crucial regulator of notochordal development, is a novel biomarker for chordomas. J Pathol 2006;209(2):157–65.

88. Miettinen M, Wang Z, Lasota J, et al. Nuclear brachyury expression is consistent in chordoma, common in germ cell tumors and small cell carcinomas, and rare in other carcinomas and sarcomas: an immunohistochemical study of 5229 cases. Am J Surg Pathol 2015;39(10):1305–12.

89. Chavez JA, Nasir Ud D, Memon A, et al. Anaplastic chordoma with loss of INI1 and brachyury expression in a 2-year-old girl. Clin Neuropathol 2014; 33(6):418–20.

90. Hasselblatt M, Thomas C, Hovestadt V, et al. Poorly differentiated chordoma with SMARCB1/INI1 loss: a distinct molecular entity with dismal prognosis. Acta Neuropathol 2016;132(1):149–51.

91. Yang XR, Ng D, Alcorta DA, et al. T (brachyury) gene duplication confers major susceptibility to familial chordoma. Nat Genet 2009;41(11):1176–8.

92. Pillay N, Plagnol V, Tarpey PS, et al. A common single-nucleotide variant in T is strongly associated with chordoma. Nat Genet 2012;44(11):1185–7.

93. Presneau N, Shalaby A, Ye H, et al. Role of the transcription factor T (brachyury) in the pathogenesis of sporadic chordoma: a genetic and functional-based study. J Pathol 2011;223(3):327–35.

94. Marucci G, Morandi L, Mazzatenta D, et al. MGMT promoter methylation status in clival chordoma. J Neurooncol 2014;118(2):271–6.

95. Amary MF, Bacsi K, Maggiani F, et al. IDH1 and IDH2 mutations are frequent events in central chondrosarcoma and central and periosteal chondromas but not in other mesenchymal tumours. J Pathol 2011;224(3):334–43.

96. Arai M, Nobusawa S, Ikota H, et al. Frequent IDH1/2 mutations in intracranial chondrosarcoma: a possible diagnostic clue for its differentiation from chordoma. Brain Tumor Pathol 2012;29(4):201–6.

97. Rosenberg AE, Nielsen GP, Keel SB, et al. Chondrosarcoma of the base of the skull: a clinicopathologic study of 200 cases with emphasis on its distinction from chordoma. Am J Surg Pathol 1999;23(11):1370–8.

98. Matloob SA, Nasir HA, Choi D. Proton beam therapy in the management of skull base chordomas: systematic review of indications, outcomes, and implications for neurosurgeons. Br J Neurosurg 2016;30(4):382–7.

99. Almefty K, Pravdenkova S, Colli BO, et al. Chordoma and chondrosarcoma: similar, but quite different, skull base tumors. Cancer 2007;110(11):2457–67.

100. Bloch OG, Jian BJ, Yang I, et al. A systematic review of intracranial chondrosarcoma and survival. J Clin Neurosci 2009;16(12):1547–51.

101. Di Maio S, Temkin N, Ramanathan D, et al. Current comprehensive management of cranial base chordomas: 10-year meta-analysis of observational studies. J Neurosurg 2011;115(6):1094–105.

102. Bloch OG, Jian BJ, Yang I, et al. Cranial chondrosarcoma and recurrence. Skull Base 2010;20(3):149–56.

103. Mitchell A, Scheithauer BW, Unni KK, et al. Chordoma and chondroid neoplasms of the spheno-occiput. An immunohistochemical study of 41 cases with prognostic and nosologic implications. Cancer 1993;72(10):2943–9.

104. Jian BJ, Bloch OG, Yang I, et al. A comprehensive analysis of intracranial chordoma and survival: a systematic review. Br J Neurosurg 2011;25(4):446–53.

105. Forsyth PA, Cascino TL, Shaw EG, et al. Intracranial chordomas: a clinicopathological and prognostic study of 51 cases. J Neurosurg 1993;78(5):741–7.

106. Koch BB, Karnell LH, Hoffman HT, et al. National cancer database report on chondrosarcoma of the head and neck. Head Neck 2000;22(4):408–25.

107. Hogendoorn PCW, Bovee JVMG, Nielsen GP. Chondrogenic tumours: chondrosarcoma (grades I–III), including primary and secondary variants and periosteal chondrosarcoma. In: Fletcher CDM, Bridge JA, Hogendoorn PCW, et al, editors. WHO classification of tumours of soft tissue and bone. 4th edition. Lyon (France): IARC; 2013. p. 264–8.

108. Thompson LD, Gannon FH. Chondrosarcoma of the larynx: a clinicopathologic study of 111 cases with a review of the literature. Am J Surg Pathol 2002;26(7):836–51.

109. Tien N, Chaisuparat R, Fernandes R, et al. Mesenchymal chondrosarcoma of the maxilla: case report and literature review. J Oral Maxillofac Surg 2007;65(6):1260–6.

110. Garrington GE, Scofield HH, Cornyn J, et al. Osteosarcoma of the jaws. Analysis of 56 cases. Cancer 1967;20(3):377–91.

111. Knott PD, Gannon FH, Thompson LD. Mesenchymal chondrosarcoma of the sinonasal tract: a clinicopathological study of 13 cases with a review of the literature. Laryngoscope 2003;113(5):783–90.

112. Nakashima Y, de Pinieux G, Ladanyi M. Chondrogenic tumours: mesenchymal chondrosarcoma. In: Fletcher CDM, Bridge JA, Hogendoorn PCW, et al, editors. WHO classification of tumours of soft tissue and bone. 4th edition. Lyon (France): IARC; 2013. p. 271–2.

113. Frezza AM, Cesari M, Baumhoer D, et al. Mesenchymal chondrosarcoma: prognostic factors and outcome in 113 patients. A European Musculoskeletal Oncology Society study. Eur J Cancer 2015;51(3):374–81.

114. Evans HL, Ayala AG, Romsdahl MM. Prognostic factors in chondrosarcoma of bone: a clinicopathologic analysis with emphasis on histologic grading. Cancer 1977;40(2):818–31.

115. Inwards C, Hogendoorn PCW. Chondrogenic tumours: dedifferentiated chondrosarcoma. In: Fletcher CDM, Bridge JA, Hogendoorn PCW, et al, editors. WHO classification of tumours of soft tissue and bone. 4th edition. Lyon (France): IARC; 2013. p. 269–70.

116. Mokhtari S, Mirafsharieh A. Clear cell chondrosarcoma of the head and neck. Head Neck Oncol 2012;4:13.

117. Wehrli BM, Huang W, De Crombrugghe B, et al. Sox9, a master regulator of chondrogenesis, distinguishes mesenchymal chondrosarcoma from other small blue round cell tumors. Hum Pathol 2003;34(3):263–9.

118. Wang L, Motoi T, Khanin R, et al. Identification of a novel, recurrent HEY1-NCOA2 fusion in mesenchymal chondrosarcoma based on a genome-wide screen of exon-level expression data. Genes Chromosomes Cancer 2012;51(2):127–39.

119. Batsakis JG. Osteogenic and chondrogenic sarcomas of the jaws. Ann Otol Rhinol Laryngol 1987;96(4):474–5.

120. Kumar R, Moser RP Jr, Madewell JE, et al. Parosteal osteogenic sarcoma arising in cranial bones: clinical and radiologic features in eight patients. AJR Am J Roentgenol 1990;155(1):113–7.

121. Roca AN, Smith JL Jr, Jing BS. Osteosarcoma and parosteal osteogenic sarcoma of the maxilla and mandible: study of 20 cases. Am J Clin Pathol 1970;54(4):625–36.

122. Wang GD, Zhao YF, Liu Y, et al. Periosteal osteosarcoma of the mandible: case report and review of the literature. J Oral Maxillofac Surg 2011;69(6):1831–5.

123. Mosalleum E, Afrogheh A, Stofberg S, et al. A review of primary osteosarcoma of the larynx and case report. Head Neck Pathol 2015;9(1):158–64.

124. Rosenberg AE, Cleton-Jansen AM, de Pinieux G, et al. Osteogenic tumours: conventional osteosarcoma. In: Fletcher CDM, Bridge JA, Hogendoorn PCW, et al, editors. WHO classification of tumours of soft tissue and bone. 4th edition. Lyon (France): IARC; 2013. p. 282–8.

125. Hoshi M, Matsumoto S, Manabe J, et al. Malignant change secondary to fibrous dysplasia. Int J Clin Oncol 2006;11(3):229–35.

126. Huvos AG. Osteogenic sarcoma of bones and soft tissues in older persons. A clinicopathologic

analysis of 117 patients older than 60 years. Cancer 1986;57(7):1442–9.

127. Torres FX, Kyriakos M. Bone infarct-associated osteosarcoma. Cancer 1992;70(10):2418–30.

128. Guadagnolo BA, Zagars GK, Raymond AK, et al. Osteosarcoma of the jaw/craniofacial region: outcomes after multimodality treatment. Cancer 2009;115(14):3262–70.

129. Givol N, Buchner A, Taicher S, et al. Radiological features of osteogenic sarcoma of the jaws. A comparative study of different radiographic modalities. Dentomaxillofac Radiol 1998;27(6): 313–20.

130. Thariat J, Schouman T, Brouchet A, et al. Osteosarcomas of the mandible: multidisciplinary management of a rare tumor of the young adult a cooperative study of the GSF-GETO, Rare Cancer Network, GETTEC/REFCOR and SFCE. Ann Oncol 2013;24(3):824–31.

131. Smith RB, Apostolakis LW, Karnell LH, et al. National cancer data base report on osteosarcoma of the head and neck. Cancer 2003;98(8): 1670–80.

132. Okada K, Hasegawa T, Yokoyama R, et al. Osteosarcoma with cytokeratin expression: a clinicopathological study of six cases with an emphasis on differential diagnosis from metastatic cancer. J Clin Pathol 2003;56(10):742–6.

133. Dujardin F, Binh MB, Bouvier C, et al. MDM2 and CDK4 immunohistochemistry is a valuable tool in the differential diagnosis of low-grade osteosarcomas and other primary fibro-osseous lesions of the bone. Mod Pathol 2011;24(5):624–37.

134. Yoshida A, Ushiku T, Motoi T, et al. Immunohistochemical analysis of MDM2 and CDK4 distinguishes low-grade osteosarcoma from benign mimics. Mod Pathol 2010;23(9):1279–88.

135. Park HR, Jung WW, Bertoni F, et al. Molecular analysis of p53, MDM2 and H-ras genes in low-grade central osteosarcoma. Pathol Res Pract 2004; 200(6):439–45.

136. Heinsohn S, Evermann U, Zur Stadt U, et al. Determination of the prognostic value of loss of heterozygosity at the retinoblastoma gene in osteosarcoma. Int J Oncol 2007;30(5):1205–14.

137. Wunder JS, Gokgoz N, Parkes R, et al. TP53 mutations and outcome in osteosarcoma: a prospective, multicenter study. J Clin Oncol 2005;23(7):1483–90.

138. Nielsen GP, Burns KL, Rosenberg AE, et al. CDKN2A gene deletions and loss of p16 expression occur in osteosarcomas that lack RB alterations. Am J Pathol 1998;153(1):159–63.

139. Tabareau-Delalande F, Collin C, Gomez-Brouchet A, et al. Chromosome 12 long arm rearrangement covering MDM2 and RASAL1 is associated with aggressive craniofacial juvenile ossifying fibroma and extracranial psammomatoid fibro-osseous lesions. Mod Pathol 2015;28(1):48–56.

140. Thariat J, Julieron M, Brouchet A, et al. Osteosarcomas of the mandible: are they different from other tumor sites? Crit Rev Oncol Hematol 2012; 82(3):280–95.

141. Clark JL, Unni KK, Dahlin DC, et al. Osteosarcoma of the jaw. Cancer 1983;51(12):2311–6.

142. Patel SG, Meyers P, Huvos AG, et al. Improved outcomes in patients with osteogenic sarcoma of the head and neck. Cancer 2002;95(7):1495–503.

143. Nora FE, Unni KK, Pritchard DJ, et al. Osteosarcoma of extragnathic craniofacial bones. Mayo Clin Proc 1983;58(4):268–72.

144. Kassir RR, Rassekh CH, Kinsella JB, et al. Osteosarcoma of the head and neck: meta-analysis of nonrandomized studies. Laryngoscope 1997; 107(1):56–61.

Printed and bound by CPI Group (UK) Ltd, Croydon, CR0 4YY

03/10/2024

01040302-0006